Procedures
in Phlebotomy

5th Edition

BD Vacutainer® Venous Blood Collection
Tube Guide

For the full array of BD Vacutainer® Blood Collection Tubes, visit www.bd.com/vacutainer.
Many are available in a variety of sizes and draw volumes (for pediatric applications). Refer to our website for full descriptions.

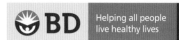

Helping all people live healthy lives

BD Vacutainer® Tubes with BD Hemogard™ Closure	BD Vacutainer® Tubes with Conventional Stopper	Additive	Inversions at Blood Collection*	Laboratory Use	Your Lab's Draw Volume/Remarks
Gold	Red/Gray	• Clot activator and gel for serum separation	5	For serum determinations in chemistry. May be used for routine blood donor screening and diagnostic testing of serum for infectious disease.** Tube inversions ensure mixing of clot activator with blood. Blood clotting time: 30 minutes.	
Light Green	Green/Gray	• Lithium heparin and gel for plasma separation	8	For plasma determinations in chemistry. Tube inversions ensure mixing of anticoagulant (heparin) with blood to prevent clotting.	
Red	Red	• Silicone coated (glass) • Clot activator, Silicone coated (plastic)	0 5	For serum determinations in chemistry. May be used for routine blood donor screening and diagnostic testing of serum for infectious disease.** Tube inversions ensure mixing of clot activator with blood. Blood clotting time: 60 minutes.	
Orange		• Thrombin-based clot activator with gel for serum separation	5 to 6	For stat serum determinations in chemistry. Tube inversions ensure mixing of clot activator with blood. Blood clotting time: 5 minutes.	
Orange		• Thrombin-based clot activator	8	For stat serum determinations in chemistry. Tube inversions ensure mixing of clot activator with blood. Blood clotting time: 5 minutes.	
Royal Blue		• Clot activator (plastic serum) • K_2EDTA (plastic)	8 8	For trace-element, toxicology, and nutritional-chemistry determinations. Special stopper formulation provides low levels of trace elements (see package insert). Tube inversions ensure mixing of either clot activator or anticoagulant (EDTA) with blood.	
Green	Green	• Sodium heparin • Lithium heparin	8 8	For plasma determinations in chemistry. Tube inversions ensure mixing of anticoagulant (heparin) with blood to prevent clotting.	
Gray	Gray	• Potassium oxalate/sodium fluoride • Sodium fluoride/Na_2 EDTA • Sodium fluoride (serum tube)	8 8 8	For glucose determinations. Oxalate and EDTA anticoagulants will give plasma samples. Sodium fluoride is the antiglycolytic agent. Tube inversions ensure proper mixing of additive with blood.	
Tan		• K_2EDTA (plastic)	8	For lead determinations. This tube is certified to contain less than .01 μg/mL(ppm) lead. Tube inversions prevent clotting.	

			Additive	Inversions*	Laboratory Use	
	Yellow		• Sodium polyanethol sulfonate (SPS)	8	SPS for blood culture specimen collections in microbiology.	
			• Acid citrate dextrose additives (ACD): **Solution A -** 22.0 g/L trisodium citrate, 8.0 g/L citric acid, 24.5 g/L dextrose	8	ACD for use in blood bank studies, HLA phenotyping, and DNA and paternity testing.	
			Solution B - 13.2 g/L trisodium citrate, 4.8 g/L citric acid, 14.7 g/L dextrose	8	Tube inversions ensure mixing of anticoagulant with blood to prevent clotting.	
Lavender	Lavender		• Liquid K_3EDTA (glass) • Spray-coated K_2EDTA (plastic)	8 8	K_2EDTA and K_3EDTA for whole blood hematology determinations. K_2EDTA may be used for routine immunohematology testing, and blood donor screening.*** Tube inversions ensure mixing of anticoagulant (EDTA) with blood to prevent clotting.	
White			• K_2EDTA and gel for plasma separation	8	For use in molecular diagnostic test methods (such as, but not limited to, polymerase chain reaction [PCR] and/or branched DNA [bDNA] amplification techniques.) Tube inversions ensure mixing of anticoagulant (EDTA) with blood to prevent clotting.	
Pink	Pink		• Spray-coated K_2EDTA (plastic)	8	For whole blood hematology determinations. May be used for routine immunohematology testing and blood donor screening.*** Designed with special cross-match label for patient information required by the AABB. Tube inversions prevent clotting.	
Light Blue Clear	Light Blue		• Buffered sodium citrate 0.105 M (≈3.2%) glass 0.109 M (3.2%) plastic • Citrate, theophylline, adenosine, dipyridamole (CTAD)	3-4 3-4	For coagulation determinations. CTAD for selected platelet function assays and routine coagulation determination. Tube inversions ensure mixing of anticoagulant (citrate) to prevent clotting.	
Clear	New Red/ Light Gray		• None (plastic)	0	For use as a discard tube or secondary specimen tube.	

Note: BD Vacutainer® Tubes for pediatric and partial draw applications can be found on our website.

BD Diagnostics
Preanalytical Systems
1 Becton Drive
Franklin Lakes, NJ 07417 USA

BD Global Technical Services: 1.800.631.0174
BD Customer Service: 1.888.237.2762
www.bd.com/vacutainer

* Invert gently, do not shake
** The performance characteristics of these tubes have not been established for infectious disease testing in general; therefore, users must validate the use of these tubes for their specific assay-instrument/reagent system combinations and specimen storage conditions.
*** The performance characteristics of these tubes have not been established for immunohematology testing in general; therefore, users must validate the use of these tubes for their specific assay-instrument/reagent system combinations and specimen storage conditions.

Courtesy Becton, Dickinson and Company, Franklin Lakes, New Jersey

Procedures
in Phlebotomy

Fifth Edition

JOHN C. FLYNN, JR., PhD, MT(ASCP)SBB
Adjunct Instructor, Medical Laboratory
  Technician Program
Harcum College
Bryn Mawr, Pennsylvania

ELSEVIER

Elsevier
3251 Riverport Lane
St. Louis, Missouri 63043

Notice

Practitioners and researchers must always rely on their own experience and knowledge in evaluating and using any information, methods, compounds or experiments described herein. Because of rapid advances in the medical sciences, in particular, independent verification of diagnoses and drug dosages should be made. To the fullest extent of the law, no responsibility is assumed by Elsevier, authors, editors or contributors for any injury and/or damage to persons or property as a matter of products liability, negligence or otherwise, or from any use or operation of any methods, products, instructions, or ideas contained in the material herein.

Previous editions copyrighted 2012, 2005, 1999, and 1994

Content Strategist: Laura Klein
Content Developmental Specialist: Meredith Madeira
Publishing Services Manager: Deepthi Unni
Project Manager: Nayagi Anandan
Design Direction: Brian Salisbury

Printed in India

Last digit is the print number: 9   8   7   6   5   4   3   2   1

Working together
to grow libraries in
developing countries

www.elsevier.com • www.bookaid.org

I dedicate this, as I do all positive things in my life, to my family. Especially:

Dylan

Shayla

Johnny

Desmond

Torin

Finn

Zeke

Leon

Myles

Cashel

Rowan

Lucius

Also, this book is dedicated to those phlebotomists and other front-line health care workers who sacrificed personal concerns and helped the nation through the COVID-19 pandemic. We will always be grateful.

CONTRIBUTORS

Jeanne Gable, PBT, (ASCP)^{cm}
Phlebotomy Instructor
Lab Sciences
Harcum College
Bryn Mawr, Pennsylvania
United States;
Certified Phlebotomist
Mobile Services Department
Abington Jefferson Health
Abington, Pennsylvania
United States

Kristy Matulevich, MEd, MLS, (ASCP)^{cm}
Associate Professor/Clinical Coordinator
Laboratory Science
Harcum College
Bryn Mawr, Pennsylvania
United States

Robert Rehfuss, PhD
Adjunct Professor
STEM Department
Bucks County Community College
Newtown, Pennsylvania
United States

Linda R. Rehfuss, PhD
Professor Emeritus
Biology and Biotechnology
Bucks County Community College
Newtown, Pennsylvania
United States

Leticia M. Rodríguez, BA, MS, PhD
Director
Human Resources
Colonial SD
Plymouth Meeting, Pennsylvania
United States

Patricia Tille, PhD, MLS(ASCP), AHI (AMT), FACSc
Graduate Program Director/Professor
Medical Laboratory Science
University of Cincinnati
Cincinnati, Ohio
United States

COSMETICS

REVIEWERS

Danyel Anderson, MT(ASCP), MPH, EdD
Medical Laboratory Technician Program
    Clinical Coordinator
Ozarks Technical Community College
Springfield, Missouri
United States

Marc Davis, Esq.
Partner, Fox Rothschild, LLP
Blue Bell, Pennsylvania
United States
Reviewed Chapter 14: Medical-Legal Issues and
Health Law Procedures

Kelsey Dodson, BS, MLS(ASCP)^{cm}, PBT (ASCP)^{cm}
Phlebotomy Program Director and Instructor
Saint Paul College
Saint Paul, Minnesota
United States

**Judith   NCPT,
NCCS**
Medic   ent Lead
Miami-Dade County Public School
D. A. Dorsey Technical College
Miami, Florida
United States

**Petra M. York, BS, AAS, CPT, CET, CMAA,
CMA-AAMA, AHI, CPhT**
Program Director
Western Technical College
EL Paso, Texas
United States

PREFACE

While robotics and nanotechnology continue to expand and take over many functions in today's world, phlebotomists continue to be an essential component of health care. Phlebotomists are often the first interaction a patient may have with our health care system and may be the only direct interaction. Thus, being a good practitioner in the art of phlebotomy is as essential as ever!

When I was first approached by WB Saunders in 1990 about writing a phlebotomy book, I never imagined that 20+ years later, the 5th edition of *Procedures in Phlebotomy* would be in publication. This book, like the previous editions, continues to be aimed at students in phlebotomy programs to assist in their training and certification. It will also be an asset to medical laboratory technicians and medical assisting and nursing students who have phlebotomy in their respective curricula. It will also help current phlebotomists who may wish to have a quick, updated reference book. Lastly, those phlebotomists who have been out of the field for a bit will find *Procedures in Phlebotomy* useful for refreshing their skills and knowledge. It continues to be straightforward and focused on phlebotomy and does not try to be "all things to all people" while continuing to be affordable in a time when the costs of textbooks continue to skyrocket. We've worked hard to provide the most current information available, including web links to relevant sources. These links were active at the time of publication.

ORGANIZATION

The book continues to be organized into two parts: The Practice of Phlebotomy and Professional Issues. Several new contributors have been instrumental in updating this edition. All other chapters have been updated or modified to ensure currency with modern phlebotomy practice. One chapter, Chapter 10, has been updated and renamed to better reflect what is happening in the profession.

Other updates to this edition include an expanded practice examination, additional end-of-chapter review questions, an expanded glossary, and an updated tube guide.

Procedures in Phlebotomy, 5th edition, will be a useful textbook addition to anyone who is interested in studying phlebotomy and in improving their skills and staying current with this critical aspect of health care.

ACKNOWLEDGMENTS

This 5th edition of *Procedures in Phlebotomy* has several new contributors. Without them, this edition would never have come to fruition. However, I would be remiss if I did not acknowledge and vigorously thank the numerous contributors that allowed the first four editions to be successful. I would like to thank the staff at Elsevier for their support. I would also like to thank Harcum College and the Medical Laboratory Science program for support. Special thanks goes to Kristy Matulevich of Harcum for going above and beyond expectations to review chapters other than her own as well as helping recruit contributors.

CONTENTS

---

*This chapter has been edited from a contribution to the fourth edition by Shirley E. Greening.

1

Introduction to Phlebotomy

John C. Flynn, Jr.

"Medicine, the only profession that labors incessantly to destroy the reason for its own existence."

—*James Bryce (1838–1922)*

OBJECTIVES

At the conclusion of this chapter, the student should be able to:
- Identify health care professionals that may perform phlebotomy.
- Name important factors in collecting a blood specimen.
- List the locations where a phlebotomist may work.
- State the difference between *certification* and *licensure*.
- Explain the purpose of a code of ethics.

OUTLINE

KEY TERMS

certification
electrocardiographs
ethical behavior
HIPAA

licensure
phlebotomy
protected health information

HISTORY

"Bleed in the acute affections, if the disease appear strong, and the patients be in the vigor of life, and if they have strength." These were the thoughts of Hippocrates, recorded nearly 25 centuries ago, regarding the usefulness of phlebotomy. He proposed that

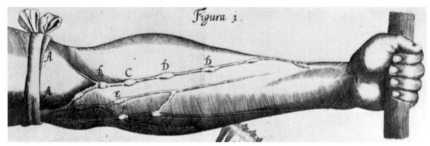

Fig. 1.1 Drawing originally published in 1628 depicting the location of veins in the arm. From Harvey, W. Exercitio anatomica de mortu cordis et sanguinis in animalibus. Frankfurt, G. Fitzer, 1628. (Courtesy Wellcome Institute Library, London.)

phlebotomy be used as a treatment for acute disease conditions.

Later, during the 11th century, when the first school of medicine was founded in Salerno in present-day Italy, "blood letting" was still a popular curative. In fact, well into modern times (that is, the 17th and 18th centuries), phlebotomy was used as a treatment for diseases ranging from mental illness to fever to convulsions (Fig. 1.1). However, as the practice of medicine and the understanding of the human body progressed, phlebotomy as a routine treatment fell into disuse.

CURRENT PHLEBOTOMY PRACTICE

Today **phlebotomy,** although no longer considered a curative, is a necessary aid in the diagnosis and treatment of disease. In ancient times, witch doctors, barbers, and, later, physicians performed phlebotomies (Fig. 1.2), but in modern times, trained professionals perform this vital function. These professionals, who traditionally were trained on the job, are increasingly being trained in formal programs and becoming certified by national certifying agencies (Box 1.1). However, formally trained phlebotomists are not the only health care personnel who may perform a venipuncture. Others include nurses, physicians, emergency medical personnel, and medical assistants. This trend will continue as hospital, laboratories, and clinics cross-train employees to perform this vital function. Unfortunately, the degree of training may not always be consistent.

Advances in modern medicine allow for marvelous treatments to be administered to patients. For example, advances in bionanotechnology allow for safer and more effective medical treatment and in many cases allow the patient to avoid major open-incision surgery

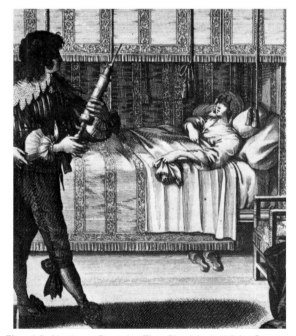

Fig. 1.2 Abraham Bosse's *The Physician's Visit.* Courtesy Trustees of the British Museum, London.

and recover more quickly. Additionally, with the growth of modern medicine and the increasingly wide range of diagnostic and screening tests available, the role of the phlebotomist has become increasingly important and complex. As can be seen in Box 1.2, which lists the primary functional areas and some of the tests common to most clinical laboratories, phlebotomists collect blood for a vast array of tests. The list of tests is not all-inclusive but gives the reader a sampling of the hundreds of assays performed in a laboratory. No

BOX 1.1   Phlebotomy Certifying Agencies

Association of Schools Advancing Health Professions (ASAHP): www.asahp.org
American Medical Technologists (AMT): americanmedtech.org
American Society for Clinical Pathology (ASCP): www.ascp.org
American Society of Phlebotomy Technicians (ASPT): www.aspt.org
National Phlebotomy Association (NPA): www.nationalphlebotomy.org

BOX 1.2   Some Common Tests in the Primary Functional Areas of a Clinical Laboratory

Hematology
Complete blood cell count (CBC)
White blood cell differential
Prothrombin time (PT)
Activated partial thromboplastin time (APTT)

Chemistry
Chemistry profiles
Glucose
Cholesterol
Electrolytes
Bilirubin
Blood urea nitrogen (BUN)
Creatinine
Enzymes
Prostate specific antigen (PSA)
Human immunodeficiency virus (HIV)
Urinalysis (may be in hematology)

Blood Bank
Blood types
Antibody screening
Prenatal testing

Microbiology and Serology
Gram stains
Plating of culture
Sensitivity testing
Pregnancy tests
Monospots
Rheumatoid arthritis screen
Rapid plasma reagin (RPR)
C-reactive protein

longer is it a matter of simply collecting a blood specimen; the modern phlebotomist must also be aware of the type of test requested, medications the patient is taking that may interfere with the testing, the importance of the timing of the blood collection, and the effect of the patient's diet.

The modern phlebotomist may also be called on to perform other functions such as measuring bleeding times, collecting donor blood, performing therapeutic phlebotomies, conducting bedside testing (known as *point-of-care testing*), and preparing specimens. Also, a category of clinical assays known as waived tests may be performed by phlebotomists (see Chapter 10). Thus the phlebotomist may be the only contact a patient has with the laboratory, and therefore it is critical that all phlebotomists conduct themselves in a professional and competent manner at all times. Furthermore, phlebotomists today must communicate and interact with the entire laboratory team (Fig. 1.3A). They must be familiar with both routine and special specimen requirements, including collection and transportation procedures for each section of the laboratory. Lately, because of changes in health care management, phlebotomists are being called on to perform such tests as **electrocardiographs,** simple laboratory tests, and some nursing functions, to name a few. This process, as noted earlier, is known as *cross-training* or *multiskilling* (see Chapter 10). Just as others are being trained to perform phlebotomy, phlebotomists are being trained to perform other functions.

Additionally, phlebotomists must also interact and communicate with the entire health care team, in addition to the laboratory team and patients' families (see Fig. 1.3B). This means they must be able to "speak the language" of medicine and communicate professionally, both in writing and orally. Although the majority of the communication will be with the clinical pathology laboratory (the formal name of hospital laboratories), phlebotomists may be called on to interact with other specialty laboratories, hospital functional areas (e.g., emergency room, x-ray) and offices. See Table 1.1 for a list of some specialty areas in health care.

Furthermore, phlebotomists are not confined to working exclusively in a hospital setting. They may work in physician office laboratories; blood collection centers, such as those operated by the American Red Cross; research institutes; commercial laboratories; or

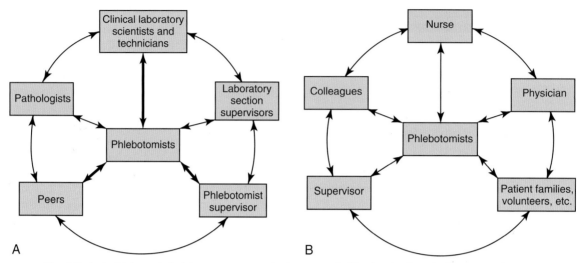

Fig. 1.3 *A,* A phlebotomist's laboratory communication network. The heavier lines indicate more frequent communication pathways. *B,* A phlebotomist's hospital communication network.

TABLE 1.1	Specialty Areas in Health Care		
Specialty Area	**Description**	**Personnel Title**	**Possible Related Blood Test**
Anesthesiology	Pain management; often assists in the operating room	Anesthesiologist	Arterial blood gases
Cardiology	Heart health	Cardiologist	Cardiac enzymes
Endocrinology	Studying and maintaining hormone related diseases	Endocrinologist	Hormone level
Gerontology or geriatrics	Maintaining the health of older adults	Gerontologist	General laboratory tests
Neurology	Study of the nervous system	Neurologist	General laboratory tests
Obstetrics (and gynecology)	Women's health	Obstetrician or gynecologist	Blood type
Oncology	Managing cancer, primarily tumors	Oncologist	Cancer markers
Orthopedics	Managing joint and bone disorders	Orthopedist	General laboratory tests
Pediatrics	Care of children	Pediatrician	Phenylketonuria (PKU) and related pediatric and newborn tests
Psychiatry	Mental health	Psychiatrist	Drug levels
Urology	Urinary tract diseases (also kidneys) and male reproductive organs	Urologist or nephrologist	Blood urea nitrogen and urinalysis; also, prostrate markers

veterinary offices. Additionally, they may be hired to visit patients in their homes or places of employment. Given all the aforementioned, it is imperative that phlebotomists must be able to handle stress (their own and the stress patients may feel) and stressful situations.

PROFESSIONAL RECOGNITION

Fig. 1.4 illustrates the organizational structure of modern laboratories, with the position of the phlebotomist highlighted; phlebotomists are an integral part of every laboratory section and play a vital role in the health maintenance team. (It should be noted that for discussion purposes, clinical laboratory scientists and medical technologists are regarded as equivalent, as are clinical laboratory technicians and medical laboratory technicians.) This partially explains the increasing number of phlebotomy training programs and the increasing number of phlebotomists becoming certified. Currently there are dozens of approved phlebotomy programs in the United States, with more than 15,000 phlebotomists certified. As shown in Box 1.1, there are several different accrediting agencies that certify phlebotomists, and although the examination fees and frequency of examination administration may vary, the underlying goal of all such programs is the same: to assure employers that the phlebotomists they are hiring meet a minimally acceptable standard of practice.

It is important for phlebotomists and all health care workers to understand the difference between **certification** and **licensure.** *Certification* is the result of successfully passing an examination or test that indicates a minimum level of knowledge. *Licensure* is a state or local requirement needed for phlebotomists to perform their duties. This is similar to an individual needing a license to operate a restaurant or drive a car.

Ethical behavior is paramount in any profession but perhaps even more so in the health care professions. Without ethical behavior as a professional cornerstone, the public will not be able to trust the people who may play an important role in their lives. Therefore all professionals should adhere to a pledge of conduct or a code of ethics. Early physicians followed the Hippocratic Oath, and in fact most still do today, and although there is no specific pledge or code for phlebotomists, there is one for the field of medical laboratory professionals, to which phlebotomists belong. This pledge is endorsed by the American Society for Clinical Laboratory Science:

As a Medical Laboratory Professional, I pledge to uphold my duty to Patients, the Profession, and Society by:

- *Placing patients' welfare above my own needs and desires.*
- *Ensuring that each patient receives care that is safe, effective, efficient, timely, equitable, and patient-centered.*

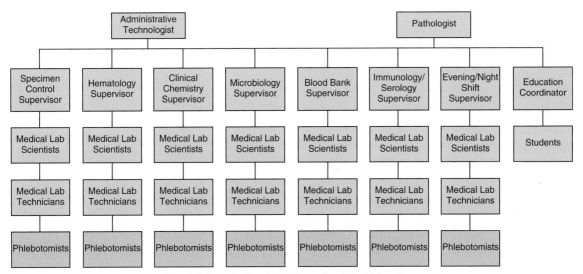

Fig. 1.4 Organizational structure of a clinical laboratory.

- *Maintaining the dignity and respect for my profession.*
- *Promoting the advancement of my profession.*
- *Ensuring collegial relationships within the clinical laboratory and with other patient care providers.*
- *Improving access to laboratory services.*
- *Promoting equitable distribution of health care resources.*
- *Complying with laws and regulations and protecting patients from others' incompetent or illegal practice*
- *Changing conditions where necessary to advance the best interests of patients.*

Phlebotomists must also be familiar with the Health Insurance Portability and Accountability Act, commonly referred to as **HIPAA.** This act is in place to protect a patient's **protected health information,** such as their name, medical condition, and treatment. Phlebotomists may have access to some of this information, and they must be trusted to maintain confidentiality and trustworthiness.

Lastly, the future of health care in the United States is in flux. The implementation of government health plan(s), in whatever form it takes, combined with an overall aging society, will likely result in an increased need for medical services for the population. This increased work will lead to an even greater need for valuable phlebotomy professionals.

SUMMARY

This brief introductory chapter is designed to provide a broad overview of the history of phlebotomy. It also serves to describe phlebotomy in the context of the clinical laboratory and introduces new phlebotomy students to the importance of professionalism and ethical behavior.

REVIEW QUESTIONS

1. Phlebotomy is a necessary aid in the _____ and _____ of disease.
2. Before formal phlebotomy training programs existed, phlebotomists were trained _____.
3. Name some places other than hospitals that may employ phlebotomists.
4. What is the purpose of certification for phlebotomists?
5. A code of conduct that can apply to phlebotomists is published by the _____.
6. The changes that are likely for health care in the United States will likely result in _____ work for phlebotomists.
7. What does it mean to act in an ethical manner?

BIBLIOGRAPHY

American Society for Clinical Laboratory Science: Pledge to the profession. Available at www.ascls.org/?page=code.

Castiglioni A. *A History of Medicine.* New York: Jason Aronson; 1969.

Haggard HW. *Devils, Drugs, and Doctors.* New York: Harper and Brothers; 1929.

Hippocrates. *The Theory and Practice of Medicine.* New York: Philosophical Library; 1964.

Inglis BA. *A Brief History of Medicine.* Cleveland: The World Publishing Company; 1965.

Anatomy and Physiology

Robert Rehfuss

"[The body is] a marvelous machine . . . a chemical laboratory, a power-house. Every movement, voluntary or involuntary, full of secrets and marvels!"

—*Theodor Herzl (1860−1904)*

OBJECTIVES

At the conclusion of this chapter, the student should be able to:

- Define all key terms included in this chapter.
- Identify body planes and describe directional terms.
- Classify the four types of tissues based on structure and function.
- Define *homeostasis*.
- Describe the organs, major structures, and functions of each body system.
- List diagnostic tests and disorders related to each body system.
- Describe how blood circulates within the heart to the lungs and tissues.
- Describe how to take a blood pressure measurement and factors that influence blood pressure readings.
- Identify the three types of blood vessels and describe their structure and function.
- Name and identify the three common veins used for venipuncture.
- List the major components of blood and describe the function of each formed element.
- Differentiate between whole blood, serum, and plasma.
- Briefly explain clot formation, fibrinolysis, and the principles of blood typing.

OUTLINE

INTRODUCTION

The human organism is the most fascinating scientific entity that exists. It can be studied from several perspectives, including anatomical, physiological, psychological, and sociological. It can be studied from the simple level of atoms and molecules to the most complex level of the total organism—the living individual. This chapter explores the anatomy and physiology pertinent to phlebotomists.

BODY PLANES AND CELLS

The parts of the body are studied relative to the **body planes,** or imaginary flat surfaces, that pass through the body (Fig. 2.1). It is important to become familiar with these planes so one can understand the anatomical relationship of one body or organ part to another. The *sagittal plane* divides the body or an organ into right and left sides. If this plane passes through the midline or center of the body or organ, it is called the *midsagittal* or *median plane.* If it divides the organ into unequal right and left sides, it is called the *parasagittal plane.* A *frontal* or *coronal plane* divides the body or organ into front (anterior) and back (posterior) portions. A *transverse* or *horizontal plane* divides the body or organ into top (superior) and bottom (inferior) portions.

Additionally, although the body can be divided into sections, there are several levels of organization within the structural framework of the human body (Fig. 2.2). Atoms combine with each other to form molecules. Molecules join with each other to form cells. Cells are the smallest, most basic unit of life. Each type of cell has its own structure, and each performs a different function to enable growth, metabolism, transportation, and reproduction within the human body. Cells are generally classified into two groups: *somatic* cells, which compose body mass; and *gonadal* cells, which are vital for reproduction. Similar cells that work

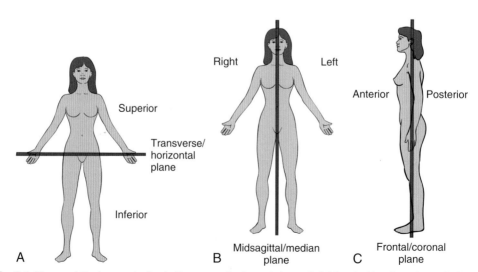

Fig. 2.1 Planes of the human body. *A,* Transverse/horizontal plane. *B,* Midsagittal/median plane. *C,* Frontal/coronal plane.

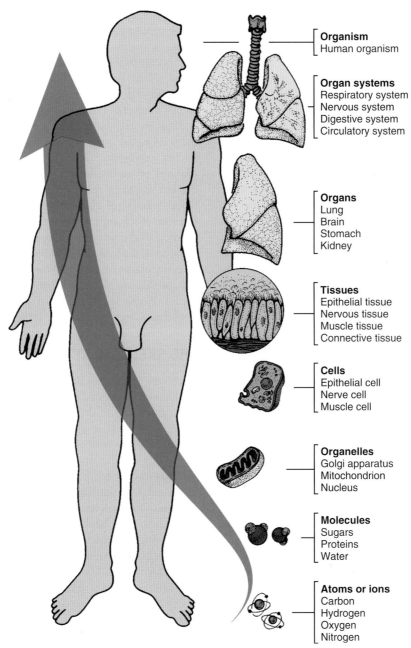

Organism
Human organism

Organ systems
Respiratory system
Nervous system
Digestive system
Circulatory system

Organs
Lung
Brain
Stomach
Kidney

Tissues
Epithelial tissue
Nervous tissue
Muscle tissue
Connective tissue

Cells
Epithelial cell
Nerve cell
Muscle cell

Organelles
Golgi apparatus
Mitochondrion
Nucleus

Molecules
Sugars
Proteins
Water

Atoms or ions
Carbon
Hydrogen
Oxygen
Nitrogen

Fig. 2.2 Levels of organization of the human body.

together to perform a particular function are called *tissues*. Tissues that work together are called *organs*, and organs that work together are called *systems*. The study of cells is **cytology**, and the study of tissues is **histology**.

TISSUES

Tissues within the body are classified into four types based on their structure and function:

1. *Epithelial tissue* forms the outer layer of skin, some internal organs, and the inner lining of blood vessels.

Additionally, epithelial cells line body cavities and cover interior structures within the body's systems. The secreting portion of glands is also composed of epithelial tissue.

2. *Connective tissue* supports and protects the body and its organs. It aids in binding organs together while also providing immunity and energy storage in the form of fat or adipose tissue. **Cartilage** and bone are examples of connective tissue.

3. *Muscle tissue* consists of fibers (cells), provides motion, and helps the body maintain posture. It forms the walls of internal organs such as the stomach, heart, and blood vessels.

4. *Nervous tissue* consists of complex, specialized cells (neurons) that transmit nerve impulses to tissues, glands, or other neurons throughout the body to help coordinate body activities.

Each organ in the body is composed of different combinations of these tissues. For example, the stomach—made mostly of epithelial and muscle tissues—contains lesser amounts of other tissues as well.

ORGAN SYSTEMS

The study of anatomy and physiology (the structure and function of the body) concentrates on the study of body systems. A body system consists of several related organs that work together to perform a common function. For example, the circulatory system, which is composed of the heart and blood vessels, provides the body with nourishment by circulating blood and nutrients through it. Usually, the organs of a system are anatomically connected; however, in some cases, the tissues are widely distributed, as seen in the endocrine system.

Body systems work together continuously and interact constantly to maintain a state of internal balance known as **homeostasis**. A disruption of this homeostasis as caused by one organ or system may affect other organ systems within the body. Each of the organ systems is discussed, with an emphasis on the cardiovascular and respiratory systems.

THE INTEGUMENTARY SYSTEM

The integumentary system, which covers the body, consists of the skin and accessory structures (Fig. 2.3). The skin, one of the largest organs in the body, consists of two principal layers. The thin, outer layer of the skin is the epidermis. Beneath this is the thicker connective tissue, or dermis, which rests on the subcutaneous layer that is composed of additional connective and adipose tissue. Fibers from the dermis connect the skin to the subcutaneous layer. The subcutaneous layer then attaches to tissues and organs. Hair follicles, nails, nerve endings, sweat glands, and **sebaceous glands** are also included in the integumentary system. This system aids in the regulation of body temperature, provides a physical protective barrier against bacteria and dehydration, contains receptors to touch and pain, houses blood vessels for circulation, and assists in the production of vitamin D within the body. The external location of the integumentary system's structures helps physicians diagnose disease because abnormalities can be easily observed. Dermatology is the medical specialty that pertains to the treatment of skin and related disorders. Please see Box 2.1 for some tests and assorted disorders associated with the integumentary system.

THE SKELETAL SYSTEM

There are 206 bones in the body (Fig. 2.4), which are grouped into axial and appendicular portions. The *axial* portion consists of the skull (cranial and facial bones), vertebral column, and thorax (sternum and ribs). The *appendicular* portion consists of the shoulder girdle, pelvic (hip) girdle, and bones of the upper and lower extremities (i.e., the arms and legs). There are 80 bones in the axial portion and 126 bones in the appendicular portion of the skeleton. The skeletal system provides the framework for the body, protects vital organs, and works with the muscular system to produce movement. Blood cells are produced within the red marrow of the bones. Orthopedics is the medical specialty that studies the skeletal system and associated structures. Please see Box 2.2 for some tests and assorted disorders associated with the skeletal system.

THE MUSCULAR SYSTEM

Muscle tissue is differentiated by its appearance, location, and function. There are three types of muscle tissue (Fig. 2.5A–C):

1. **Smooth (visceral) muscle** tissue is located in the walls of blood vessels and hollow organs such as the stomach. This tissue looks smooth or nonstriated

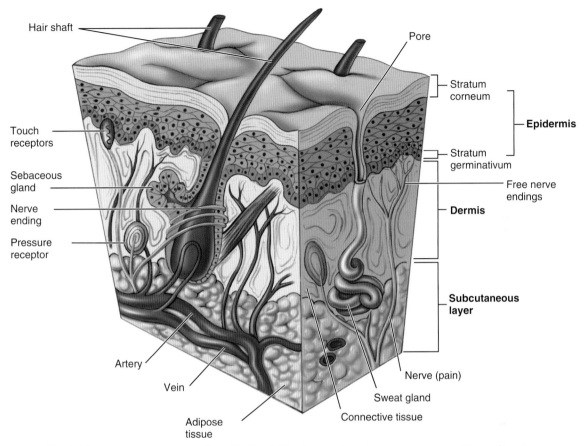

Fig. 2.3 Cross-section of the skin. From Herlihy B. (*The Human Body in Health and Illness*. 4th ed., Saunders, St. Louis, 2011.)

BOX 2.1 Integumentary System	
Diagnostic Tests	**Disorders**
Biopsies	Acne
Fungal cultures on skin	Cancer (melanoma and
scrapings	other types)
Microbiology cultures	Herpes
Tissue cultures	Impetigo or Psoriasis

because it lacks alternating light and dark bands. It is involuntary muscle tissue, which means it needs stimulation from hormones or nerve transmitter substances to function.

2. **Cardiac muscle** tissue forms most of the heart. This tissue is striated because it has varying bands and is involuntary. The contraction of the cardiac muscle is usually not under the body's conscious control and is responsible for the heart's ability to beat.

3. **Skeletal muscle** tissue primarily attaches itself to the bones and helps move the skeleton. It is striated and voluntary because it can be made to contract and relax with conscious control.

The body is composed of more than 700 muscles. Muscles need a source of energy to function. For example, glucose from the blood enters the contracting muscle, combines with oxygen (O_2), and provides energy in the form of **adenosine triphosphate (ATP).** However, O_2 is not always required for muscle function, and if this **anaerobic** process continues for an extended period, **lactic acid** accumulates in the blood and muscle tissue. This buildup soon causes muscle fatigue and the "burning" you may feel in your muscles. As skeletal muscle contracts to work, heat is generated. Much of

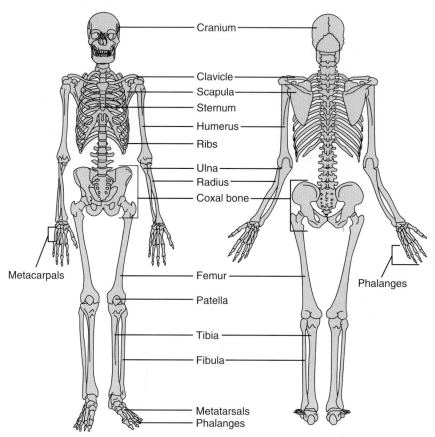

Fig. 2.4 Anterior and posterior views of the skeletal system.

BOX 2.2   Skeletal System

Diagnostic Tests	Disorders
Alkaline phosphatase (ALP)	Arthritis
Calcium	Bursitis
Complete blood cell (CBC) count	Gout
Erythrocyte sedimentation rate (ESR)	Osteoporosis
Synovial fluid analysis	Tumors
Uric acid	Kidney Disorders

the heat is used to maintain normal body temperature. For example, a football player helps keep his body warm by actively participating in the sport even in very cold weather. *Myology* is the study of muscles. Please see Box 2.3 for some tests and assorted disorders associated with the muscular system.

THE NERVOUS SYSTEM

The purpose of the nervous system is to detect changes, known as *stimuli*, from both internal and external environments. It then analyzes the information and coordinates an appropriate response. Nerve cells, or **neurons**, conduct impulses from the receptors in the body to and within the *central nervous system* (CNS). The body also uses chemicals called *neurotransmitters* to carry impulses between neurons. A common neurotransmitter is acetylcholine. The junction between two neurons is called a *synapse*.

The nervous system is divided into two sections (Fig. 2.6). The CNS consists of the brain and spinal cord. The **peripheral nervous system (PNS)** consists of all nervous tissue outside the CNS. The PNS is further divided into the somatic nervous system (SNS) and the autonomic nervous system (ANS), sometimes called the *visceral nervous system* (Fig. 2.7). The SNS conveys

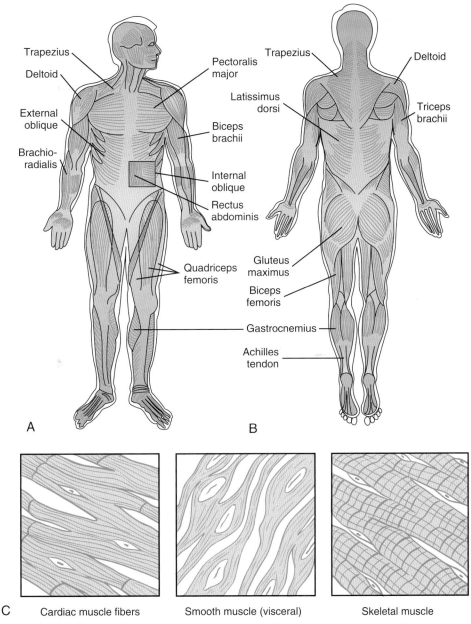

Fig. 2.5 The muscular system. *A,* Anterior view. *B,* Posterior view. *C,* Types of tissues.

information from the head, body wall, and extremities to the CNS. The CNS then sends impulses to the skeletal muscle. In contrast, the ANS conveys information from the viscera to the CNS. The CNS then sends impulses to the stomach, cardiac muscle, and glands.

The ANS is further divided into two systems: the sympathetic and the parasympathetic. The *sympathetic system* stimulates or excites the organ to start activity. This is known as the "fight or flight" response. The *parasympathetic system* decreases or inhibits activity to restore and maintain balance. Neurology is the medical

BOX 2.3   Muscular System

Diagnostic Tests	Disorders
Creatine kinase (CK) and isoenzymes	Muscular dystrophy
Lactate dehydrogenase (LD or LDH)	Myalgia
Lactic acid	Tendinitis
Myoglobin	Rhabdomyolysis

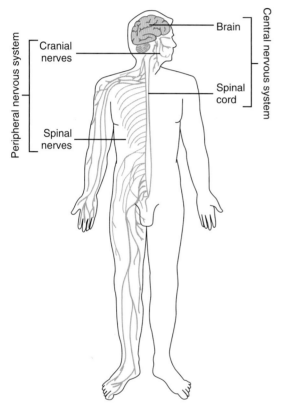

Fig. 2.6 The nervous system.

(Figure labels: Peripheral nervous system; Cranial nerves; Spinal nerves; Brain; Spinal cord; Central nervous system)

organs include the eye, ear, tongue, and nose. They are responsible for vision, hearing and equilibrium, taste, and smell, respectively. General receptors detect touch, pain, pressure, and temperature. The medical specialties that diagnose abnormalities within this system include ophthalmology (eyes) and otolaryngology (ears, nose, and throat).

THE ENDOCRINE SYSTEM

The endocrine system contains two types of glands that secrete substances that affect other cells: exocrine and endocrine. *Exocrine glands* secrete substances into ducts that are then carried to organs or body cavities or outside the body. Sweat glands are an example of this type of gland. The remainder of the discussion is devoted to *endocrine glands*, which constitute the endocrine system. Endocrine glands secrete their substances or **hormones** into the space around the secretory cells. Examples of these glands include the **pituitary**, which is regulated by the **hypothalamus** in the brain; the **thyroid**, which is located below the **larynx** or voice box; and the **adrenals**, which lie superior to each of the kidneys. Fig. 2.8 shows the major endocrine glands.

Hormones are very powerful substances. Small amounts can produce large changes in the body. They regulate metabolism and energy production, contraction of muscles, growth, and aspects of the immune system. They also help maintain homeostasis within the body and play an important role in the reproductive cycle from its initial stages of gamete production through delivery of the newborn infant. **Prolactin, insulin**, and **oxytocin** are just a few of the many hormones secreted in the human body. Endocrinology is the study of the endocrine system. Please see Box 2.5 for some tests and assorted disorders associated with the endocrine system.

THE CARDIOVASCULAR SYSTEM

All cells within the body must be constantly supplied with nutrients and oxygen. The circulatory system (Fig. 2.9) is responsible for this function. It also removes waste products and carbon dioxide (CO_2) by transporting them to the proper sites for disposal. Additionally, it helps control body temperature. The circulatory system includes the *heart*, which pumps

specialty that studies the nervous system. Please see Box 2.4 for some tests and assorted disorders associated with the nervous system.

The sensory organs, a component of the nervous system, contain many receptor cells that can detect stimuli. The receptors may be widely distributed or localized in the sense organs within the body. The sense

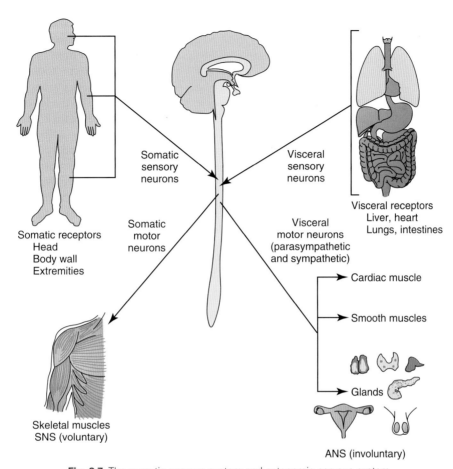

Fig. 2.7 The somatic nervous system and autonomic nervous system.

Somatic sensory neurons

Visceral sensory neurons

Somatic receptors
Head
Body wall
Extremities

Somatic motor neurons

Visceral motor neurons (parasympathetic and sympathetic)

Visceral receptors
Liver, heart
Lungs, intestines

Cardiac muscle

Smooth muscles

Glands

Skeletal muscles
SNS (voluntary)

ANS (involuntary)

BOX 2.4 Nervous System

Diagnostic Tests	Disorders
Acetylcholine receptor antibody	Amyotrophic lateral sclerosis (ALS)
Cerebral spinal fluid (CSF) analysis	Epilepsy
Cholinesterase	Meningitis
Drug levels	Multiple sclerosis (MS)
Rapid *Streptococcus* screen	Parkinson disease
RAST (allergy screens)	Shingles

---

blood through *veins* and *arteries.* The lymphatic vessels return **lymph**, which is very similar to interstitial fluid (the fluid found between cells in the body), to the blood. This makes the lymphatic vessels an auxiliary part of the circulatory system. Please see Box 2.6 for some tests and assorted disorders associated with the cardiovascular system.

The Heart

The heart is a four-chambered muscular organ (Fig. 2.10). Its main responsibility is to pump blood with sufficient pressure to meet the needs of the body's cells and to keep blood circulating in the vessels (Fig. 2.11). The heart is enclosed by the pericardium. It is a tough, white fibrous tissue. It is lined by a double-layer membrane. The inner layer or epicardium forms the outer layer of the heart itself. Beneath the epicardium is the myocardium, or the main layer of the heart, which is composed of cardiac muscle and forms most of the heart wall. The heart is divided into two parts by this wall. Each part is composed of an upper chamber

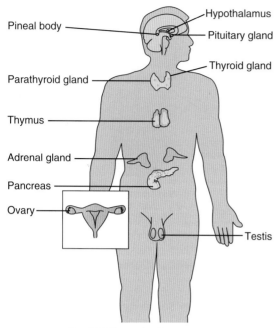

Pineal body

Hypothalamus

Pituitary gland

Parathyroid gland

Thyroid gland

Thymus

Adrenal gland

Pancreas

Ovary

Testis

Fig. 2.8 The endocrine system.

BOX 2.5   Endocrine System

Diagnostic Tests	Disorders
Adrenocorticotrophic hormone (ACTH)	Cushing syndrome
Aldosterone	Diabetes insipidus
Antidiuretic hormone (ADH)	Diabetes mellitus
Catecholamines	Dwarfism
Cortisol	Hyperthyroidism
Glucose tolerance tests	Hypothyroidism
Hemoglobin A1c	General diabetes
Insulin	General diabetes
Testosterone	Male hypogonadism
Thyroid function studies (T3, T4, thyroid stimulating hormone [TSH])	Thyroiditis

(atrium) and a lower chamber (ventricle). The right atrium receives deoxygenated blood from various parts of the body, primarily through the two veins called the *superior vena cava* and the *inferior vena cava*. The superior vena cava brings blood from the body parts superior to, or above, the heart. The inferior vena cava brings blood from the body parts inferior to, or below, the heart. The blood flows from the right atrium to the right ventricle, which pumps it to the lungs. Here in the lungs, blood cells release CO_2 and pick up O_2. The oxygenated blood returns to the left atrium in the heart. It then passes to the left ventricle and out of the heart, where it is distributed via the aorta, the largest artery, to circulate throughout the body. This pattern of blood flow is maintained by valves within the heart's chambers, which prevent any backflow from ventricles to atrium. The four valves in the heart are the tricuspid, mitral, pulmonary semilunar, and aortic semilunar. A heart murmur is caused when one of the valves does not close properly and blood leaks into it.

Blood Flow Summary

1. Deoxygenated blood enters the heart through the superior and inferior venae cavae.
2. Blood flows into the right atrium.
3. Blood passes through the tricuspid valve and enters the right ventricle.
4. Blood leaves the heart through the pulmonic semilunar valve and flows into the lungs through the pulmonary arteries where it becomes oxygenated.
5. Oxygenated blood returns to the heart through the pulmonary veins and enters the left atrium.
6. Blood moves through the mitral valve and into the left ventricle.
7. Blood flows into the aorta through the aortic semilunar valve and returns to circulation.

Heartbeat and Blood Pressure

The rhythmical nature of cardiac muscle contraction (heartbeat) originates in and through the heart with no extrinsic stimulation. Small masses, or nodes, make up the conductive system in the heart, which emits the electrical impulses. The heartbeat originates in the *sinoatrial node*, which is therefore called the "pacemaker" of the heart.

The heart is stimulated by the ANS. These nerves alter the heart rate but are not responsible for the heartbeat. At resting state, the heart beats approximately 70 to 72 times per minute. One complete contraction-relaxation cycle lasts approximately 0.8 seconds. Exercise, emotions, hormones, drugs, and body temperature are some factors that can influence heart rate. The **electrocardiogram** (ECG) records

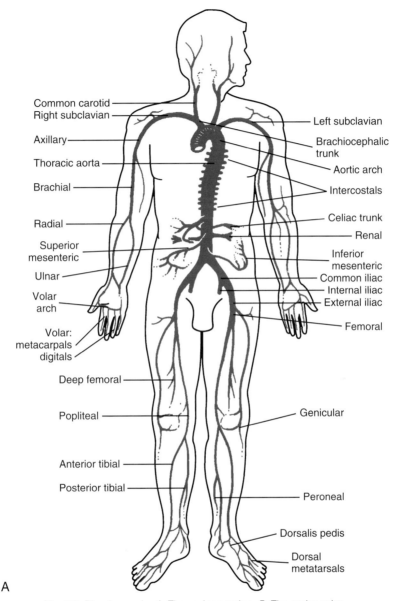

Common carotid
Right subclavian
Axillary
Thoracic aorta
Brachial
Radial
Superior mesenteric
Ulnar
Volar arch
Volar: metacarpals digitals
Deep femoral
Popliteal
Anterior tibial
Posterior tibial

Left subclavian
Brachiocephalic trunk
Aortic arch
Intercostals
Celiac trunk
Renal
Inferior mesenteric
Common iliac
Internal iliac
External iliac
Femoral
Genicular
Peroneal
Dorsalis pedis
Dorsal metatarsals

A

Fig. 2.9 Blood vessels. *A*, The major arteries. *B*, The major veins.

electrical potentials generated by the heart. Abnormalities in heartbeat can be detected with its use. More details on ECGs are in Chapter 10.

The cardiac cycle is composed of a phase of contraction (**systole**) and a phase of relaxation (**diastole**). These phases are the basis for the interpretation of blood pressure measurements. Blood pressure is produced by the contraction of the heart muscle. It is

defined as the force with which blood pushes against blood vessel walls. It is measured in terms of millimeters of mercury (mm Hg) by using a **sphygmomanometer** or blood pressure cuff. The cuff is placed around the arm and inflated to compress the brachial artery. (Note: The leg may also be used. The femoral artery is compressed in this case.) The stethoscope is placed above the bend of the elbow, and air pressure in

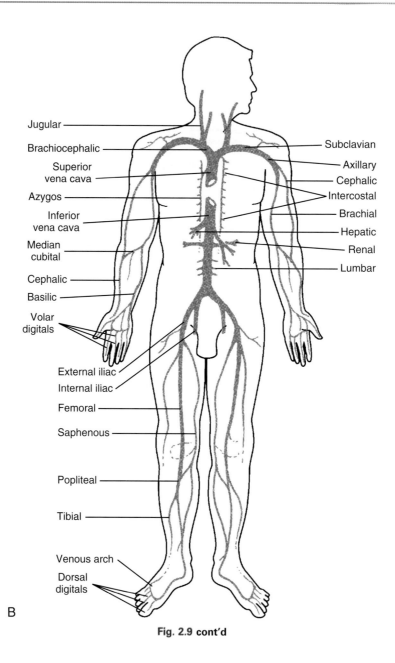

Jugular

Brachiocephalic

Superior
vena cava

Azygos

Inferior
vena cava

Median
cubital

Cephalic

Basilic

Volar
digitals

External iliac

Internal iliac

Femoral

Saphenous

Popliteal

Tibial

Venous arch

Dorsal
digitals

Subclavian

Axillary

Cephalic

Intercostal

Brachial

Hepatic

Renal

Lumbar

B

Fig. 2.9 cont'd

the cuff is released slowly. The first sound heard represents the artery beginning to open. This is recorded as systolic blood pressure. The sounds decrease in intensity until they are no longer audible as blood freely flows through the vessel. The last audible sound is the diastolic blood pressure. Normal blood pressure varies among individuals, but it is usually written as *systolic/diastolic*, or *120/80 mm Hg*.

Many factors influence blood pressure. They include total blood volume, thickness of blood, and elasticity and diameter of the blood vessels. Blood pressure is very helpful in the diagnosis of heart diseases such as **coronary heart disease**, **atherosclerosis**, and **arrhythmias**. High blood pressure (**hypertension**) is associated with a higher risk of cardiovascular accident (stroke) or myocardial infarction (heart attack). **Hypotension**, or

BOX 2.6 Circulatory System

Diagnostic Tests	Disorders
Arterial blood gases	Anemia
Bone marrow analysis	Congestive heart failure
Cholesterol	Embolus
Coagulation studies	Hemophilia
Prothrombin time (PT)	Leukemia
Activated partial thromboplastin time (APPT)	Pericarditis
Fibrin degradation products (FDP)	Polycythemia
Complete blood cell (CBC) count	Varicose veins
Creatine kinase (CK) and isoenzymes	Heart attack
Blood differential	Autoimmune diseases
Ferritin	Liver diseases
Iron (total and binding capacity)	Liver diseases
Potassium	Heart arrhythmia
Triglycerides	Coronary artery disease
Troponin	Heart attack

low blood pressure, can also cause serious medical problems. Additional factors that affect blood pressure include exercise; daily activities such as eating; stress levels; hydration; body temperature; body position; and hemodynamic stability. The medical specialty that studies the heart is cardiology.

Blood Vessels

There are three kinds of blood vessels (Fig. 2.12A):

1. *Arteries* carry oxygenated blood away from the heart. Exceptions to this include pulmonary and umbilical arteries, which carry unoxygenated blood to the lungs and placenta, respectively, for oxygenation (see Fig. 2.11). They are composed of three layers of tissue and have very thick walls. The arterial system branches out from the largest artery, the *aorta*, to the smallest of the arteries, called the *arterioles*.

2. *Capillaries* receive the flow of blood from the arteries. Capillaries are very small and narrow. They are most important to circulation because it is through their walls that all O_2, nutrients, and waste products pass between the blood and cells.

3. *Venules* receive blood flow from the capillaries. Venules empty blood into larger veins. Pressure in the veins is low, so they are equipped with valves to prevent the backflow of blood. The veins carry deoxygenated blood to the heart. Veins are also composed of three layers of tissue, but their walls are very fine.

The diameter of the blood vessels can be altered by changes in the walls of the vessels. The vessels can narrow (constrict) or widen (dilate). The changes control blood pressure in the vessels. The *pulse* is an index of the heart's actions, the elasticity of the vessels, and the resistance in the capillaries and arterioles. Arterial pulse can be taken from the brachial, femoral, and radial arteries. Pulse is evaluated by the following criteria: rate, rhythm, and strength. The normal resting pulse for an adult is 60 to 80 beats per minute. An increase is seen after exercise and in medical conditions associated with fever. Pulse is decreased during sleep.

The three major arm veins used for venipuncture are called the **antecubital veins**. They are located in the area anterior to and below the bend of the elbow (see Fig. 2.12B). The **median cubital vein** is usually large and easy to locate. It is not likely to move during insertion of the needle because it is well anchored. It is the best choice for venipuncture and will cause the least pain to the patient. The **cephalic** and **basilic veins** may be used; however, they may not be as easy to locate. The basilic vein has a tendency to roll or move when the needle is inserted, making venipuncture more difficult. One must also be careful not to inadvertently puncture the median nerve. This could be quite painful to the patient. A recent research study concluded that anatomical relationships between upper extremity superficial veins and cutaneous nerves are so intimate that needle-nerve contact during venipuncture is common. Because of these relationships, nerve injury may occur even when the venipuncture is properly performed and atraumatic.[1]

The Blood

Blood consists of the formed elements (cells and cell fragments) and a clear, pale yellow liquid component called plasma. When anticoagulants are added to blood to prevent clotting, this portion can be separated from the cells during centrifugation. **Plasma** is approximately 90% water. The other 10% consists of plasma proteins, amino acids, hormones, electrolytes, gases, antibodies,

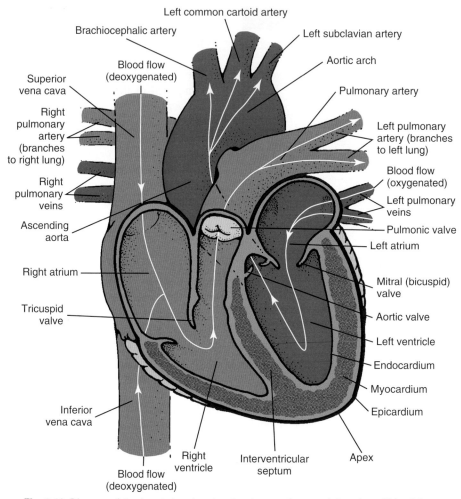

Fig. 2.10 Diagram of the heart showing the chambers, valves, and direction of blood flow.

coagulation factors, and other nutrients. If blood is collected in a tube with no anticoagulant, it will clot. After **centrifugation,** the pale-yellow liquid portion is called **serum**. It contains similar constituents as plasma, except for the coagulation, or clotting factors. Phlebotomists should refer to laboratory protocol to determine what constitutes the proper specimen. Some laboratory test methodologies may require serum, others may require plasma, and some may be completed with either serum or plasma. (In some cases, whole blood is acceptable for testing as well.)

Plasma makes up approximately 55% of total blood volume. The remaining 45% are the formed elements or cells. The three classes of formed elements are **erythrocytes** (red blood cells), **leukocytes** (white blood cells), and **thrombocytes** (platelets). After centrifugation, the white blood cells and platelets form a thin layer called the *buffy coat*. Fig. 2.13 shows the different types of cells found in the blood. Fig. 2.14 shows a comparison of centrifuged and uncentrifuged blood.

Red blood cells are biconcave disks, which allows them to be flexible when traveling through veins and capillaries. They are the most numerous of the formed elements (Table 2.1). *Erythropoiesis*, or red blood cell production, is the result of an increase in erythropoietin, a hormone produced primarily in the

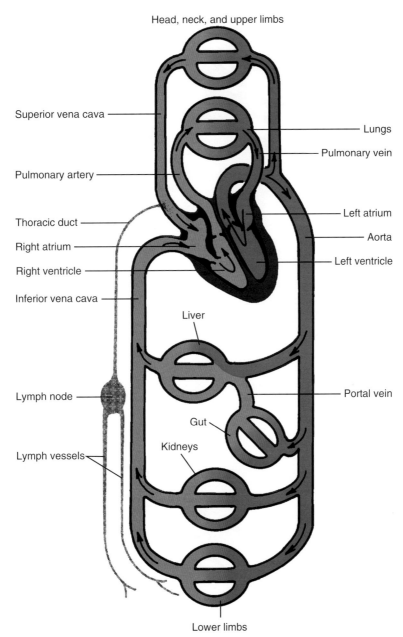

Fig. 2.11 The blood circuit.

kidneys. When body tissues become hypoxic because they are not receiving adequate O_2, the kidneys increase production of erythropoietin. This stimulates the bone marrow to produce additional red blood cells. The primary function of the red cells is to carry O_2 in the bloodstream. This is accomplished by the presence of the **hemoglobin** molecule within the cell. Hemoglobin contains iron and gives the red cell its color. Normal erythrocytes live for approximately 120 days. At the end of their life cycle, they

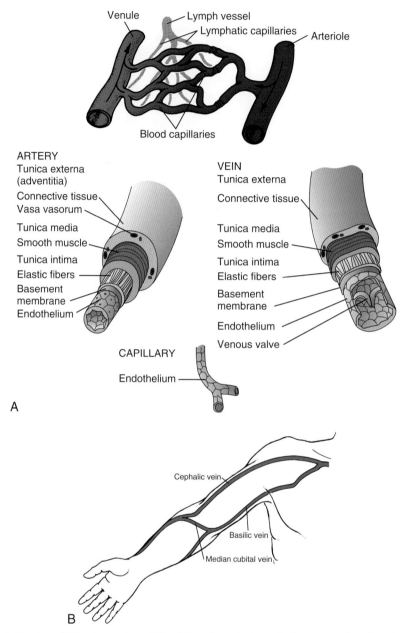

Fig. 2.12 *A,* Structure of blood vessels and blood flow through them. *B,* Common veins of venipuncture. A, Modified with permission from Applegate, EJ. *The Anatomy and Physiology Learning System.* 4th ed. St. Louis, Saunders, 2011.

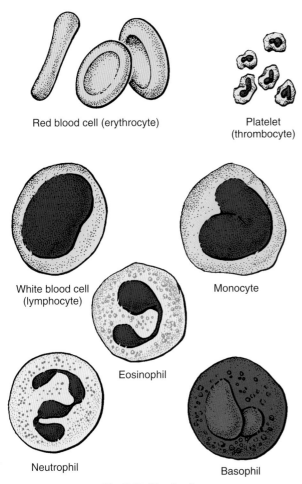

Red blood cell (erythrocyte)

Platelet
(thrombocyte)

White blood cell
(lymphocyte)

Monocyte

Eosinophil

Neutrophil

Basophil

Fig. 2.13 Blood cells.

Whole blood
(cellular and liquid
components)

Serum or
plasma

Buffy coat
(white blood
cells and
platelets)

Red blood
cells

Uncentrifuged
blood

Centrifuged
blood

Fig. 2.14 Comparison of centrifuged and uncentrifuged blood.

TABLE 2.1 Normal Blood Cell Values for an Adult	
Red blood cells	$4.50–6.00 \times 10^{12}$/L
White blood cells	$4.5–11.0 \times 10^{9}$/L
Neutrophils	45–70%
Lymphocytes	20–40%
Monocytes	3–8%
Eosinophils	2–4%
Basophils	1–2%
Platelets	$150–450 \times 10^{9}$/L

are removed from circulation by the liver or spleen. The iron and protein in the hemoglobin are recycled by the body.

There are two main classifications of white blood cells: granulocytes and agranulocytes. Granulocytes have granules in the cytoplasm, whereas agranulocytes do not. *Neutrophils* are the most common type of granulocyte (see Table 2.1). They engulf bacteria by **phagocytosis** and are significantly increased in acute infections. They are known as *polymorphonuclear leukocytes* or *segmented neutrophils* because their nucleus is multilobed, with an average of three to five lobes per cell.

Eosinophils have a bilobed nucleus and large granules that stain red-orange. They increase during allergic

reactions or parasitical infections. *Basophils* are the least common leukocyte. They also have a bilobed nucleus and large granules; however, these granules stain blue-black. They secrete histamine and heparin. Histamine increases blood flow to damaged vessels, and heparin acts as an anticoagulant.

The agranulocytes include the lymphocytes and monocytes. *Lymphocytes* protect the body and provide immunity. They are abundant in the lymphatic system. The T-lymphocytes attack bacteria and viruses, whereas the B-lymphocytes produce antibodies that react with microorganisms or their toxins. *Monocytes* are the largest white blood cells, and they engage in phagocytosis. They can leave the blood and enter the tissue. In the tissue, they are called *macrophages*. They continue the cleansing process within the tissue.

Thrombocytes, also called *platelets*, are cell fragments that aid in blood clotting. They are formed from the "pinching off" of small sections of cytoplasm from a megakaryocyte within the bone marrow. When a blood vessel is damaged, platelets adhere to the surface and begin to clump or aggregate together so clotting occurs. When not used for clotting, platelets remain in circulation for 9 or 10 days before entering the spleen.

Coagulation

The process of coagulation or **hemostasis** involves three steps that result in clot formation, thus preventing excessive blood loss:

1. The damaged blood vessels constrict to reduce flow of blood.
2. A platelet plug is formed.
3. A series of reactions occurs in a specified sequence or cascade so that a product of one reaction catalyzes the next. Many factors are necessary for clotting to occur (Fig. 2.15).

The *intrinsic pathway* contains factors found in the blood. The *extrinsic pathway* factors are stimulated from the tissue when damage occurs. The intrinsic and extrinsic pathways come together to form the common or joint pathway. The final product of these steps is fibrin, which is a meshwork that traps cells and platelets into a clot. There is a delicate balance between clot formation and fibrinolysis (dissolving of a clot) within the body to maintain hemostasis.

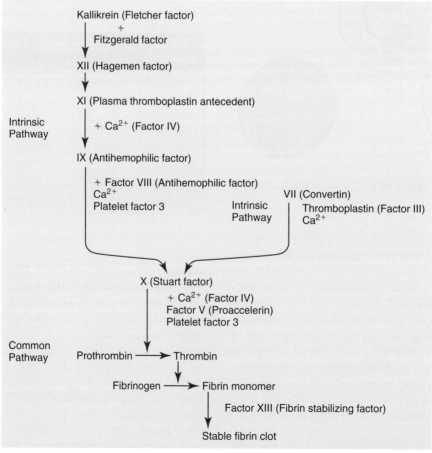

Fig. 2.15 Simplified coagulation cascade showing intrinsic, extrinsic, and common pathways.

Excessive clot formation can lead to thrombi and emboli being formed in the blood vessels. Warfarin (Coumadin) and heparin are two drugs used to prevent this. Insufficient quantities of clotting factors may also be dangerous. For example, patients with hemophilia do not produce an adequate level of factor VIII and may bleed excessively.

Blood Typing

If an individual loses a large quantity of blood, it may be necessary to give the person a transfusion of blood, plasma, platelets, or another component to replenish those lost. Serological testing for the transfusion of red blood cells is important to correctly identify blood group **antigens** located on the surface of red blood cells. Commercially prepared antisera (**antibodies**) agglutinate or clump with their corresponding antigens. There are many blood group antigens (Table 2.2); however, the ABO and Rh groups are most important. When considering the transfusion of red blood cells, antibodies in the recipient's plasma must also be considered. In the ABO blood group, these antibodies are naturally occurring, without known stimulus, whereas most other blood group antibody production is stimulated by previous transfusion or pregnancy.

The ABO blood groups are based on the presence or absence of antigens on the cells (Fig. 2.16). Table 2.3 lists the antigens and antibodies for each blood type in the ABO system. Notice that an individual cannot have the same antigen and antibody present. The body will produce antibodies to whichever antigen is not present on an individual's red blood cells.

It is best to give blood of a matching type to avoid adverse reactions called *transfusion reactions*. A **transfusion reaction** is caused when a foreign antigen from donor cells reacts with antibodies formed in the recipient. These reactions can range from mild, causing hives or a slight fever, to severe, resulting in death. In emergencies, an AB type person can receive blood of

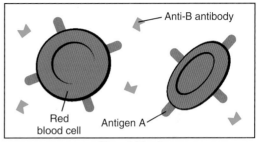

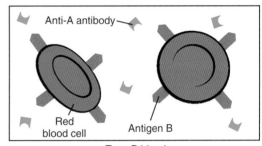

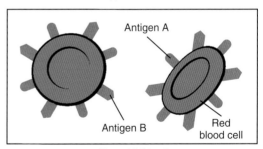

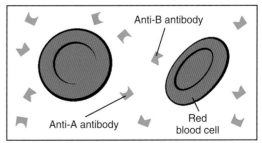

Fig. 2.16 Blood groups. Antigens and antibodies in the A, B, AB, and O blood groups.

TABLE 2.2 **Blood Group Systems and Their Common Antigens**	
Blood Group	**Antigens**
Rh	D, C, c, E, e
MNS	M, N, S, s
Kell	K, k
Duffy	Fy^a, Fy^b
Kidd	Jk^a, Jk^b
Lewis	Le^a, Le^b

TABLE 2.3 ABO Blood Group System				
Blood Type	Antigen	Antibodies	Can Receive From	Can Donate To
A	A	Anti-B	A, O	A, AB
B	B	Anti-A	B, O	B, AB
AB	A, B	None	AB, A, B, O	AB
O	None	Anti-A, anti-B	O	O, A, B, AB

any ABO type, and an O type person can give blood to any ABO type (see Table 2.3).

Rh factor, or the D antigen, is the second blood group considered when transfusing blood products. Approximately 85% of the white population is Rh or D positive, and 15% is Rh or D negative; approximately 91% of the black population is Rh positive. When transfusions are given, both ABO and Rh type should match between donor and recipient.

THE LYMPHATIC SYSTEM

The lymphatic system (Fig. 2.17), primarily a system of vessels and tissue nodules, works in conjunction with the circulatory system to carry fluid through the vessels. This system has three main functions within the body. It returns interstitial fluid (the fluid from the spaces between cells) to the blood from which it came. When this fluid passes from the spaces into the lymphatic vessels, it is called *lymph*. Lymphatic vessels are similar to veins in structure but have more valves than veins. The vessels join to form the lymphatic trunks that merge until the lymph enters two ducts. The right lymphatic duct collects lymph from the upper right quadrant of the body and empties it into the right subclavian vein. The thoracic duct, the largest lymphatic duct in the body, collects lymph from all other regions of the body and empties it into the left subclavian vein. Lymph nodes are distributed along the vessels at varying intervals. A lymph node is a mass of lymphoid tissue that filters bacteria and other foreign material from the lymph before allowing it to return to circulation.

The second function of the lymphatic system is the collection of fat and fat-soluble vitamins from the digestive process. It transports these via lymph capillaries called *lacteals* to the general circulation. The lymph in the lacteals is usually milky in appearance because it has such a high fat content.

The lymphatic system also plays an important role in immunity and defense by providing the body with lymphocytes that fight against infection and disease. These lymphocytes mature in the thymus, one of the lymphatic organs. The spleen and tonsils also serve as part of the lymphatic system. The spleen acts as a filtration system much like the lymph nodes do. Tonsils function to prevent infection by way of the nose or mouth. Please see Box 2.7 for some tests and assorted disorders associated with the lymphatic system.

THE RESPIRATORY SYSTEM

The respiratory system serves the body in three ways: respiration, circulation, and pH maintenance. The respiration process includes (1) the intake of **oxygen (O_2)** by breathing or ventilation into the lungs; (2) the exchange of gases between the lungs and blood; (3) subsequent exchange of gases from the blood to tissue; and (4) the transport of **carbon dioxide (CO_2)** back to the atmosphere. Fig. 2.18 shows the path of air flow from the nasal cavity into the lungs.

The **lungs** are the organs of respiration. The right lung has three lobes and is shorter than the left lung because the liver forces the diaphragm up. It has a greater volume than the left lung, which has only two lobes.

The blood transports the respiratory gases (O_2 and CO_2) between the lungs and tissues. Hemoglobin in the red blood cells has the ability to bind or release O_2 as the tissue cells' demand for O_2 increases and decreases within the body. Factors such as temperature, pH, O_2 levels, and CO_2 levels influence this process. CO_2, a waste product of metabolism, is carried by the blood to the lungs. It can be carried in the plasma or by the hemoglobin molecule and bicarbonate ions within the red blood cells. Because the CO_2 content in the lungs is low, the CO_2 diffuses into the lungs and is exhaled.

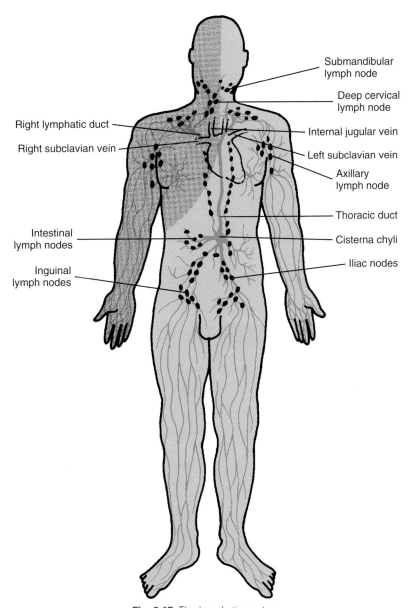

Submandibular
lymph node

Deep cervical
lymph node

Right lymphatic duct

Internal jugular vein

Right subclavian vein

Left subclavian vein

Axillary
lymph node

Thoracic duct

Intestinal
lymph nodes

Cisterna chyli

Inguinal
lymph nodes

Iliac nodes

Fig. 2.17 The lymphatic system.

The pH of the blood is regulated by the increase and decrease of CO_2. An increase in CO_2 reduces the pH of the blood, which makes the blood more acidic (acidosis). This causes a condition called **hyperventilation**. The body tries to increase O_2 levels by increasing the rate of respiration. Excess CO_2 molecules are blown off. This decrease in CO_2 increases the pH of the blood, which makes the blood more alkaline

BOX 2.7 **Lymphatic System**	
Diagnostic Tests	**Disorders**
Bone marrow biopsy	Hodgkin disease
Complete blood cell (CBC) count	Lymphadenopathy
Lymph node biopsy	Lymphoma
Mononucleosis test	Splenomegaly

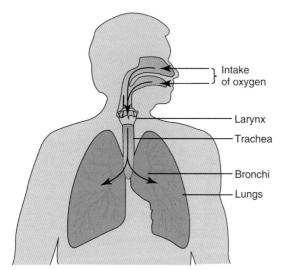

Fig. 2.18 The respiratory system showing flow of air into lungs.

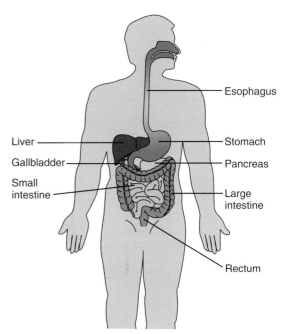

Fig. 2.19 The digestive system.

BOX 2.8 **Respiratory System**	
Diagnostic Tests	**Disorders**
Arterial blood gases	Asthma
Complete blood cell (CBC) count	Bronchitis
Electrolytes	Cystic fibrosis
Microbiological cultures	Emphysema
Sputum cultures	Pneumonia
Tuberculin test (purified	Tuberculosis
protein derivative [PPD]),	
respiratory syncytial virus (RSV)	

(alkalosis). A pulmonologist studies the lungs and related respiratory organs. Please see Box 2.8 for some tests and assorted disorders associated with the respiratory system.

THE DIGESTIVE SYSTEM

Food must be broken down into small molecules so that it can be digested, absorbed, and metabolized by the body. The digestive system (Fig. 2.19) is responsible for these functions. After food is ingested, chewed, and swallowed, it moves down the esophagus into the stomach. Gastric glands in the **stomach** secrete gastric juice, which is composed of hydrochloric acid, mucus, enzymes, and other fluids. Food particles mix with these and are then emptied into the small intestine by peristalsis.

Peristalsis is the rhythmic wave of smooth muscle contraction. It is here, in the **small intestine,** that digestion is completed. Intestinal enzymes and products produced by the **liver, gallbladder,** and **pancreas** are required elements to aid in this process. The liver produces bile, which is concentrated and stored in the gallbladder until needed. **Bile** contains bile salts, which help in the digestion of fat molecules. The pancreas produces enzymes such as amylase and lipase, which help break down complex carbohydrates and fatty acids. Nutrients are then absorbed, and the remainder is passed on to the **large intestine.**

Absorption occurs by active transport across cell membranes through villi that line the inner surface of the small intestine. Each villus contains a blood capillary and a lymphatic capillary (lacteal). Simple sugars and amino acids pass into the blood capillaries, and fatty acids enter the lacteals. In the large intestine, water and electrolytes are absorbed, and waste products are excreted via the rectum and anus.

BOX 2.9 Digestive System

Diagnostic Tests	Disorders
Amylase	Cancer
Bilirubin	Cholecystitis
Lipase	Gastritis
Occult blood test	Hepatitis
Ova and parasite analysis	Pancreatitis
Ova and parasite analysis	Parasitical infection
Ova and parasite analysis	Polyps
Ova and parasite analysis	Ulcers

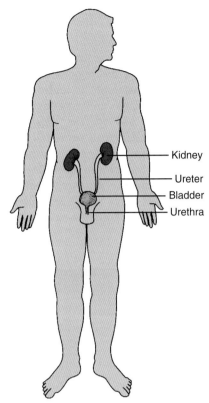

Fig. 2.20 The urinary system.

After nutrients are absorbed, they are used by the body to produce energy for all the chemical reactions that occur. These chemical reactions are called *metabolism*. Metabolic reactions are divided into two categories: anabolism and catabolism. **Anabolism** is the process of making larger molecules from smaller ones. This requires the use of chemical energy or ATP. **Catabolism** is the breakdown of large molecules into smaller ones. Energy is released during catabolism. Gastroenterology is the study of the digestive organs. A gastrologist studies diseases of the stomach. Please see Box 2.9 for some tests and assorted disorders associated with the digestive system.

THE RENAL SYSTEM

The primary function of the urinary system (Fig. 2.20) is to maintain fluid hemostasis or balance in the body and to excrete waste products. It consists of a pair of kidneys, ureters, bladder, and urethra.

The kidneys filter the blood to remove waste products and excrete them into the urine. The functional unit in the kidney is called a *nephron*. Blood flows into the kidney, where it is filtered by the glomerulus, a cluster of capillaries within the nephron. Urine then passes from the nephrons into the bladder via the ureters. The bladder is a temporary storage area for the urine. Urine exits the body through the urethra, which is controlled by voluntary skeletal muscle. In males, the urethra, which is much longer than in females, transports both urine and semen. The urethra passes through the prostate gland and **penis**.

After the filtration process, useful substances and water are moved from the filtrate in the kidney to the blood. This process is called *reabsorption*. The kidneys alter the concentration and volume of urine. This helps maintain blood concentration, volume, and pressure. Other functions of the kidneys include renin and erythropoietin production. *Renin* is an enzyme that is made in response to a low blood pressure or low sodium concentration. It stimulates **vasoconstrictor** production to increase blood pressure. Erythropoietin is a hormone that controls red blood cell production in the bone marrow. The study of the urinary system is known as *urology*. Please see Box 2.10 for some tests and assorted disorders associated with the renal system.

THE REPRODUCTIVE SYSTEM

The reproductive system involves mechanisms that work together to produce offspring. The primary reproductive organs, or **gonads**, are the **testes** in males and the **ovaries** in females (Fig. 2.21). The ovaries produce egg cells, or ova, and the testes produce spermatozoa, or sperm cells. These sex cells, or *gametes*, also produce hormones that are important in the reproductive process. **Testosterone**, an **androgen**, is necessary for the development and function of the male reproductive organs and for the development and maintenance of secondary male sex characteristics. The primary female hormones are the estrogens. They induce ovulation and the growth of female reproductive structures. **Estrogens** are also responsible for the development of secondary female sex characteristics. **Progesterone** and other hormones secreted by the pi-

tuitary gland help regulate the functions of the female reproductive system.

Sperm cell production in the testes begins at the onset of puberty and continues throughout the life of a male. Sperm are released from the testes and enter the **epididymis**—a series of ducts—where they mature and are stored. They then pass through the urethra and penis, where they exit the body. The seminal vesicles, **prostate**, and bulbourethral (Cowper) glands secrete fluids that form semen. Semen is a mixture of these secretions and sperm.

The female reproductive system includes the ovaries, **uterus**, **vagina**, uterine tubes, external genitalia, and glands. The menstrual cycle takes place from the onset of puberty until menopause. During the menstrual cycle, usually a single mature ovum is released from the ovaries. This is called *ovulation*. The lining of the uterus prepares for implantation of the egg if it should become fertilized by a sperm.

This process occurs under the influence of hormones whose levels have gradually risen during the cycle. If the egg is not fertilized during ovulation, some of these hormone levels decline and menstruation begins. Early in the menstrual cycle the ovaries produce estrogen and progesterone that stimulate the development of the uterus's lining, or endometrium. One type of pituitary hormone production is subsequently inhibited, and this cyclic pattern continues. If fertilization occurs, the zygote (fertilized egg) attaches to the wall of the uterus and begins to develop into a fetus. Please see Box 2.11 for some tests and assorted disorders associated with the reproductive system.

BOX 2.10	**Renal System**
Diagnostic Tests	**Disorders**
Albumin	Cystitis
Ammonia	Kidney stones
Blood urea nitrogen (BUN)	Nephritis
Creatinine	Renal failure
Creatinine clearance (24-hour urine)	Urinary tract infection (UTI)
Electrolytes	Renal failure
Osmolality	Renal failure
Urinalysis including microscopic examination	Urinary tract infection (UTI)
Urine cultures	Urinary tract infection (UTI)

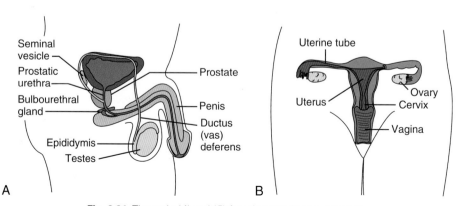

A   B

Fig. 2.21 The male (*A*) and (*B*) female reproductive systems.

BOX 2.11 Reproductive System

Diagnostic Tests	Disorders
Acid phosphatase	Cancer (cervical, ovarian,
Estrogen	prostate, testicular, uterine)
Human chorionic gonadotropin (HCG)	Infertility
Papanicolaou (PAP) smear	Ovarian cysts
Rapid plasmin reagin (RPR)	Sexually transmitted diseases (STDs)
Testosterone	Osteoporosis

SUMMARY

This chapter provided an introduction of the major body systems. It also provided some of the tests that might be ordered to monitor or diagnose conditions associated with the systems. It is important for the phlebotomist to have a general understanding of the body's systems and what blood tests might be ordered.

CASE 2.1 CRITICAL THINKING

Sally, the morning phlebotomist, was paged "stat" to the intensive care unit to collect blood from Mrs. Smith. Among the tests requested are a complete blood count, blood urea nitrogen and creatinine, amylase, and troponin. The respiratory therapist also asks Sally to transport an arterial blood gas sample he has just collected to the laboratory. What organ systems are being evaluated by these tests?

CASE 2.2 CRITICAL THINKING

Mr. Black is receiving a unit of blood for a low hemoglobin level when Jim, the phlebotomist, is called "stat" to the floor to collect samples. Mr. Black is partially unresponsive when Jim arrives at his room. Mr. Black has also spiked a temperature and appears to have labored breathing.
1. What could be causing Mr. Black's rise in temperature and unresponsiveness?
2. Why might this type of reaction occur?
3. Why was Jim called "stat" to the floor to collect blood?

▮ REVIEW QUESTIONS

1. The _____ is the smallest unit of life.
2. A group of organs working together to perform related functions is defined as a _____.
3. _____ muscle makes up the heart.
4. The _____ are responsible for producing gametes.
5. _____ aids in the coagulation process by forming a plug to stop blood flow.
6. The digestion process is completed in the _____.
7. Blood transports the respiratory gases of _____ and _____ between the lungs and the tissues.
8. The _____ system plays an important role in immunity and defense against infection.
9. The _____ alter the concentration and volume of urine.
10. The three kinds of blood vessels are _____, _____, and _____.
11. A _____ plane divides the body or organ into superior and inferior portions, and a _____ divides the body or organ into anterior and posterior planes.
12. The skin, one of the largest organs in the body, is part of the _____ system.
13. Chemicals used by the body to carry impulses between neurons are called _____.
14. The five types of white blood cells are _____, _____, _____, _____, and _____.

15. _____ is released during the process of catabolism.

16. The alkaline phosphatase test is used to evaluate the _____ system.

17. Polycythemia is a condition associated with the _____ system.

18. Deoxygenated blood enters the heart through the:
  a. Superior vena cava
  b. Aorta
  c. Pulmonary artery
  d. Left ventricle

19. Which arm vein is usually large, easy to locate, and not likely to move during a venipuncture?
  a. Cephalic
  b. Basilic
  c. Median cubital
  d. Aorta

20. The liquid portion of anticoagulated whole blood is called:
  a. Cells
  b. Thrombi
  c. Serum
  d. Plasma

21. Which of the following is **not** one of the main functions of the lymphatic system?
  a. Collection of fat and vitamins from the digestive system
  b. Production of erythropoietin
  c. Production of lymphocytes
  d. Transportation of interstitial fluid from cells to blood

22. All of the following directly affect blood pressure except:
  a. Exercise
  b. Body temperature
  c. Body position
  d. White blood cell count

REFERENCES

Horowitz SH. Venipuncture-induced causalgia: anatomic relations of upper extremity superficial veins and nerves, and clinical considerations. _Transfusion._ 2000;40.

BIBLIOGRAPHY

Barrett KE, Barman SM, et al. _Ganong's Review of Medical Physiology._ 26th. New York: McGraw-Hill Companies; 2019.
Loukas M, Tubbs R, et al. _Gray's Anatomy Review._ 3rd. St. Louis: Elsevier; 2010.
Patton KT. _Anatomy & Physiology._ 10th. St. Louis: Mosby; 2018.

Infectious Diseases and Their Prevention

Patricia Tille

"Infectious disease is one of the few genuine adventures left in the world."

—*Hans Zinsser, Physician (1878–1940)*

OBJECTIVES

At the conclusion of this chapter, the student should be able to:
- Discuss bloodborne pathogens—hepatitis B, hepatitis C, and human immunodeficiency virus (HIV)—and their significance.
- Describe the routes of transmission for infectious diseases.
- Describe the chain of infection.
- Describe the symptoms and routes of transmission for common viral and bacterial diseases.
- Discuss the importance of common viral and bacterial diseases for phlebotomists.
- Discuss the importance of multidrug-resistant organisms (MDRO) in a hospital setting.
- Identify personal protective equipment (PPE) that phlebotomists use on the job.
- Describe the proper technique for putting on and taking off PPE.
- Describe Standard Precautions and Transmission-Based Precautions used to protect health care workers from infectious diseases.

OUTLINE

KEY TERMS

airborne transmission
bloodborne pathogens
communicable

direct contact transmission
droplet transmission
hepatitis B

human immunodeficiency virus (HIV)
indirect contact transmission
infection
infectious microorganisms
methicillin-resistant *Staphylococcus aureus* (MRSA)
multidrug-resistant organism (MDRO)
nosocomial

pathogen (pathogenic)
personal protective equipment (PPE)
respiratory and cough etiquette
sequelae
Standard Precautions
Transmission-Based Precautions Virulence factors

INTRODUCTION

Phlebotomists encounter patients with many different diseases. Some diseases are **communicable** or infectious, meaning that they can be transmitted or spread from the patient to another individual. This chapter describes common infectious diseases found in inpatient and outpatient settings, infection control principles used by health care professionals, and isolation procedures recommended by the Centers for Disease Control and Prevention (CDC) to prevent infection of health care workers.

Infectious microorganisms capable of causing disease **(pathogenic)** that can be transmitted through blood or body fluids are classified as **bloodborne pathogens** and include viruses and bacteria. In 1991, Congress passed the Occupational Safety and Health Administration (OSHA) regulation (29 CFR 1910.1030) titled *Occupational Exposure to Bloodborne Pathogens*. This regulation required employers to provide certain safeguards to health care workers with guidelines for the prevention of occupational exposure to **hepatitis B, human immunodeficiency virus (HIV),** and other bloodborne pathogens.

In addition to bloodborne pathogens, health care workers can also be exposed to many other pathogenic viruses and bacteria that may cause disease. This chapter examines several pathogens encountered in the health care environment, including viral agents such as influenza, rubella, and measles and bacteria such as **methicillin-resistant *Staphylococcus aureus* (MRSA),** meningitis, and tuberculosis (TB).

Knowing what type of pathogen a health care worker may encounter is important, but it is also important to know the common practices that can prevent a health care worker from becoming infected. These include immunization, **personal protective equipment (PPE),** sharps injury prevention, hand hygiene, standard precautions, and transmission-based precautions. Lastly,

this chapter highlights special populations of individuals or environments, such as specific hospital units, ambulatory care settings, and long-term care settings, with unique challenges related to potential exposure to infectious disease.

INFECTIOUS DISEASES ENCOUNTERED IN A HEALTH CARE SETTING

Bloodborne Pathogens

Bloodborne pathogens or **infectious microorganisms** may be bacterial or viral. In either case, they are transmitted via blood and body fluids and can lead to serious and potentially fatal conditions.

Hepatitis B

By definition, hepatitis is the inflammation of the liver. There are several forms of hepatitis; the key types are discussed in the following sections.

Route of infection. Hepatitis B is transmitted through blood transfusions or contaminated blood products (rare in the United States), needle sticks (including acupuncture, tattoos, or piercings), sexual contact, needles shared among drug abusers, and occupational exposure of health care workers. The concentration of hepatitis B is very high in blood and semen. Hepatitis B is present in very high quantities in the semen of an infected individual and can be transmitted through sexual contact as can other bacterial, viral, and infectious diseases. Before blood products were routinely screened for hepatitis B, blood transfusion was the most common cause of hepatitis. The risk of contracting hepatitis B from exposure to a patient's blood greatly increases when an individual is accidentally stuck with a contaminated needle. Contaminated needles are found in hospitals, acupuncture clinics, and tattoo parlors and among needles shared by drug abusers. The CDC estimates that at least 1000 needle sticks with dirty (blood-containing) needles occur to health care workers every day.

Health care workers can be occupationally exposed to hepatitis B when an infected individual's blood comes into contact with broken skin or mucous membranes. Blood can be splashed or otherwise spread through contact with a patient's saturated clothing or body surfaces in the emergency room or operating room after a serious accident or injury. Blood can be splashed into one's eyes or mouth (mucous membranes) during medical procedures in these settings and in the dental clinic or acute care setting. Although the amount of patient blood present during a routine dental procedure is small, many dental professionals have contracted hepatitis B from a blood splatter and exposure through an open wound or mucous membrane (eyes or mouth).

Symptoms. Once a person is exposed to hepatitis B, it takes 2 to 6 months for an infection to be evident and for symptoms to appear. Infection with hepatitis B may be asymptomatic, acute, chronic, or fulminant. In asymptomatic hepatitis B infection, the virus is introduced into an individual's bloodstream, and the virus is cleared from the bloodstream before it can do enough damage to produce symptoms. Although there are no symptoms present, hepatitis B can lead to liver damage if left undetected or treated. Acute infection with the hepatitis B virus may produce jaundice, nausea, vomiting, joint pain, rashes, and marked elevation in liver function tests. These signs and symptoms are because of the inflammation that occurs in the liver from the virus replicating in the cells. In chronic hepatitis, the virus is replicating at a low level within the cells of the liver. The pathology or liver damage is caused by the patient's immune system (defense against viruses and bacteria) attempting to clear the virus. The chronic infection eventually leads to cirrhosis, portal hypertension, or hepatocellular carcinoma. Diagnosis of chronic infection requires laboratory tests to detect the virus and monitor liver function. Fulminant hepatitis B infection is characterized by severe tissue damage followed by liver failure. It is diagnosed when a patient develops hepatic encephalopathy within 8 weeks of the onset of disease symptoms.

Sequelae. Individuals who recover from a hepatitis B infection may not have any **sequelae** until years later. The most common sequelae associated with hepatitis B

infection include cirrhosis, portal hypertension, hepatocellular carcinoma, and dementia.

Hepatitis C

Route of infection. The routes of infection for hepatitis C are similar to hepatitis B. The virus is transmitted by blood, blood products, or tissue. Health care workers, intravenous drug abusers, children whose mothers are infected at the time of birth, and individuals who may be exposed to contaminated needles used for tattoos and body piercing are at a higher risk for hepatitis C. Health care workers can be exposed to the hepatitis C virus through the same types of exposures as the hepatitis B virus: contaminated accidental needle sticks, blood and blood products, and splashing of blood onto mucous membranes or into open cuts or wounds on the skin.

Symptoms. Hepatitis C also causes inflammation of the liver, but infected individuals do not usually experience the severe symptoms associated with an acute infection of hepatitis B. Hepatitis C produces a milder acute disease than hepatitis B. In fact, people infected with hepatitis C usually discover the infection after repeated elevated liver function tests and elevation in antibodies to the virus in the bloodstream. Many individuals infected with hepatitis C develop a long-term, chronic infection. A long-term infection occurs when there are necrotic changes to the liver for more than 6 months.

Sequelae. Long-term infection eventually leads to cirrhosis and liver cancer. See Table 3.1 for a summary of the various forms of hepatitis.

Human Immunodeficiency Virus

HIV is a retrovirus that was discovered in 1983. The virus causes a loss of immune function, which leads to opportunistic infections, other diseases, and complications. Infection with HIV may also lead to the development of systemic disease referred to as *acquired immune deficiency syndrome* (AIDS). HIV infection is a worldwide epidemic. According to the World Health Organization (WHO), "in 2020 there were 37.7 million people living with HIV, 1.5 million new HIV infections, and 680,000 AIDS-related deaths."[1] Approximately 40,000 people are diagnosed with HIV in the United States annually, with an "estimated 1,189,700 people in the United States" living with HIV at the end of 2019.[2]

TABLE 3.1	Characteristics of Viral Hepatitis				
	Hepatitis A	**Hepatitis B**	**Hepatitis C**	**Hepatitis D**	**Hepatitis E**
Source of virus	Feces	Blood or blood-derived body fluids	Blood or blood-derived body fluids	Blood or blood-derived body fluids	Feces
Route of transmission	Fecal-oral	Percutaneous permucosal	Percutaneous permucosal	Percutaneous permucosal	Fecal-oral
Incubation period (days)	15–45	7–160	15–160	28–45	2–9 weeks
Severity	Mild	Moderate	Variable	Often severe	Variable
Chronic infection	No	Yes	Yes	Yes	No
Prevention	Pre- or postexposure immunization	Pre- or postexposure immunization	Blood donor screening; risk behavior modification	Pre- or postexposure immunization; risk behavior modification	Ensure safe drinking water

In 1999, new drugs that slow the replication of the HIV virus were introduced, resulting in fewer people developing AIDS and dying. More people are living with HIV. This is because of the treatment advances that are slowing the progression of the disease. However, people infected with HIV represent a larger pool of people that can infect others. As more vulnerable populations become infected with HIV, the epidemic is moving throughout the country and across the globe. Smaller, more rural communities are seeing an increase in individuals infected with the virus, especially minorities, females, and the younger population.

Route of infection. HIV is spread through contact with the blood or body fluids of an infected individual. Some of the common routes for transmission of the virus include having unprotected sex with an infected individual; having multiple sex partners; having sex with a partner who has another sexually transmitted disease; sharing needles, syringes, rinse water, or other equipment used to prepare or deliver illegal drugs for injection; or being born to an HIV-infected mother. There are other uncommon ways to become infected with HIV, such as from an accidental needle stick contaminated with HIV-infected blood; from receiving blood transfusions, blood products, or an organ transplant from an HIV-infected donor; by being bitten by an HIV-infected person; and from tattooing or body piercing with a needle contaminated with HIV-infected blood.

Between 1985 and 2022, the CDC received 58 confirmed cases of HIV and 150 suspected cases of HIV through occupational exposure.[3] Most of the time (99.7%), a needle stick with a dirty needle does not lead to HIV infection. The risk of contracting HIV from mucous membrane exposure or blood entering through broken skin is 0.1% or less. Nonetheless, all health care workers must continue to use proper safety precautions to prevent exposure and spread of HIV and other bloodborne pathogens.

Symptoms. Once the HIV virus enters the body, it attacks the lymphocytes and begins replicating. Viral replication leads to an increase in infected lymphocytes that travel throughout the body, seeding themselves in various organs, especially the lymph nodes, thymus, and spleen. In the initial stage of infection, the individual will have very few symptoms, but 3 to 6 weeks after infection, 50% to 70% of infected individuals will experience flulike symptoms, such as fever, headache, tiredness, and enlarged lymph nodes in the neck and groin area. The individual may be misdiagnosed with a viral illness like influenza because the symptoms disappear in 1 week to 1 month. At this point, the individual's blood and body fluids contain large amounts of HIV. Some individuals experience a more severe bout of symptoms that may be present for a longer period, whereas others remain asymptomatic. After this symptomatic period, the virus lies latent or dormant for many years. Even though the individual has no symptoms, the virus is still replicating inside the body. During the late stage of infection, the individual develops AIDS.

Acquired immune deficiency syndrome. AIDS is the late stage of HIV infection. Symptoms of AIDS include rapid weight loss; recurring fever; profuse night sweats; extreme and unexplainable fatigue; swelling of the lymph glands in the armpits, groin, or neck for long periods; diarrhea that lasts for more than 1 week; sores of the mouth, anus, or genitals; *Pneumocystis* pneumonia or other secondary infectious diseases; red, brown, pink, or purplish blotches on or under the skin or inside the mouth, nose, or eyelids (Kaposi patches); and memory loss, depression, and other neurological disorders.

Other Bloodborne Pathogens

Although hepatitis B, hepatitis C, and HIV are the most frequently transmitted bloodborne pathogens, other bloodborne pathogens are also important. These include malaria and the West Nile virus in the United States. Technically, any disease in which the infectious agent is present in the blood can be considered a bloodborne pathogen. See Box 3.1 for a list of infectious bloodborne pathogenic diseases.

Communicable Diseases

Bloodborne pathogens pose a threat to phlebotomists, but these exposures can be prevented through engineering controls, PPE, education, awareness, and adherence to procedures. There are, however, other diseases that can be transmitted to the phlebotomists through other routes. These routes of infection include direct contact, indirect contact, and the droplet and airborne routes. Infection control practices and procedures can help minimize the exposure of phlebotomists to other communicable diseases.

Route of Infection

The concept of route of transmission is very important because it lays out the chain of infection. For example, there needs to be a source of pathogens for an individual to become infected. These sources include humans (patients, health care workers, family members,

> ### BOX 3.1 Infectious Diseases
>
> **Bloodborne Pathogens***
> - Chickenpox (varicella)
> - Prions (Creutzfeldt-Jakob disease [CJD])
> - Viral hemorrhagic fevers (Ebola, Lassa, or Marburg)
> - Gastrointestinal infections (*Clostridioides difficile, Escherichia coli* O157-H7, *Shigella,* rotavirus)
> - Hantavirus
> - Hepatitis A, B, C
> - Human immunodeficiency virus (HIV)/acquired immune deficiency syndrome (AIDS)
> - Influenza
> - Methicillin-resistant *Staphylococcus aureus* (MRSA)
> - Parvovirus
> - Poliovirus
> - Respiratory pathogens (pneumonia)
> - Rubella (measles)
> - Coronaviruses (Severe acute respiratory syndrome [SARS], SARS-CoV2, or COVID-19)
> - Tuberculosis
> - Vancomycin-intermediate or -resistant S. *aureus*
> - Vancomycin-resistant enterococcus (VRE)
> - Any multidrug-resistant microorganism
> - Skin microorganisms (lice, scabies, varicella zoster [chickenpox], bacteria)

visitors) who may have an active infection, a chronic infection, or be asymptomatic. An individual's normal bacteria (*normal microbiota*) found on an individual can also cause infections in others. Other sources for pathogens can be inanimate objects or fomites. Inanimate objects can include pens (especially if inserted into someone's mouth), telephones, and tabletops. If there is no source of pathogens, then an individual cannot be infected. Next, there needs to be a susceptible individual (*host*) with a portal of entry for the pathogen. Exposure to a pathogen does not mean someone is infected. An **infection** is characterized by growth or multiplication of a microorganism within or on the host (*colonization*) resulting in harm. Infection of an individual is a complicated process involving the number of organisms transmitted to the person, the **virulence factors** (characteristics that permit a microorganism to cause disease) of the pathogen, and interaction between the organism and the individual's immune system. Stated simply, if a critical mass of the pathogen possesses virulence factors and overcomes the host's defense system, an infection will result. An individual infected with a pathogen may appear asymptomatic, acutely ill, severely ill, or deathly ill. The latter part of the chapter discusses special patient populations.

Lastly, a pathogen requires a mode of transmission to cause an infection. Sneezing and coughing are two of the most common modes of transmission for the influenza virus. If any of these three links in the infection chain are missing, chances are very good that infection can be prevented. This section discusses the four modes of transmitting microorganisms from one person to another. See Fig. 3.1 for the chain of infection. The key to preventing infection is to "break" the chain.

Contact Transmission

Direct contact transmission occurs when a pathogen is transmitted from one individual to another. The Guideline for Infection Control in Health Care Personnel (1998) summarizes a few examples of instances in which direct contact transmission can occur between patients and health care workers:

1. A health care worker's mucous membrane or nonintact skin comes in contact with blood or other blood-containing body fluids from a patient.
2. A scabies-infected patient's mites are transferred to the unprotected skin of a health care worker.

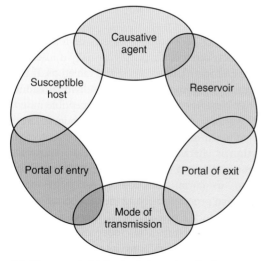

Fig. 3.1 The spread of infection is best described as a chain of several links.

3. Herpes virus is passed to a health care worker after the ungloved worker provides care to a patient's herpetic lesion.

There are several microorganisms that can be transmitted by direct contact through these instances or similar conditions. When an infection is passed through a direct-contact transmission route, the three links of the infection control chain can usually be identified—source, susceptible host, and a route of entry.

Indirect Contact Transmission

The **indirect contact transmission** route may be more difficult to determine how the transmission of the infection occurred. Indirect contact transmission occurs through an intermediate source, such as an object or another person. The Guideline for Hand Hygiene in Health Care Settings cites evidence pointing to the contamination of a health care worker's hands as the possible source for this type of transmission. The following are examples of how this type of transmission might occur in the health care setting:

- A health care worker may be processing blood specimens in the laboratory and pick up the telephone receiver to answer a phone call without taking off gloves.
- Patient-care devices may be shared between patients without cleaning or disinfecting first.
- Pediatric patients may transmit infectious agents through shared toys.
- Instruments that are not cleaned well in between patients can transmit infectious organisms.

Even though soiled clothing, uniforms, laboratory coats, or isolation gowns have not been implicated in transmitting infectious organisms, the possibility does exist. As a result, clothing items other than the health care worker's personal uniform are now primarily constructed of synthetic materials and are a single-use item that can be immediately discarded if soiled or damaged.

Droplet Transmission

Technically, **droplet transmission** can be considered a form of contact transmission because large respiratory droplets from one individual must land on the mucous membranes of another individual to give the organism an opportunity to cause an infection. Interestingly, some infectious organisms that are transmitted through contact transmission are also transmitted through droplet transmission. Sneezing, coughing, or even talking generates small respiratory droplets that can carry enough organisms to cause an infection if they land on a susceptible host. Respiratory droplets can also be formed during suctioning, endotracheal intubation, and cardiopulmonary resuscitation. Although the exact distance that the respiratory droplets travel is not yet at consensus, a good rule of thumb is 3 feet. If a health care worker is within 3 feet of an individual who is producing respiratory droplets, additional PPE beyond gloves and gowns should be worn—especially masks (certified N-95), face shields (eye protection), or a powered air-purifying respirator (PAPR).[4] PPE should also be worn when entering any patient's room. Patients are generally placed in a special negative air-pressure room where the air is discharged outdoors and monitored through a filtration system if the patient is infected with a known virulent respiratory pathogen. The room air must circulate through a high-efficiency particulate air (HEPA) filter or a series of HEPA filters before it is vented outdoors. Respiratory droplets are heavy compared with air and do not travel very long distances. Organisms that are transmitted via respiratory droplets cannot infect another host over long distances. Organisms transmitted by droplet transmission include *Bordetella pertussis,* influenza virus, adenovirus rhinovirus, *Mycoplasma pneumoniae,* severe acute respiratory syndrome (SARS)—associated coronavirus (SARS-CoV and COVID-19), group A streptococcus, and *Neisseria meningitidis.*

Airborne Transmission

For a pathogen to be transmitted through the air, small droplets or particles must be generated that contain infectious agents that remain infective over longer distances. It is important to note that some respiratory infectious diseases are capable of being transmitted via large droplets or smaller airborne particles.[5] These infectious agents must be able to retain their infective nature for a distance outside of the source. An example is fungal spores. The spores released by a mature fungus are infective and can remain infective for a long period and a long distance. Pathogens that are transmitted by this route can infect individuals far away that have never had face-to-face contact with the infected individual. Because respiratory pathogens may be spread either via droplet or **airborne transmission,** the infection control procedures have become more

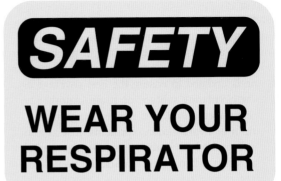

Fig. 3.2 Airborne Precaution signage should be displayed outside the patient room. Airborne Precautions indicate the use of an N-95 or higher respirator. (Courtesy Occupational Safety and Health Administration.)

standardized, including the use of PPE and specialized patient rooms to prevent the spread of infection. Pathogens transmitted through airborne transmission routes include *Mycobacterium* TB, rubeola virus (measles), coronavirus (COVID-19) and varicella-zoster virus (chickenpox; Fig. 3.2). On rare occasions, smallpox, monkey pox, and avian flu have been transmitted through the airborne route.

Common Viral Diseases

This section reviews several of the common viral diseases.

Influenza

There are three types of influenza viruses—A, B, and C. Types A and B cause the seasonal flu, and type C causes a mild respiratory illness but not epidemics. The subtypes of influenza A are classified based on two surface proteins—hemagglutinin (H) and neuraminidase (N). Identified subtypes of this virus are known to have 18 different hemagglutinin and 11 different neuraminidase proteins (e.g., H1N1 or H3N2).[6] In addition, influenza A viruses are subdivided into strains. Influenza B viruses do not have subtypes, but they do have strains. In addition to the different subtypes and strains, influenza viruses tend to mutate about every year so that the body's immune system will not recognize the new virus. Because the virus is capable of changing the structure of the subtype or strain, the virus is able to reinfect individuals that were previously infected by a different strain or subtype. There are two ways an influenza virus mutates: antigenic drift and antigenic shift. Antigenic drift occurs when the virus changes only a little but enough to appear as a "new" virus to the body. Antigenic drift is monitored annually, and each year a new vaccine is updated to ensure the best coverage against the new circulating subtype or strain. Another type of change, antigenic *shift*, is a major change in the hemagglutinin or neuraminidase proteins. Just as antigenic drift affects the body's ability to recognize a viral subtype or strain, when a shift occurs, the population that was protected with the old vaccine is now susceptible to infection with the new virus. Influenza A viruses undergo both antigenic shift and drift, whereas influenza B viruses undergo only antigenic drift.

Seasonal influenza. Although winter is when the flu cases peak, the outbreak can begin as early as October and continue into May. Most of the influenza cases peak in January or February. There are sporadic cases that occur during the other calendar months. These cases are used to formulate the influenza vaccine for the current year.

Symptoms. Symptoms include fever, muscle aches, headache, malaise, dry cough, sore throat, and runny nose. The fever, muscle aches, and headache can last for 3 to 5 days. The dry cough, sore throat, runny nose, and malaise can last for 2 weeks or more. There are many diseases with these types of symptoms, so diagnosing influenza can be difficult. These symptoms come on suddenly. Depending on the health of the host, influenza may cause severe disease that is followed by complications. People who are 65 years and older, people with chronic medical conditions (asthma, diabetes, or heart disease), pregnant females, and young children are more prone to complications from an influenza infection. In fact, complications from the flu (pneumonia, bronchitis, and sinus and ear infections) can be life-threatening or lead to death.

Transmission route. All types of influenza (A, B, and C) are transmitted by person-to-person contact. Respiratory droplets from one person adhere to another person's mucous membranes, and infection results. Individuals that present with symptoms should stay home from work and out of public places to prevent spread of the infection. However, most individuals feel fine until the symptoms suddenly appear and may transmit the virus unknowingly early during infection. These individuals can begin infecting others 1 day before symptoms begin and 5 to 7 days after becoming ill. Even those individuals who are infected with the influenza virus but have no symptoms (*asymptomatic*) can still infect others during this time.

H1N1 influenza. H1N1 is the serotype of a novel influenza A virus that appeared in the spring of 2009.

Cycle. H1N1 first appeared in March of 2009 and peaked in November of that same year. The cycle did not recur during 2010.

Symptoms. The symptoms of H1N1 influenza A include fever of 101°F or higher, malaise, extreme fatigue, headache, vomiting, nausea, sore throat, cough, and body aches. These symptoms can last for 2 to 4 weeks.

Transmission route. Influenza A is transmitted from person-to-person through respiratory droplets.

Coronavirus (SARS-CoV2)

Coronaviruses are known respiratory pathogens that are capable of infecting the upper and lower respiratory tract. Rhinoviruses and coronaviruses cause approximately 55% of all upper respiratory tract illnesses. Three genotypes of coronovirus have been identified that cause severe disease in humans: SARS-CoV, Middle Eastern respiratory syndrome–related coronavirus (MERS-CoV), and SARS-CoV2.[6] SARS-CoV2, also known as COVID-19, was first identified in 2019. The virus rapidly spread and became a worldwide pandemic. In May 2022, the CDC reported a total of 83,278,995 cases of COVID-19 in the United States, resulting in 999,785 deaths.[2,7]

Various treatments have been used to lessen the disease severity of symptoms and mortality associated with COVID-19. These include convalescent plasma from an individual who has recovered from COVID-19, remdesivir, steroids to minimize the cytokine storm, and anticoagulants to prevent disseminated intravascular coagulation and organ damage. More recently, Paxlovid, an antiviral experimental medication, was authorized by the Food and Drug Administration (FDA) for emergency use only in patients with mild to moderate COVID who are at risk for serious comorbidities. Paxlovid is the commercial name for the antiviral nirmatrelvir, a protease inhibitor that targets the viral polyprotein, preventing the virus from biosynthesis and maturation of virions.[11,13] Paxlovid, an experimental Pfizer drug, has demonstrated 89% effectiveness in preventing serious illness, hospitalizations and death in COVID-19 patients (statnews.com).[12]

A series of vaccines for COVID-19 have been developed and are available for individuals 5 years of age and older. Because of the replication mechanism for the nucleic acid in COVID-19, the virus can rapidly undergo mutation, altering the protein structure of the virus and rendering current vaccines less effective. The CDC and other commercial organizations monitor the strain types and genomic sequences of the virus to continually develop new and effective vaccines. The most recent vaccine is a bivalent vaccine that contains a sequence to the original COVID-19 strain as well as a sequence to the recent omicron BA.4 and BA.5 variants. However, as new strains are continually coming to the forefront, the CDC recommends that individuals receive COVID-19 vaccinations and remain current with updated and new vaccines as the virus mutates and they become available.[14] https://www.cdc.gov

Symptoms. Symptoms of a coronavirus infection may initially appear similar to influenza. However, infection can rapidly progress to SARS or severe acute respiratory syndrome, which requires hospitalization and supportive care or mechanical ventilation. After the initial incubation period of 2 to 14 days and the onset of flu-like symptoms, an individual may develop a dry cough and shortness of breath. Additional symptoms may include diarrhea, low oxygen saturation, anosmia (loss of smell), and dysgeusia (distortion of taste).[6]

Transmission route. COVID-19 is transmitted person-to-person via respiratory secretions or aerosols.

Rubella

Rubella was discovered in the eighteenth century in Germany and is thought to be a variant of the measles (rubeola). The virus is a member of the *Togavirus* family. It is a ribonucleic acid virus and has one antigenic type. The virus replicates in the nasopharynx and regional lymph nodes, and 5 to 7 days after exposure, the virus has replicated enough to cause a viremia that can spread to the tissues. This is an acute viral disease that is characterized by a fever and distinctive maculopapular rash. In pregnant females, this is the period when the virus crosses the placenta and causes damage to the unborn fetus. The rubella virus has been implicated in many birth defects, including deafness, cataracts, heart defects, microencephaly, mental retardation, bone alterations, and liver and spleen damage. In fact, if a female is infected early in pregnancy, there is a 20% chance of the fetus becoming damaged by this virus. To prevent the birth defects caused by this virus, in the 1960s the U.S. government highly recommended that all children be vaccinated against the disease. The measles, mumps, and rubella vaccine is on the list of childhood vaccines recommended by the CDC.

Symptoms. In children and young adults, rubella is a mild disease. The incubation period for the virus is approximately 14 days before producing symptoms. During this period, the infected person may have a low-grade fever and is able to infect others. The distinctive maculopapular rash appears 14 to 17 days after exposure to an infected individual. During the second week of the disease, the infected individual experiences lymphadenopathy. After some individuals have recovered from the infection, complications such as arthritis (adult females), arthralgia, thrombocytic purpura, encephalitis, neuritis, and orchitis can occur.

Transmission route. This virus is spread through droplet transmission when an infected individual coughs and sneezes or by transplacental transfer from mother to fetus.

Measles

Infections with measles are rare because of the concerted effort of industrialized countries to eradicate the virus through aggressive vaccination programs. The virus is in the *Paramyxoviridae* family, genus *Morbillivirus*. Although measles can be moderate to moderately severe, the complications from infection include pneumonia, encephalitis, and death. A vaccine was introduced in 1963 to protect children from the disease but was ineffective. In 1968, a new vaccine was developed using live attenuated virus. In 1989, a second dose of the vaccine was recommended, and by 2001, a second dose was required. One of the reasons for this second dose was that close to one third of all infections resulted in complications and sequelae. The complications and sequelae included pneumonia (and hospitalization), encephalitis, death, and subacute sclerosing panencephalitis (SSPE). SSPE is a fatal disease of the nervous system that develops 7 to 10 years after infection with the measles virus.

Symptoms. Once an individual is infected with the measles virus, the virus undergoes a 14-day incubation period. During this time, the person has a fever ($\geq 101°F$), malaise, cough, runny nose, and conjunctivitis. These symptoms are followed by the distinct maculopapular rash that lasts for more than 3 days.

Transmission route. The measles virus is spread through droplet transmission when an infected person coughs and sneezes.

Mumps

Mumps is an acute viral illness and, in the prevaccine era, was the primary cause of aseptic meningitis and deafness in children. The mumps virus is of the family *Paramyxoviridae*. The virus replicates in the nasopharynx and regional lymph nodes, which produces a viremia in about 12 to 25 days. This viremia lasts for 3 to 5 days. The viremia allows the virus to spread to the meninges, salivary glands, testes, and ovaries. These tissues become inflamed and produce the parotitis and aseptic meningitis. A combination vaccine is used for the prevention of the highly transmissible respiratory viruses, including the measles, mumps, and rubella. The vaccine is given in two doses and is referred to as the MMR vaccine.

Symptoms. The typical incubation period for the mumps virus is 14 to 18 days and during this time, the infected individual may experience muscle aches, anorexia, malaise, headache, low-grade fever, otitis (earache), and parotitis. Parotitis is the most common symptom, and it may include one or both sides. This lasts for approximately 10 days. Like the measles, the mumps have serious complications, which include aseptic meningitis, encephalitis, orchitis, oophoritis, pancreatitis, deafness, myocarditis, arthritis, and nephritis, as well as a risk of fetal death in pregnant females during the first trimester. Aseptic meningitis is the most common complication. Adults are more at risk for this condition than children, and males more commonly than females. Orchitis is also a common complication in males. The other complications are rare.

Transmission route. The mumps virus is spread through droplet transmission when an infected individual coughs and sneezes.

COMMON BACTERIAL INFECTIONS

Methicillin-Resistant *Staphylococcus aureus*

Methicillin-resistant *Staphylococcus aureus* (MRSA) is a bacterium resistant to penicillin, methicillin, amoxicillin, oxacillin, and most other antibiotics. MRSA is well known for skin infections but can also cause infections in other areas of the body (e.g., pneumonia).

When patients, especially individuals with weakened immune systems, become infected with MRSA, mortality may be increased because of the limited number of antibiotics available to treat the infections. MRSA infections are found in a variety of settings including health care—acquired (HA-MRSA), community-acquired (CA-MRSA), and livestock-acquired (LA-MRSA).[6] It is important to remember that MRSA is a serious infection; however, nonmethicillin-resistant *S. aureus* are also capable of causing infections. Additional species within the *Staphylococcus* genus are also capable of carrying the methicillin-resistant gene determinant and have been associated with serious infections such as methicillin-resistant *Staphylococcus epidermidis* (MRSE).[6]

Symptoms

The most common *Staphylococcus* infection is a skin infection. The skin may appear red, swollen, painful, warm to the touch, full of pus, and accompanied by a fever. *S. aureus* is the most common cause of boils.

Transmission Route

The microorganism that causes infection can be spread by direct contact with lesions or sores on an infected individual. The organism may also spread by indirect contact, such as by using an infected individual's personal item or touching a surface that has been contaminated. Direct and indirect transmission of the organism is capable of causing infections.

Meningococcal Meningitis

Meningococcal meningitis is caused by *Neisseria meningitidis*. A more severe form of the disease is called *meningococcemia* with sepsis and rash. This form of disease has also been referred to as *invasive meningococcal disease*.[8] Rates of infection with *N. meningitidis* have dropped significantly to approximately 0.12/100,000 in the United States because of the availability of a quadrivalent vaccine that prevents infection with the four most common serotypes (capsular types A, C, W, and Y) of the bacterium. An additional vaccine is also available for the more recently identified capsular type B.[8]

Symptoms

Meningitis symptoms vary significantly and may include fever, headache, confusion, photophobia (sensitivity to light), and stiff neck.[8]

Transmission Route

Transmission is via respiratory droplets. The bacterium can colonize the nasal passages with no symptoms. Colonized individuals can infect others without knowing it. Approximately 10% of the population may be colonized with the organism on the mucosal surfaces of the oropharynx and nasopharynx.[8]

Tuberculosis

Tuberculosis (TB) is usually a respiratory disease caused by the slow-growing bacterium *Mycobacterium tuberculosis.* The bacterium can also attack the kidney, spine, and brain. Infection with the microorganism can be fatal and was once the most frequent cause of death in the United States. A TB infection is treatable with antibiotics. *M. tuberculosis* grows very slowly, and the antibiotics are effective during the active dividing stages of the bacterium. Because of the slow growth, some organisms may avoid death by developing antibiotic resistance to the drug. To effectively treat the infection, the drugs must be taken for 6 months to 1 year. Because the antibiotic therapy covers such a long period, many individuals will stop taking the medication after the symptoms begin to improve. Patients are typically treated with a combination of isoniazid and rifampin to prevent the development of multidrug-resistant TB (MDR TB).[8] When a patient fails to complete the required antibiotic treatment, the organism can develop resistance to the drugs before being completely killed. Unfortunately, MDR TB, extensively drug-resistant TB (XDR-TB), and now strains of clinically unmanageable totally drug-resistant TB (TDR-TB) have appeared.[8,9] MDR TB may be resistant to the antibiotics isoniazid, rifampicin, pyrazinamide, and/or ethambutol.[9,10] The development of antibiotic resistance makes it difficult to treat TB infections.

Symptoms

Symptoms of people infected with pulmonary TB include a bad cough that lasts 3 weeks or longer, pain in the chest, coughing up blood or sputum, weakness or fatigue, weight loss, loss of appetite, chills, fever, and night sweats. A skin or blood test for TB will be positive, and the person may have a positive sputum smear, culture, or abnormal chest x-ray examination.

Transmission Route

The transmission route for TB is airborne, from one individual to another. When a person with active TB coughs, sneezes, speaks, or sings, TB bacteria are introduced into the air. Anyone who breathes this contaminated air may become infected.

Pneumonia

Pneumonia is a lung infection that can be mild or severe in people of all ages. Adults 65 years of age and older and children younger than 5 years old are more susceptible to infectious agents that cause pneumonia. Also, people who are immunocompromised (e.g., who have HIV or AIDS), have chronic diseases (e.g., asthma, chronic obstructive pulmonary disease [COPD]), and who smoke are more prone to develop pneumonia. To fight the respiratory infection, the body will mount a white blood cell (WBC) response in an attempt to kill the organisms causing the infection. These WBCs will migrate toward the lungs in the bloodstream causing the lungs to fill with fluid. If untreated, the fluid will totally fill the lungs, and the person may die. There are many drugs that can treat the infection and help clear the lungs of fluid.

Symptoms

Pneumonia is caused by many different organisms that produce the common symptoms of coughing, fever, fatigue, nausea, vomiting, rapid breathing, shortness of breath, chills, or chest pain. Most cases of pneumonia are considered community acquired. This means that someone who has not been recently hospitalized or in a health care facility develops pneumonia. The most common cause of pneumonia is the bacterium *Streptococcus pneumoniae* (pneumococcus). Other common causes of pneumonia include influenza, parainfluenza, respiratory syncytial virus, *Staphylococcus aureus, Pneumocystis jirovecii,* and adenovirus.

Transmission Route

Pneumonia is transmitted through respiratory droplets, direct contact, and indirect contact. Person-to-person transmission occurs when the infected individual coughs or sneezes, and susceptible hosts inhale the pathogen. Pneumonia can also be contracted through hard surfaces where the respiratory droplets have landed and are picked up by a susceptible host. A vaccine is available for streptococcal pneumonia.

Multidrug-Resistant Organisms

Multidrug-resistant organisms (MDROs) are defined as bacteria that are resistant to one or more classes of antibiotics. Some of the names may imply that the organism is resistant to only one antibiotic, but many times the bacteria are found to be resistant to many antibiotics. Some of these organisms are especially important in health care settings, including MRSA, vancomycin-resistant enterococcus (VRE), multidrug-resistant *Streptococcus pneumoniae* (MDRSP), MDR TB, and gram-negative bacteria that are resistant to multiple classes of antibiotics including extended-spectrum β-lactamase producing organisms and carbapenem-resistant bacteria.

Challenges

A patient infected with an MDRO exhibits the same symptoms as an individual infected with the same non-MDRO organism. The patient infected with the non-MDRO organism usually is treated with common oral antibiotics that are able to kill the organism and allow the patient to recover. The patient infected with the MDRO organism cannot be treated with the common antibiotics because these will not kill the organism. Instead, the organism continues to grow, and the infection worsens. Many of the more potent antibiotics must be given intravenously. Sometimes the antibiotics do not kill the organism but may slow the infection significantly permitting the individual's protective mechanisms to kill the infecting agent. When the organism cannot be killed by antibiotics or the patient's immune system is compromised and unable to manage the infection, the patient may die. Infections with MDRO organisms must be reported to public health agencies. These agencies track the organisms in an attempt to control the spread and mitigate the development of new antibiotics.

INFECTION CONTROL PRACTICES TO PREVENT INFECTION

Sharps Injury Prevention

Protecting the phlebotomist from a sharps injury, such as accidentally sticking oneself with a clean or dirty needle, has become more sophisticated during the past couple of decades. Later in the text, the numerous safety devices and precautions are discussed.

Occupational Safety and Health Administration Law

In 1991, when OSHA passed the bloodborne pathogen standard, control measures were introduced to reduce

the number of needlestick injuries. An update to this regulation was enacted in 2001, mandated by the Needlestick Safety and Prevention Act, and signed into law in November 2000. Among the provisions of this Act was the update to the definition of engineering controls, exposure control plans that annually document consideration of devices to minimize occupational exposure, input from frontline workers for identification, evaluation, and selection of devices with engineering controls, and a sharps injury log. The CDC estimates that 385,000 needlesticks happen to hospital-based health care workers, and phlebotomy is categorized as one of the highest-risk sharps procedures (Fig. 3.3). Needlesticks and sharps injuries are instrumental in occupational transmission of hepatitis B, hepatitis C, and HIV. The prevention of these injuries has been an essential feature of Standard Precautions. Health care service providers are required to use safety-engineered sharps devices and develop a comprehensive injury prevention program.

Education

Education of health care workers is essential to breaking the chain of infection and reducing the spread of infectious organisms. Infection control principles should be taught during a health professional's initial training and annually thereafter. This is especially true for health care workers who have contact with patients, such as phlebotomists, nurses, therapists, and technicians.

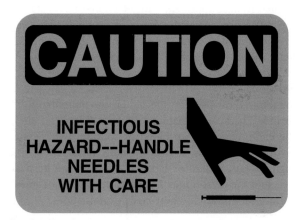

Fig. 3.3 The Centers for Disease Control and Prevention has categorized phlebotomy as one of the highest-risk sharps procedures. (Courtesy Occupational Safety and Health Administration.)

Facility-specific training on Standard and Transmission-Based Precautions are usually provided during orientation and periodically thereafter to maintain competency. It is important to note that if the policies and procedures change, all health care workers need additional training to ensure compliance.

Hand Hygiene

The connection between transmission of infectious agents and handwashing was discovered by Joseph Lister. Lister found that if midwives washed their hands after assisting on one birth before going to another mother, the incidence of infections dropped significantly. Hand hygiene (i.e., handwashing) is still believed to be the *single most important factor in reducing the transmission of infectious agents in health care settings.* Hand hygiene refers to both handwashing and use of disinfectant alcohol-based gels. If a health care worker is not able to wash hands between patients, the gel should be used. Artificial fingernails harbor infectious agents and should not be worn while providing patient care or drawing blood.

The standard procedure for washing hands gets rid of most of the pathogens on your skin. The proper technique for washing hands is illustrated in Procedure 3.1.

PROCEDURE 3.1 Handwashing

Materials
- Hand soap
- Sink
- Paper towel

1. Wet hands with warm water. All jewelry should be removed (Fig. 3.4).

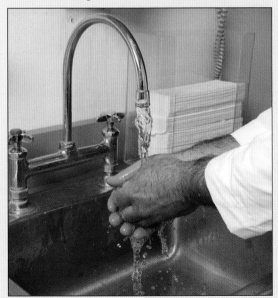

Fig. 3.4 (Courtesy Rick Davis.)

2. Use a generous portion of soap (Fig. 3.5).

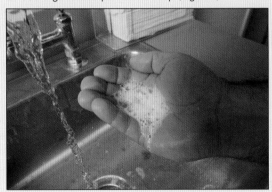

Fig. 3.5 (Courtesy Rick Davis.)

3. Thoroughly scrub hands for at least 15 seconds; work up a lather. Be sure to clean between fingers and wrist (Fig. 3.6).

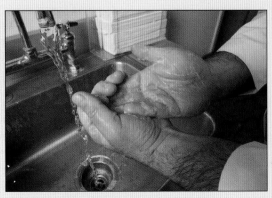

Fig. 3.6 (Courtesy Rick Davis.)

PROCEDURE 3.1   Handwashing—cont'd

4. Completely rinse hands under warm water. Keep hands in downward position (Fig. 3.7).

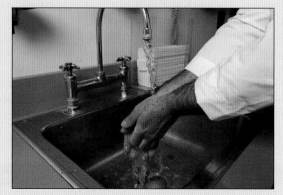

Fig. 3.7 (Courtesy Rick Davis.)

5. Thoroughly dry hands and use a paper towel to turn water off (Fig. 3.8).

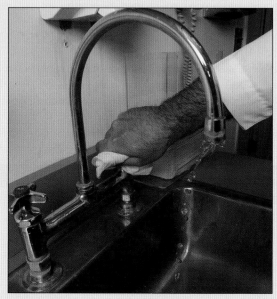

Fig. 3.8 (Courtesy Rick Davis.)

Personal Protective Equipment

Personal protective equipment (PPE) is a variety of barriers and respirators that a health care worker can wear to keep mucous membranes, airways, skin, and clothing from coming into contact with infectious organisms. The PPE used depends on the patient's condition and the interaction the health care worker has with the patient. Procedures for donning and removing PPE can be found in Tables 3.2 and 3.3.

Locations that require health care workers to don PPE also provide biohazardous containers to collect the soiled PPE outside the door. Handwashing is a must after leaving a contaminated room and touching an infectious patient.

Gloves. Gloves protect the hands of a health care worker when there is a potential for exposure to the blood or body fluids of a patient, the health care worker has nonintact skin, there is direct contact with a patient who has a confirmed infectious disease, or when handling visibly contaminated objects. The best gloves to use are nitrile because they protect the health care worker well without sensitization to latex. Gloves should be worn for every phlebotomy procedure without exception.

Isolation gowns. The need for health care workers to wear an isolation gown is based on the Standard and Transmission-Based Precautions. The gown is worn to protect the health care worker's arms and exposed body areas and to prevent the contamination of clothing with blood or body fluids. The type of gown needed to protect health care workers depends on the nature of the patient's disease and the amount of anticipated contact with the patient and infectious material. The OSHA Bloodborne Pathogens Standard mandates the wearing and use of PPE to protect health care workers. Gowns are the first piece of PPE to be donned and should fully cover the arms and the body from the neck to midthigh. Gloves and other PPE can be worn alone, but gowns are always worn in combination with other PPE. To help contain the spread of infectious material, always turn the inside of the gown inward when removing and

TABLE 3.2 Proper Personal Protective Equipment Donning Technique

Example of Safe Donning of Personal Protective Equipment	Illustration
Gown • Fully cover torso from neck to knees, arms to end of wrist, and wrap around the back. • Fasten in back at neck and waist.	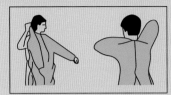
Mask or Respirator Secure ties or elastic band at middle of head and neck. • Fit flexible band to nose bridge. • Fit snug to face and below chin. • Fit-check respirator.	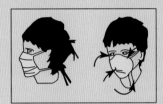
Goggles or Face Shield • Put on face and adjust to fit.	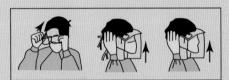
Gloves • Use nonsterile for isolation. • Select according to hand size. • Extend to cover wrist of isolation gown.	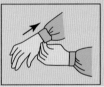
Safe Work Practices • Keep hands away from face. • Work from clean to dirty. • Limit surfaces touched. • Change when torn or heavily contaminated. • Perform hand hygiene.	

Adapted from Casanova L, Alfano-Sobsey E, Rutala WA, Weber DJ, Sobsey M. Virus transfer from personal protective equipment to health care employees' skin and clothing. *Emerg Infect Dis* [serial on the Internet]. 2008 Aug. Available from http://wwwnc.cdc.gov/eid/article/14/8/08-0085.htm.

roll it into a bundle. Place it in the contaminated linen receptacle.

Masks. There are three primary purposes for mask use in health care settings. They can be worn by health care workers to protect them from infectious material, worn by health care workers to protect patients from infectious agents on health care workers, and worn by a coughing patient to contain the potential respiratory droplet and airborne particles. Masks can be used in combination with goggles to protect the eyes, nose, and mouth, or a face shield may be worn. Do not confuse masks with particulate respirators (i.e., N-95) that

TABLE 3.3   Proper Personal Protective Equipment Removal Technique

Example of Safe Removal of Personal Protective Equipment	Illustration
Gloves • Outside of gloves is contaminated! • Grasp outside of glove with opposite gloved hand; peel off. • Hold removed glove in gloved hand. • Slide fingers of ungloved hand under remaining glove at wrist.	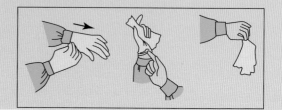
Goggles or Face Shield • Outside of goggles or face shield is contaminated! • To remove, handle by "clean" headband or earpieces. • Place in designated receptacle for reprocessing or in waste container.	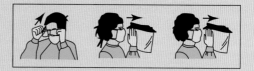
Gown • Gown front and sleeves are contaminated! • Unfasten neck, then waist ties. • Remove gown using a peeling motion; pull gown from each shoulder toward the same hand. • Gown will turn inside out. • Hold removed gown away from body, roll into a bundle and discard into waste or linen receptacle.	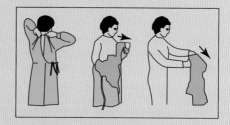
Mask or Respirator • Front of mask or respirator is contaminated—DO NOT TOUCH! • Grasp ONLY bottom then top ties or elastics and remove. • Discard in waster container.	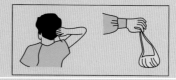
Hand Hygiene Perform hand hygiene immediately after removing all PPE!	
Safe Work Practices Remove PPE at doorway before leaving patient room or in anteroom	

Adapted from Casanova L, Alfano-Sobsey E, Rutala WA, Weber DJ, Sobsey M. Virus transfer from personal protective equipment to healthcare employees' skin and clothing. *Emerg Infect Dis.* [serial on the Internet]. 2008 Aug. Available from http://wwwnc.cdc.gov/eid/article/14/8/08-0085.htm.

prevent inhalation of small airborne infectious agents. Standard Precautions require that the mouth, nose, and eyes, as well as other skin surfaces, need to be covered to provide protection to the health care worker from contracting infectious agents. Use of masks, eye protection, and face shields is mandated by the OSHA Bloodborne Pathogens Standard if blood or body fluids may be splashed or sprayed.

Goggles and face shields. Transmission of pathogens from infectious body fluids splashing or spraying has been documented. To prevent infection, health care workers must wear goggles or face shields when there is a possibility of blood or body fluid splashing into the face. Personal eyeglasses and contact lenses are not adequate to protect an eye from infectious body fluids. One of the most reliable forms of eye protection is a pair of indirectly vented goggles with an antifog coating. There are goggles that fit over the top of prescription eyeglasses. Because face shields cover not only the eyes but also the mouth, nose, and facial skin, these are considered a better protection for splashes and sprays of body fluids.

Respiratory protection. Respiratory protection provides a barrier to airborne infectious agents. Because these agents can be very small, use of a respirator with N-95 filtration or higher is needed to filter out the infectious agents. Respiratory protection is regulated by OSHA. The regulation relates to health care, and the standard requires employers to implement a program to protect workers.

Standard Precautions

Standard Precautions are practices for preventing the health care–associated transmission of infectious agents to anyone, regardless of the infectious agent and the route of transmission. The major tenet of Standard Precautions is that all blood, body fluids, secretions, excretions except sweat, nonintact skin, and mucous membranes may contain transmissible infectious agents. Therefore, when handling any blood or body fluid, the following infection control principles are used as appropriate: hand hygiene and use of gloves, gown, mask, eye protection, or face shield. If a health care worker is handling equipment or items in a patient environment that may have been contaminated with body fluids, these must be handled in such a way as to prevent transmission of an infectious agent. Additional features of Standard Precautions that are recommended to protect patients include **respiratory and cough etiquette,** safe injection practices, and use of

masks for insertion of catheters or injection of material into spinal or epidural spaces via lumbar puncture procedures. The most relevant feature for phlebotomists is respiratory etiquette.

Respiratory etiquette. This strategy is incorporated into Standard Precautions and serves as a method of preventing the spread of respiratory illnesses. In a hospital setting, this strategy targets patients and visitors with cough, congestion, runny nose, or increased respiratory secretions. This strategy includes education of staff, patients, and visitors; posting signs in several languages stating recommendations (covering mouth and nose with a tissue when coughing, then disposing of the tissue); and requiring a coughing person to wear a surgical mask, practice hand hygiene after coughing or touching the mouth and secretions, and stand more than 3 feet away from another person.

Transmission-Based Precautions

Transmission-Based Precautions are used in addition to Standard Precautions for diseases that have multiple routes of infection. These precautions can also be used in conjunction with one another to ensure that maximum protection is provided for the health care worker. Maximum protection can be provided by applying the precautions if the pathogen is suspected. Precautions can always be discontinued if the pathogen is not confirmed. There are three types of Transmission-Based Precautions: Contact Precautions, Droplet Precautions, and Airborne Precautions. See Table 3.4 for recommendations from CDC.

Contact Precautions. The purpose of Contact Precautions is to prevent the spread of pathogens transmitted through direct and indirect contact. In addition, Contact Precautions can be used for excessive wound drainage, fecal incontinence, and other discharges that produce an increased risk for the environmental contamination and disease transmission. Health care workers are required to wear a gown and gloves for all patient interactions. The PPE is donned before entering the patient's room and is removed and discarded when leaving the patient's room.

Droplet Precautions. The purpose of Droplet Precautions is to prevent the spread of pathogens that are transmitted through respiratory secretions. These patients can be roomed with other patients, but because of the mode of transmission of the disease, the curtain between the patients should be drawn to prevent transmission of

TABLE 3.4 Recommendations for Application of Standard Precautions for the Care of All Patients in All Health Care Settings

Component	Recommendations
Hand hygiene	Use after touching blood, body fluids, secretions, excretions, contaminated items; immediately after removing gloves; between patient contacts.
Personal Protective Equipment	
Gloves	Use when touching blood, body fluids, secretions, excretions, contaminated items; when touching mucous membranes and nonintact skin.
Gown	Use during procedures and patient-care activities when contact of clothing or exposed skin with blood, body fluids, secretions, and excretions is anticipated.
Mask, eye protection (goggles), face shield	Use during procedures and patient-care activities likely to generate splashes or sprays of blood, body fluids, secretions, especially suctioning, endotracheal intubation.
Soiled patient care equipment	Handle in a manner that prevents transfer of microorganisms to others and to the environment; wear gloves if visibly contaminated, perform hand hygiene.
Environmental control	Develop procedures for routine care, cleaning, and disinfection of environmental surfaces, especially frequently touched surfaces in patient-care areas.
Needles and other sharps	Do not recap, bend, break, or hand-manipulate used needles; always use needles with safety features; place used sharps in a puncture-resistant container.
Respiratory hygiene and cough etiquette (source containment of infectious respiratory secretions in symptomatic patients, beginning at initial point of encounter [e.g., triage and reception areas in emergency departments and physician offices])	Instruct symptomatic persons to cover mouth and nose when sneezing or coughing; use tissues and dispose in no-touch receptacle; observe hand hygiene after soiling of hands with respiratory secretions; wear surgical mask if tolerated or maintain spatial separation, >3 feet if possible.

the disease to the other patient. Health care workers must wear a mask when close contact with the patient is expected. The mask is donned before entering the room and removed and discarded when leaving the room.

Airborne Precautions. The purpose of Airborne Precautions is to prevent the spread of pathogens transmitted through the air for long distances. These patients should be placed in a single-occupancy room with special air handling and ventilation systems to prevent release of infectious air to the outside environment. Examples of organisms that require this type of precautions include rubeola, varicella, *M. tuberculosis*, H1N1 influenza, and SARS-CoV. Health care workers entering the room of a patient with any of these pathogens are required to wear a

respirator with filtration of N-95 or higher. Facilities that have the specially equipped rooms must also have a respiratory protection program that includes training on the use of respirators, fit testing, and seal checks.

Environmental Infection Control
Some pathogens are transmitted through an airborne route, then settle in the environment. Fungi are notorious for spreading spores through the air, and these spores disperse throughout the environment. Susceptible hosts can inhale these spores and become infected. This type of an infection is not transmitted from a person. Contracting disease from pathogens that are transmitted from the environment is distinct from contracting the disease from an infected person. All environmental

surfaces should be cleaned daily with an appropriate disinfectant, as mandated by Standard Precautions.

Patient care equipment. Medical equipment is always cleaned and maintained as specified by the manufacturer's instructions to prevent patient-to-patient transmission of infectious agents. In health care settings, providing patients on Transmission-Based Precautions with dedicated equipment such as a blood pressure cuff, thermometer, tourniquet, or stethoscope can assist in preventing transmission of the infectious agent.

Special Precautions

Many factors increase the risk of disease transmission in the various health care settings. Some of these factors include increased susceptibility to infections (immunocompromised); presence of indwelling devices; level of care; exposure to environmental sources; length of stay; and frequency of interaction of patients, residents, and health care workers. Every institution adapts transmission prevention guidelines according to their needs. These needs are driven by data on institutional, local, regional, and national epidemiology and emerging infectious diseases.

Special Considerations in the Hospital Setting

Because the hospital is where sick people go to receive treatment, it should come as no surprise that hospitals carry an inherent increased risk of transmission for infectious diseases. Vulnerable populations such as trauma patients, burn patients, children, transplant patients, and health care workers who handle blood and other infectious materials daily can serve as new transmission sites or may allow an infectious agent to be transmitted from one area to another area in the hospital. These areas include the intensive care unit (ICU), burn unit, pediatric unit, transplant unit, and the clinical laboratory.

Intensive care unit. Patients with the most severe and life-threatening conditions are treated in the intensive care unit (ICU). Patients in the ICU are immunocompromised by life-threatening disease states (e.g., thyroid toxicity, diabetic ketoacidosis, encephalitis), major trauma, major surgical procedures, respiratory failure, myocardial infarction, congestive heart failure, overdoses, strokes, bleeding, renal failure, hepatic failure, multiorgan system failure, and so on. These patients usually have multiple in-dwelling devices, extended stays, many interactions with health care workers, and prolonged exposure to antibiotics.

This area usually has one of the highest health care–acquired (nosocomial) infection rates in the hospital. Unfortunately, when these fragile patients acquire a **nosocomial** infection, the infection is usually more severe and often results in death. The infections are transmitted by direct contact—environmental factors and person-to-person.

Burn unit. One of the largest defenses the human body mounts against environmental pathogens is the skin. The skin helps keep the inside of the body free of outside pathogenic organisms. Trauma to the skin allows pathogens to enter and cause disease. In a burn unit, many patients have a significant amount of damaged skin caused by burning. People who have more than 30% of the body covered in burns have a significantly increased chance of contracting an infection while in the hospital. People who have less than 30% of their body covered with burns usually contract an infection through the placement of invasive devices. The most common pathogens found on a burn unit include *S. aureus*, MRSA, enterococci, VRE, gram-negative bacteria, and *Candida* spp.

Pediatric and neonatal intensive care units. The pediatric and neonatal ICUs have reported high rates of central venous catheter–associated bloodstream infections. These are serious infections because bacteria is circulating throughout the child's bloodstream. These hospital units can also have a high incidence of community-acquired infections because the children do not have immunity because of their young age or lack of vaccinations. Because of the patient population, these units lend themselves to close physical contact between the health care personnel, infants, and young children—cuddling, feeding, playing, changing soiled diapers, and cleaning respiratory secretions. This personal contact increases transmission risks to both patients and health care workers.

Clinical laboratory. Clinical laboratory workers are exposed to blood and body fluids from patients daily. Phlebotomists are also exposed to patients when drawing blood in an outpatient drawing room or from admitted patients. The interaction with sick patients can increase the risk of transmission to the phlebotomist. Clinical laboratory workers also handle infectious secretions, body fluids, and tissues to be screened for infectious agents, such as cerebral spinal fluid, respiratory secretions and lavages, feces, semen, peritoneal fluid, and ascites fluid for culture of infectious agents.

Although procedures exist for handling all specimens, an increased transmission risk exists because of the daily handling of these specimens.

Special Considerations for Outpatient (Ambulatory) Care

Because there are many more outpatient clinics than hospitals, it follows that many health care services are delivered at outpatient clinics. Examples include hospital-based outpatient clinics, nonhospital-based clinics, physician offices, public health clinics, free-standing dialysis centers, occupational health clinics, school clinics, ambulatory surgical centers, and urgent care centers. These settings include a sick patient sitting in a waiting room. This permits exposure to other patients from respiratory droplets or airborne pathogens. The patient is then brought back to a room, seen by the provider, and sent home with a treatment. The rooms are cleaned quickly between patients. Immunocompromised patients can also wait for extended periods, mingling with sick and healthy patients.

Special Considerations for Long-Term Care

Long-term care is available in facilities such as nursing homes, homes for the developmentally disabled, behavioral health care settings, rehabilitation centers, hospices, and assisted-living facilities. Facilities such as nursing homes represent a huge transmission risk because most of the residents are older adults. As a result, the residents share common eating and living areas and are encouraged to participate in facility-sponsored activities. Although residents are usually confined to the building, they can freely mingle with each other and the health care workers. This means that residents who are colonized or infectious can spread disease to other residents. Some of the risk factors associated with long-term care facility residents include weakened immune system caused by age, immobility, incontinence, chronic diseases, poor functional status, fragile skin, medications, and invasive devices. This population is extremely vulnerable to infectious diseases.

SAFETY SUMMARY

- Always wear appropriate personal protective equipment (PPE) for phlebotomy.

- Know the route of transmission and precautions of common diseases and conditions.
- Wash hands between patients or after handling potentially infectious material.
- Properly dispose of contaminated phlebotomy and PPE.

SUMMARY

This chapter discusses the potential for exposure to infectious bacterial and viral diseases to phlebotomists and other health care workers. The chapter also discusses the symptoms and routes of transmission for selected uncommon pathogens, sharps injury prevention, PPE, hand hygiene, Standard Precautions, and Transmission-Based Precautions. Also highlighted are specific hospital areas where prevention of disease transmission is very important. Special considerations for outpatient clinics and long-term care facilities are also discussed. Phlebotomists can be a link in the infection chain by transmitting disease to others, but not if they follow infection control principles and are alert for infectious diseases.

CASE 3.1   Critical Thinking

A phlebotomist goes to the emergency room to draw a patient. The phlebotomist finds out the patient is a child who has a widely spread skin rash. The emergency room clerk said the doctor mentioned that the child may have meningococcemia. What type of personal protective equipment should the phlebotomist wear and why?

CASE 3.2   Critical Thinking

A fellow phlebotomist confides in a colleague that they were stuck with a dirty needle about a month ago. The phlebotomist tells you that they are feeling really tired lately and their urine looks like tea. The individual didn't bother to go to the Employee Health Department when it happened because they were embarrassed. What advice would you give to the phlebotomist? What disease does the phlebotomist appear to have contracted? What treatment is available for the disease?

REVIEW QUESTIONS

1. What is a bloodborne pathogen, and why is it important for phlebotomists to learn about these organisms?
2. Why is it important for a phlebotomist to learn about infectious diseases?
3. What are the various routes of transmission for medically important pathogens?
4. What is malaria?
5. What is HIV?
6. What is AIDS?
7. How would you know if a patient had tuberculosis?
8. What are the symptoms for meningitis? How do they differ from meningococcemia?
9. Why would phlebotomists want to protect themselves from getting infected with MRSA or VRE?
10. What are Standard Precautions, and why are they important?
11. What are Transmission-Based Precautions? Explain the three different types.
12. Why is it important to disinfect the patient's environment and patient-care equipment?
13. When should gloves be worn?
14. When should gowns be worn?
15. When should masks be worn?
16. What did the OSHA Bloodborne Standard of 1991 do?
17. What did the Needlestick Safety and Prevention Act do?
18. What are the symptoms and sequelae of hepatitis C?
19. Why are patients in the ICU immunocompromised and easy to infect?
20. Why is handwashing so important?

REFERENCES

1. World Health Organization. https://www.who.int/news/item/01-12-2021-world-aids-day-2021—step-up-be-bold-end-aids-end-inequalities-and-end-pandemics. [accessed 5-23-2022].
2. Centers for Disease and Control. Basic statistics, https://www.cdc.gov/hiv/basics/statistics.html. [accessed 5-23-2022].
3. Centers for Disease and Control. Occupational Exposure to HIV. https://www.cdc.gov/hiv/workplace/healthcare-workers.html. [accessed 5-23-2022].
4. Verbeek JH, Rajamaki B, Ijaz S, et al. Personal protective equipment for preventing highly infectious diseases due to exposure to contaminated body fluids in healthcare staff. *Cochrane Database Syst Rev.* 2020;4(4):CD011621. https://doi.org/10.1002/14651858.CD011621.pub4. Published 2020 Apr 15.
5. Wang CC, Prather KA, Sznitman J, et al. Airborne transmission of respiratory viruses. *Sci.* 2021;373(6558):eabd9149. https://doi.org/10.1126/science.abd9149.
6. Tille PM. *Bailey and Scott's Diagnostic Microbiology.* 15th ed. Elsevier; 2022
7. Centers for Disease and Control. Covid Data Tracker, https://covid.cdc.gov/covid-data-tracker/#datatracker-home. [accessed 5-23-2022].
8. Carroll KC, Pfaller MA, Landry ML, et al. *Manual of Clinical Microbiology.* 12th ed. Washington D.C: ASM Press; 2019.
9. Khawbung JL, Nath D, Chakraborty S. Drug resistant Tuberculosis: a review. *Comp Immunol Microbiol Infect Dis.* 2021;74:101574. https://doi.org/10.1016/j.cimid.2020.101574. Epub 2020 Nov 16. PMID: 33249329.
10. Miotto P, Zhang Y, Cirillo DM, Yam WC. Drug resistance mechanisms and drug susceptibility testing for tuberculosis. *Respirology.* 2018;23(12):1098—1113. https://doi.org/10.1111/resp.13393. Epub 2018 Sep 6. PMID: 30189463.
11. Pillaiyar T, Manickam M, Namasivayam V, Hayashi Y, Jung SH. "An overview of severe acute respiratory syndrome-coronavirus (SARS-CoV) 3CL protease inhibitors: peptidomimetics and small molecule chemotherapy". *J Med Chem.* 2016;59(14):6595—6628. https://doi.org/10.1021/acs.jmedchem.5b01461. PMC 7075650. PMID 26878082.
12. Mahase E. Covid-19: Pfizer's paxlovid is 89% effective in patients at risk of serious illness, company reports. *BMJ.* 2021;375:n2713. https://doi.org/10.1136/bmj.n2713. PMID: 34750163.
13. Wen W, Chen C, Tang J, et al. Efficacy and safety of three new oral antiviral treatment (molnupiravir, fluvoxamine and Paxlovid) for COVID-19 : a meta-analysis. *Ann. Med.* 2022;54(1):516—523. https://doi.org/10.1080/07853890.2022.2034936. PMID: 35118917; PMCID: PMC8820829.
14. Centers for Disease and Control. https://www.cdc.gov. [accessed 10-27-2022].

BIBLIOGRAPHY

Belay ED, Schonberger LB. The public health impact of prion diseases. *Ann Rev Public Health*. 2005;26:191–212. https://doi.org/10.1146/annurev.publhealth.26.021304.144536. Retrieved from www.cdc.gov/ncidod/dvrd/prions/resources/BelayE_Annu_Rev_Public_Health.pdf.

Bolyard EA, Tablan OC, Williams WW, Pearson ML, Shapiro CN, Deitchman SD. Guideline for infection control in health care personnel. *Infect Control Hosp Epidemiol*. 1998;19:407–463. Retrieved from http://www.cdc.gov/hicpac/pdf/InfectControl98.pdf.

Centers for Disease Control and Prevention (CDC): Abstract: consensus statement: tularemia as a biological weapon: medical and public health management. Abstracted from Dennis DT, Inglesby TV, Henderson DA, et al: *JAMA* 285(21): 2763–2773. (Full article available at: http://jama.ama-assn.org/cgi/content/full/285/21/2763.) Access date July 27, 2011.

Centers for Disease Control and Prevention (CDC): Diphtheria. *Epidemiology and Prevention of Vaccine-Preventable Diseases*. 12th ed. (The Pink Book), April 2011, (Chapter 6). Centers for Disease Control and Prevention (CDC). *Exposure to blood: what healthcare personnel need to know*, July 2003. Retrieved from http://www.cdc.gov/ncidod/dhqp/pdf/bbp/Exp_to_Blood.pdf. Access date July 27, 2011.

Centers for Disease Control and Prevention (CDC). Guideline for hand hygiene in health-care settings: recommendations of the healthcare infection control practices advisory committee and the HICPAC/SHEA/APIC/IDSA Hand Hygiene Task Force. *MMWR (Morb Mortal Wkly Rep)*. 2002;51(RR16). Retrieved from http://www.cdc.gov/mmwr/PDF/rr/rr5116.pdf.

Centers for Disease Control and Prevention (CDC). *Influenza Vaccination of Health-Care Personnel: Recommendations of the Healthcare Infection Control Practices Advisory Committee (HICPAC) and the Advisory Committee on Immunization Practices (ACIP)* 55; 2006. Retrieved from www.cdc.gov/mmwr/PDF/rr/rr5502.pdf.

Centers for Disease Control and Prevention (CDC). *Management of Multidrug-Resistant Organisms in Healthcare Settings*; 2006. Retrieved from www.cdc.gov/ncidod/dhqp/pdf/ar/MDROGuideline2006.pdf.

Centers for Disease Control and Prevention (CDC). Mumps. *Epidemiology and Prevention of Vaccine-Preventable Diseases*. 12th ed. The Pink Book; 2011 (Chapter 14). Access date July 27, 2011.

Centers for Disease Control and Prevention (CDC). Pertussis. *Epidemiology and Prevention of Vaccine-Preventable Diseases*. 12th ed. The Pink Book; 2011 (Chapter 15). Access date July 27, 2011.

Centers for Disease Control and Prevention (CDC). Rubella. *Epidemiology and Prevention of Vaccine-Preventable Diseases*. 12th ed. The Pink Book; 2011 (Chapter 19). Access date July 27, 2011.

Centers for Disease Control and Prevention (CDC): Smallpox. http://www.emergency.cdc.gov/agent/smallpox/

Centers for Disease Control and Prevention (CDC). *Types of Influenza Viruses*. Retrieved from http://www.cdc.gov/flu/about/viruses/types.htm.

Centers for Disease Control and Prevention (CDC). *Vaccine Preventable Diseases Surveillance Manual*. 4th ed.; 2008. Washington, D.C. Retrieved from http://www.cdc.gov/vaccines/pubs/surv-manual/chpt07-measles.htm.

Centers for Disease Control and Prevention. *Infectious Diseases Related to Travel. CDC Health Information for International Travel 2012*. New York: Oxford University Press; 2012. Retrieved from http://wwwnc.cdc.gov/travel/page/yellowbook-2012-home.htm.

Jabra-Rizk MA, Falkler WA, Meiller TF. Fungal biofilms and drug resistance. *Emerg Infect Dis*; 2004. Retrieved from http://www.cdc.gov/ncidod/EID/vol10no1/03-0119.htm.

Rutala WA, Weber D. *Healthcare Infection Controls Practices Advisory Committee HICPAC, Centers for Disease Control and Prevention (CDC): Guideline for Disinfection and Sterilization in Health Care Facilities*; 2008. Retrieved from http://www.cdc.gov/hicpac/pdf/guidelines/Disinfection_Nov_2008.pdf.

Sehulster L, Chinn RYW. Guidelines for environmental infection control in health-care facilities: recommendations of CDC and the healthcare infection control practices advisory committee (HICPAC). *MMWR (Morb Mortal Wkly Rep)*. 2003;52(RR10):1–42. Retrieved from http://www.cdc.gov/mmwr/preview/mmwrhtml/rr5210a1.htm.

Siegel JD, Rhinehart E, Jackson M, Chiarello L: *Healthcare Infection Control Practices Advisory Committee: 2007 Guideline For Isolation Precautions: Preventing Transmission of Infectious Agents in Healthcare Settings*. Retrieved from http://www.cdc.gov/hicpac/pdf/isolation/Isolation2007.pdf.

Tablan OC, Anderson LJ, Besser R, Bridges C, Hajjeh R. *Guidelines for Preventing Health-Care-Associated Pneumonia: Recommendations of CDC and the Healthcare Infection Control Practices Advisory Committee*; 2003. Retrieved from http://www.cdc.gov/mmwr/preview/mmwrhtml/rr5303a1.htm.

Medical Terminology

Leticia M. Rodríguez

"Knowledge of Languages is the doorway to wisdom"

—*Roger Bacon*

OBJECTIVES

At the conclusion of this chapter, the student should be able to:
- Identify the parts of medical words.
- Define prefix, suffix, and word root.
- Explain the purpose of a combining vowel.
- Discuss how plural medical terms are formed.

OUTLINE

KEY TERMS

combining vowel
prefix
suffix
word root

INTRODUCTION

Learning medical terminology can be somewhat like learning a new language. Unless you are immersed in the language daily, it is often difficult to become fluent. Phlebotomists are not expected to be fluent in medical terminology, but they are expected to be familiar with several common terms. For example, *venipuncture* (*veni* = vein, *puncture* = puncture) means to puncture a vein. This is an obvious and easy example of a medical term.

The purpose of this chapter is to provide some common medical terms that phlebotomists may encounter when performing their job duties and explain specific parts of these terms and how they are placed together for specific meanings. Medical terms are used frequently in most health care professions, and having a good base knowledge of these terms will assist a practicing phlebotomist. The more experience one receives in the medical professions, the easier it becomes to learn medical terminology because terms are universal and overlap in several disciplines.

MEDICAL TERMINOLOGY: THE BASICS

Medical terms are derived from Latin and ancient Greek. Because of the origin of the *word root*, changing the prefix or the suffix of a word root can change the entire meaning of the word. Medical terms contain a number of specific components:

- The **word root** is the word that gives the most important meaning of the word, or the basis for the word.
- The **prefix** alters the specific definition at the *beginning* of the word. For example, *hist* is a prefix meaning "tissue." When added to the suffix *logy*, meaning the study of a specific field, the prefix and suffix make the new word *histology*, meaning the study of tissue. (The extra "o" will be discussed later in this chapter.)
- The **suffix** alters the specific definition at the *ending* of the word. For example, *pod* is the word root pertaining to the foot and *iatry* is the suffix for a specific body component; together they make the new word *podiatry*: the study of the foot (it also means the diagnosis and treatment of foot ailments).
- A **combining vowel** is a vowel added in a word between two word roots or a word root and a suffix to make pronunciation easier. The most commonly used combining vowel is the vowel "o." For example, *lip* is the word root for fat and *suction* is the suffix for removal; the combining vowel "o" makes the new word *liposuction*.

Using the previous criteria, we identify the parts of the following medical terms as follows:

Venipuncture
Vein (word root: "vein") "i" (combining vowel) puncture (suffix: "to draw blood from")

Phlebotomy
Phleb (prefix: vein) "o" (combining vowel) tomy (suffix: "to cut")

Histology
Hist (prefix: "tissue") "o" (combining vowel) logy (suffix: "the study of")

Podiatry
Pod (word root: "foot") iatry (suffix: "study of specific body part")

Liposuction
Lip (word root: "fat") "o" (combining vowel) suction (suffix: "to remove")

PREFIXES

A prefix is a word element that is placed in front of a word. A prefix changes the meaning of the word root by adding information about the context of the word *before* its root meaning. For example, the prefix *epi-* is the prefix meaning *on* or *over*. An example is the word *epicardium*: covering over the heart. Table 4.1 lists examples of prefixes used in common medical terms.

TABLE 4.1	Prefixes	
Prefix	**Meaning**	**Examples**
a-	absence	apathy
ante-	before	antepartum
anti-	opposed	anticoagulant
bio-	life	biology
cata-	under	cataract
cerebello-	pertaining to the cerebellum	cerebellum
chlor-	green in color	chlorophyll
cryo-	cold	cryoablation
dis-	separation	dissection
dys-	bad	dyspnea
endo-	inside	endoscope
hemat-	pertaining to blood	hematology
hyper-	above	hypertension
hypo-	below	hypodermic needle
intra-	within	intramuscular
iso-	same	isotonic
irid-	iris	iridectomy
kin-	movement	kinesthesia
lei-	smooth	leiomyoma
lipo-	fat	liposuction
lute-	yellow	corpus luteum
masto-	pertaining to the breast	mastectomy
mega-	large	megakaryocyte
mero-	part	merocrine
neo-	new	neoplasm

TABLE 4.1   Prefixes—cont'd

Prefix	Meaning	Examples
neuro-	pertaining to nerves	neurological
optico-	pertaining to the eyes	opticochemical
peri-	around	pericardium
poly-	many	polymyositis
post-	after	postmortem
quadri-	four	quadriceps
rhino-	pertaining to the nose	rhinoplasty
sarco-	muscular	sarcoma
schiz-	double-sided	schizophrenia
semi-	half	semilunar
tachy-	rapid	tachycardia
trache-	trachea	tracheotomy
tri-	three	tricuspid
uro-	pertaining to urine	urology
xen-	foreign	xenograft

TABLE 4.2   Word Roots

Word Root	Meaning	Examples
adip	fat	adipose
aer	air	aerobic
angi	vessel	angiogram
arteri	artery	arteriosclerosis
arthr	joint	arthritis
bili	bile	bilirubin
bronch	bronchus	bronchitis
cardi	heart	cardiogram
cephal	head	cephalic
chondr	cartilage	chondrocalcinosis
colo	colon	colonoscopy
cry	cold	cryoablation
cubitum	elbow	antecubital fossa
cutane	skin	percutaneous
cyst	bladder	cystitis
cyt	cell	cytology
derm	skin	dermis
encephal	brain	encephalitis
enter	intestines	enteritis
erythr	red	erythrocyte
esophagi	esophagus	esophagitis
estr	female	estrogen
fibrin	fiber	fibrinolysis
gastr	stomach	gastrointestinal
gluc	sugar	glucose
hem	blood	hematocrit
hepat	liver	hepatitis
lipid	fat	lipernia
leuk	white	leukocyte
my	muscle	myalgia
necr	death	necrosis
nephr	kidney	nephritis
onc	tumor	oncology
or	mouth	oral
oste	bone	osteoporosis
path	disease	pathogen
phleb	vein	phlebotomy
pnea	breath	pneumatic
pulmon	lung	pulmonary
ren	kidney	renal

WORD ROOTS

A word root is the main component of a medical term that establishes the *initial meaning* of the word. The suffix and prefix used with the word root establish the *actual meaning* of the word and are critical to understanding the context of a medical term. Nearly all word roots point toward an organ, body system, structure, tissue, condition, or substance. For example, *phleb-* is the word root for vein, so each time a medical term has the root word *phleb-*, it involves veins. Medical roots tend to match their language. Latin prefixes go with Latin suffixes, and Greek prefixes go with Greek suffixes. Table 4.2 lists examples of word roots used in common medical terms.

SUFFIXES

A suffix is a word element that is placed at the end of a word. A suffix changes the meaning of the word root or adds information about the context of the word *after* its root meaning. For example, the suffix *-oma* is the suffix

TABLE 4.2   Word Roots—cont'd

Word Root	Meaning	Examples
sclera	hard	sclerotic
spleno	spleen	splenomegaly
stetho	chest	stethoscope
thromb	clot	thrombosis
thorac	chest	thoracic
tox	poison	toxicology
vas	vessel	vascular
ven	vein	venipuncture

TABLE 4.3   Suffixes

Suffix	Meaning	Examples
-algia	pain	myalgia
-ary	pertaining to	biliary tract
-ase	enzyme	lactase
-cele	hernia	hydrocele
-crine	to secrete	endocrine
-desis	binding	arthrodesis
-dynia	pain	vulvodynia
-emia	blood condition	anemia
-ectomy	surgical removal	appendectomy
-iatry	study of specific body part	podiatry
-itis	inflammation	arthritis
-ium	structure	pericardium
-lepsy	attack	epilepsy
-lysis	destruction	paralysis
-metry	measuring	optometry
-oma	tumor	hematoma
-osis	condition	tuberculosis
-pathy	disease	cardiopathy
-penia	deficiency	thrombocytopenia
-plasty	shape	angioplasty
-plegia	paralysis	tetraplegia
-poiesis	formation	hemopoiesis
-rrhea	flowing	diarrhea
-scopy	viewing	endoscopy
-stasis	stopping	hemostasis
-stomy	opening	colostomy
-tension	pressure	hypertension
-tomy	cut	phlebotomy
-tripsy	crushing	lithotripsy

meaning "growth" or "tumor." It demonstrates this in the word *hematoma*: a swelling or collection of blood. Table 4.3 lists examples of suffixes used in common medical terms.

PLURALS

When learning medical terminology, keep in mind the structure of plural words, which mean "more than one." Plural words are created using the source language of the word. In the English language this can usually be done by adding an "-s" or "-es" to the end of a word. In Greek or Latin languages, plural words have their own rules. You will most commonly have to use a resource for forming these words, and they can usually also be found in a medical dictionary. Table 4.4 lists plural endings.

ABBREVIATIONS

It is common for various professions and occupations to have abbreviations that are commonly used in a given field. For example, ft^2 means "square feet," a common unit in carpentry. Abbreviations are also commonly used in the medical profession. Table 4.5 has a partial list of the abbreviations commonly used in the medical field.

TABLE 4.4   Examples of Plurals

Word Ending	Plural Form	Example
-a	-ae	vertebrae
-ax	-ces	thoraces
-en	-ina	foramina
-ex	-ices	cortices
-is	-es	diagnoses
-ix	-ices	appendices
-ma	-ta	sarcomata
-nx	-ges	larynges
-um	-a	ilea
-us	-i	alveoli
-on	-a	spermatozoa
-y	-ies	deformities
-yx	-yces	calyces

TABLE 4.5 Common Abbreviations	
Abbreviation	**Meaning**
ABGs	arterial blood gases
ABO	ABO blood group system
bid	Latin: *bis in die* (twice a day)
BUN	blood urea nitrogen
CBC	complete blood count
CL⁻	chloride
CO_2	carbon dioxide
COVID	Coronovirus disease
CSF	cerebrospinal fluid
Diff	white blood cell count differential
DOB	date of birth
FBS	fasting blood sugar
FUO	fever of unknown origin
Hgb/Hb	hemoglobin
Hct	hematocrit
H&H	hemoglobin and hematocrit
HDL	high-density lipoprotein
K^+	potassium
LDL	low-density lipoprotein
Lytes	electrolytes
MI	myocardial infarction
Na^+	sodium

TABLE 4.5 Common Abbreviations—cont'd	
Abbreviation	**Meaning**
O_2	oxygen
PCR	polymerase chain reaction
pH	measure of the acidity and alkalinity of a fluid based on hydrogen ion content
PP	postprandial: after a meal
PT	protime or prothrombin time
PTT	partial thromboplastin time
QNS	quantity not sufficient
RBC	red blood cell: usually referring to red blood cell count
RA	rheumatoid arthritis
RPR	rapid plasma regain
STD	sexually transmitted disease
T&C	type and crossmatch blood for transfusion
Trig	triglycerides
UA	urinalysis
UTI	urinary tract infection
WBC	white blood cell: usually referring to white blood cell count
y/o or yo	years old

SUMMARY

This chapter serves to provide the basic elements of medical terminology. When studying the meanings and components of medical terminology, keep in mind these specific details: the word root, a possible prefix, a possible suffix, and a possible combining vowel. Also remember that the language of origin will assist when changing a medical term from singular to plural. Most medical terms are formed from the Greek or Latin language.

▌ REVIEW QUESTIONS

1. _____ is added between some suffixes and word roots to make the word easier to pronounce.
2. _____ is added before a word root to assist in defining the word or giving the word context.
3. Most word roots originate from which languages? _____
4. Break down the following words into their parts and define the words:
   a. Cytopenia
   b. Osteopathy

  c. Lipase
  d. Intrarenal
  e. Phlebitis
5. Define the following abbreviations:
  a. FUO

  b. Lytes
  c. QNS
  d. PTT
  e. PP
  f. FBS

5

Equipment

John C. Flynn, Jr.

"A chain is only as strong as its weakest link."

Anonymous

OBJECTIVES

At the conclusion of this chapter, the student should be able to:

- Identify the various blood collection tubes, their additive, and common clinical tests.
- Discuss the various types of needles and microcollection devices.
- Explain the importance of proper needle disposal.
- Explain the use of tube holders.
- Discuss the various ways to locate a vein for venipuncture.
- Identify and properly use gloves and goggles.
- Discuss the use of training aids.
- List additional equipment that a phlebotomist should carry.

OUTLINE

KEY TERMS

activated partial thromboplastin time (aPTT)

complete blood cell (CBC) count

ethylenediaminetetraacetate (EDTA)

heparin

needle gauge

personal protective equipment

prothrombin time (PT)

specific gravity

white blood cell (WBC) differential

INTRODUCTION

Phlebotomists often hear that a blood test result is only as good as the collected specimen. This includes, in addition to proper collection technique, a proper evacuated tube, proper needle selection, and adequate transport and storage to the laboratory. If a hematological specimen is collected in a chemistry tube, then the sample is going to be worthless for hematological analysis. Therefore it is very important that the correct tube, along with the proper additive (if appropriate), is used in every blood collection.

This chapter discusses the various tubes, their anticoagulants, and the other common equipment associated with phlebotomy and microcollection procedures. The use of vacuum tubes, commonly called *evacuated tubes*, is nearly universal. It should be noted that traditionally, evacuated tubes were made of glass. It is becoming commonplace for tubes to be made of plastic. The immediate benefit is obvious: less chance of breaking and contaminating the surrounding environment or harming the phlebotomist and exposing them to a bloodborne pathogen. Also, the maximum amount of blood collected is determined by the vacuum and although it is easy to underfill an evacuated tube, it is much harder to overfill an evacuated tube.

Before proceeding, however, the phlebotomist must understand the difference between plasma, serum, and whole blood. Plasma and serum are the liquid portion of a centrifuged blood sample. Plasma, which is collected in anticoagulated tubes, contains all coagulation factors. Serum is the liquid that remains after blood has clotted. It lacks some coagulation factors that were used during the clotting process. Whole blood is anticoagulated blood that has not been separated into plasma and cells via centrifugation. For example, blood collected into lavender-stoppered tubes and used for a complete blood cell (CBC) count is whole blood.

TUBES AND ANTICOAGULANTS

The tubes are discussed in the general order of collection. There is more discussion regarding the order of draw in Chapter 6. It is important that all tubes used for venipuncture are within their expiration date. Tubes that are beyond their expiration date may result in an unsuccessful venipuncture because of loss of vacuum. Also, the additive may no longer be optimally active, which could result in erroneous laboratory results.

YELLOW-STOPPERED TUBES

Yellow-stoppered tubes often contain acid-citrate-dextrose (ACD). In addition to inhibiting the coagulation process, ACD maintains red blood cell viability. Yellow-stoppered tubes may also contain sodium polyanetholesulfonate (SPS). Tubes with SPS are often the tubes of choice for blood culture collections, but increasingly the blood culture bottles used are those that have been adapted for insertion into the tube holder and a winged collection device. As noted above, at one time the tubes were made of glass, but they are now made of plastic, thus rendering them safer (Fig. 5.1). Another point about collecting for blood cultures is that a special skin preparation solution is used to sterilize the area of the blood culture collection. The skin preparation is often a combination of alcohol and iodine or povidone-iodine or chlorhexidine gluconate. These all do a better job of cleansing the site than simply isopropyl alcohol. This, in turn, reduces the risk of contaminating the sample with skin flora. Collection for blood cultures will be further explored in Chapter 7.

BLUE-STOPPERED TUBES

Another common tube used for the hematology laboratory (or, more precisely, the coagulation laboratory) is

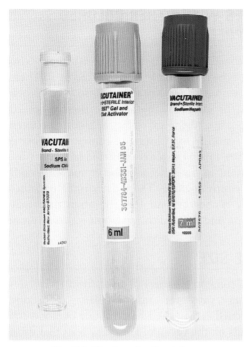

Fig. 5.1 Plastic collection tubes.

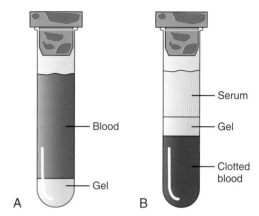

Fig. 5.2 Blood collection tube with gel separator. *A,* Before centrifugation. *B,* After centrifugation. (From Bonewit-West K. *Clinical Procedures for Medical Assistants,* 8th ed. St. Louis, Saunders, 2011.)

the *blue-stoppered* tube. Sodium citrate is used as the primary ingredient in these tubes to prevent coagulation. Sodium citrate, like ethylenediaminetetraacetate (EDTA), binds calcium and thus prevents coagulation. Blue-stoppered tubes are used for coagulation studies such as prothrombin time (PT) and activated partial thromboplastin time (aPTT). Blood from these tubes cannot be used for CBC counts or differentials because of the effects of citrate on the cellular components. It is also critical with these tubes to maintain the proper blood/anticoagulant ratio; therefore the tubes must be filled to the "fill line" indicated on the tube. If not filled properly, erroneous laboratory results may occur. They also must be inverted several times after collection to adequately mix the blood and anticoagulant.

RED-STOPPERED TUBES

Tubes with *red stoppers* are used frequently. These tubes generally have no additive and are used when serum is required for testing, such as in blood banking and many serological procedures. Some red top tubes may contain a clot activator that is not apparent to the naked eye so be sure to check which tube you are using. A tube with

a clot activator will need to be inverted several times after collection.

"TIGER TOPS" AND GOLD TUBES

A special type of red-stoppered tube contains a serum-cell separator. These tubes have red stoppers and are often referred to as "tiger tops," "speckled reds," or "mottled tops." The separator, which is a gel, works by settling between the clot and the serum during centrifugation, based on the specific gravity, thereby making it easier for the laboratory worker to access the serum. The gel separates the two components of the specimen because its density or specific gravity is between that of the clot and serum (Fig. 5.2). The tubes are used often in chemistry for a variety of tests, such as enzymes, liver screening tests, and electrolytes. Becton, Dickinson, and Company (Franklin Lakes, NJ) has marketed a gold-stoppered tube with a serum-cell gel separator and a dry clot enhancer coated on the inside of the tube. Although the stopper is red, it has a gold plastic cap over it. Apart from the variation of the cap, this tube is used like the more traditional "tiger-top" tube. This cap is referred to as a *Hemoguard* and is discussed further at the end of this section.

GREEN-STOPPERED TUBES

Green-stoppered tubes contain the anticoagulant sodium heparin or lithium heparin. Heparin is a natural anticoagulant and stops the coagulation process by inactivating thrombin and thromboplastin. Blood collected in these tubes is assayed when plasma or whole blood is needed—as, for example, in tests for ammonia. Green-stopped tubes are also the tubes of choice when doing human leukocyte antigen typing or chromosome analysis. A light-green heparinized tube is also available that has a gel separator when heparinized plasma is required.

LAVENDER-STOPPERED TUBES

In the hematology laboratory, the majority of specimens are collected in *lavender-stoppered* (also known as *purple-stoppered*) tubes. The primary additive in these tubes is the anticoagulant EDTA. EDTA prevents blood from clotting by chelating or binding calcium that, in turn, allows the cells to be counted and studied. Calcium is needed for clot formation, and by binding calcium, coagulation can be prevented.

Lavender-stoppered tubes are used for general hematological studies such as the CBC count, white blood cell (WBC) differential, and platelet count and function tests. Occasionally, the blood smear for the WBC differential can be made from a drop of blood collected via a finger stick. However, this is usually not practical, and the EDTA tube is used. In fact, if platelets are to be evaluated, the EDTA tube is preferred. The smear should be made within a half hour of the collection because EDTA may cause some distortion of WBC morphological findings.

GRAY-STOPPERED TUBES

To inhibit glycolytic action, sodium fluoride or sodium fluoride with thymol may be used. One of these ingredients is often combined with potassium oxalate, which inhibits the clotting process by binding calcium. These ingredients are found in *gray-stoppered* evacuation tubes. Blood collected in these tubes is generally used for glucose and alcohol analysis.

PINK TUBES

Pink tubes contain spray-dried EDTA and are used for whole-blood hematological analysis and may be used for blood bank testing.

TUBES WITH OTHER COLORED STOPPERS

Occasionally tubes with other colored stoppers, such as black, brown, and dark blue, may be used. These may come with a variety of additives, so the phlebotomist should be aware of the additive these tubes contain before using them to collect a blood specimen. See pages ii and iii for a listing of common stopper colors, additives, mixing requirements, and laboratory use. It is important to note that all tubes come with expiration dates clearly marked. These dates must be adhered to strictly. Tubes beyond the expiration date may lose vacuum, and the additive may not function properly.

TUBE SIZE

Tubes come in a variety of sizes, from 15 mL down to capillary sizes for microcapillary collections. As mentioned earlier, the actual volume of blood collected depends on the vacuum. For many tests that use a tube with an anticoagulant, a minimum amount of blood must be drawn into the tube. Otherwise, the blood/anticoagulant ratio will not be ideal, and this could adversely affect the test. The phlebotomist should check the manufacturer's specifications regarding the minimum acceptable amount of blood that can be drawn into an anticoagulated tube.

Most tubes used for adults range from 3 to 10 mL. Pediatric evacuated tubes generally range from 2 to 4 mL. Blood-holding devices for microcapillary collection hold less than 1 mL of blood. Fig. 5.3 shows some examples of blood-collecting devices for microcapillary collection. Please note that microcapillary collection does not depend on vacuum but rather capillary action.

SPLASHGUARDS

In an effort to reduce the aerosol mist that may be generated when a stopper is removed from a tube, Becton, Dickinson, and Company (Franklin Lakes, NJ) has manufactured a stopper that has a splashguard placed over it. A tube with this type of stopper is known as a *Hemoguard* (Fig. 5.4). Hemoguard tubes are available as replacements for all of the commonly used traditional tubes. The splashguard decreases the aerosol

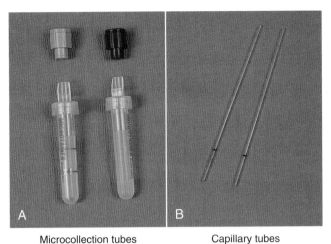

Microcollection tubes   Capillary tubes

Fig. 5.3 *A,* Microcollection tubes. *B,* Capillary tubes.

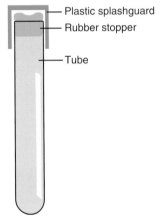

— Plastic splashguard
— Rubber stopper

— Tube

Fig. 5.4 Cross-section of a collection tube with a splashguard, which is used to reduce the potentially infectious aerosol mist that may be generated when the stopper is removed from the tube.

mist, which may be infectious. Also, some tubes are designed so that certain instruments can access the specimen directly, thus entirely eliminating the need to remove the stopper.

NEEDLES

A very important part of the blood collection system is the needle. Needles are hollow, stainless-steel shafts with a beveled end tapered to a point. The tube-end of the needle is also honed to a point if it is part of the

evacuated tube system. Each needle is sterilized and individually packaged. In some countries, needles are reused after cleaning and sterilization, but in the United States, all needles are used once and then disposed of properly.

NEEDLE SIZE

Needles come in a variety of sizes; the size is referred to as the **needle gauge**. The gauge is a measurement of the diameter of the needle: the larger the gauge number, the smaller the diameter of the needle. For routine phlebotomy, most needles are 21 or 22 gauge; however, during blood donation, an 18-gauge needle is common. If a patient has small or fragile veins, the phlebotomist often elects to use a small-gauge needle (e.g., 22 gauge).

Needles are generally 1 or 1.5 inches in length. The needle selected depends on the individual patient and on the depth of the vein from which blood is to be collected.

MULTIPLE-DRAW NEEDLES

Another variable in needle choice is whether the needle will be used for a single draw or multiple draw. In other words, will one or more than one tube of blood be collected? The multiple-draw needle has a retractable sheath over the part of the needle that extends into the evacuated tube. This sheath prevents blood from leaking out while the phlebotomist is changing tubes.

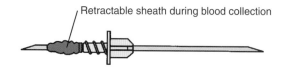
Retractable sheath during blood collection

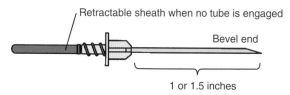
Retractable sheath when no tube is engaged

Bevel end

1 or 1.5 inches

Fig. 5.5 Multidraw needle demonstrating the retractable sheath. (Courtesy Rick Davis.)

Fig. 5.5 demonstrates how a multiple-draw needle works. Today the most common needle of choice, regardless of the number of tubes collected, is a multidraw needle.

WINGED INFUSION NEEDLES

Although generally used as part of an intravenous set to administer fluids or medicine to patients, the winged infusion needle (sometimes referred to as a *butterfly needle*; Fig. 5.6) is generally used to collect blood from patients presenting a difficult draw, but it is not uncommon for some phlebotomists to use these needles to collect blood during routine draws. Once the butterfly needle is in place, a syringe or evacuated tube, with a tube holder, is used to withdraw blood from the vein (see Chapter 6).

BLOOD LANCETS

For difficult patients and in situations that normally call for microcapillary techniques, a blood lancet may be used. This is a small, sterile, disposable instrument used for skin puncture (Fig. 5.7). Semiautomated lancets are available with a variety of point lengths and blade widths to help control the depth of puncture or incision, which is especially important in children and infants and is further discussed in Chapter 8. The semiautomated lancet automatically and permanently retracts after activation for enhanced safety. A variety of semiautomated lancet devices are commercially available, and although the manual lancet was the most

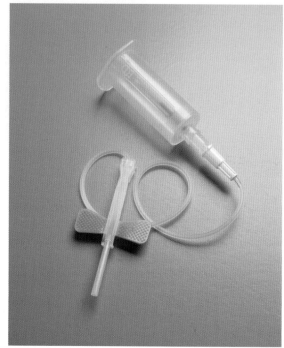

Fig. 5.6 Winged infusion set, commonly referred to as a *butterfly*. (Courtesy Rick Davis.)

commonly used device for microcapillary puncture in the past, semiautomated devices are now employed.

NEEDLE DISPOSAL EQUIPMENT

Needle disposal equipment has evolved over time from manually recapping and then unscrewing needles, to cutting off the needle, to unscrewing the needle directly into a puncture-resistant container. Disposal has evolved to the point of discarding both the needle and tube holder. In addition to being puncture-resistant, the container has a biohazard symbol clearly displayed, is leak proof, and has a locking lid to seal the container once it reaches three-fourths full. In light of the Federal Needlestick Safety and Prevention Act, which states that employees must review and implement safer medical devices as they become available, more advanced needle safety and disposal safeguards are becoming more commonly used. The purpose is to avoid any accidental needle punctures; the less the phlebotomist has to directly manipulate the needle, the less possibility there is of needle puncture. The puncture-resistant containers come in a

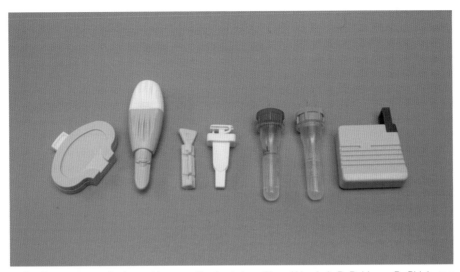

Fig. 5.7 Capillary puncture devices with two collection tubes. (From Warekois R, Robinson R. *Phlebotomy*, 3rd ed. St. Louis, Saunders, 2012.)

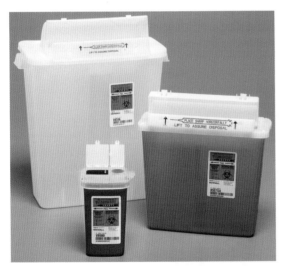

Fig. 5.8 Three types of needle-disposal units. (Courtesy Rick Davis.)

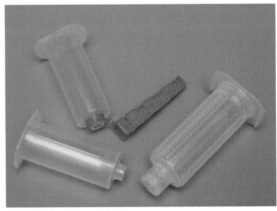

Fig. 5.9 Various tube holders. (*A*, Reproduced with permission from H1-A4, "Evacuated Tubes and Additives for Blood Specimen Collection—Fourth Edition; Approved Standard," 1996, NCCLS; *B*, Courtesy Rick Davis.)

TUBE HOLDERS

The tube holder or, as it is sometimes called, the *barrel* or *adapter*, allows the phlebotomist to safely and securely manipulate the evacuated tubes and draw blood from a patient. Holders come in a variety of sizes to accommodate normal- and pediatric-sized evacuated tubes (Fig. 5.9). Fig. 5.10 shows a fully assembled needle, tube, and tube holder. Given the current concern for safety, as discussed previously, one-time-use needle holders, in which the needle and tube holder are disposed of simultaneously, are becoming commonplace.

variety of sizes; some are small enough to fit conveniently on the phlebotomist's tray. As noted above, at one time, the needle was unscrewed into a disposal container; however, the current acceptable practice is to discard the entire needle and its holder. Therefore other needle safety and disposal devices are commercially available to prevent accidental needle punctures. These devices range from sheaths that enclose the used needles to retractable needles, and both the needle and holder are discarded with such devices (Fig. 5.8).

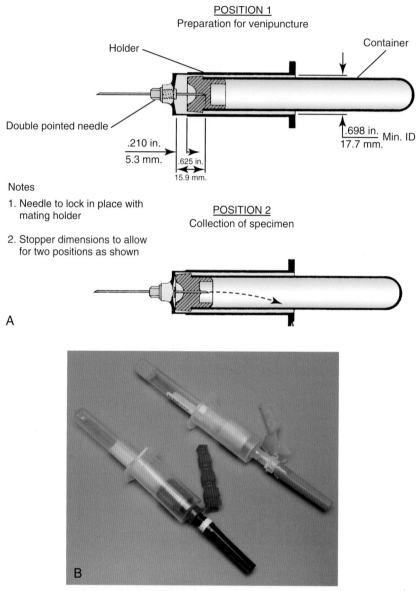

POSITION 1
Preparation for venipuncture

Holder

Container

Double pointed needle

.210 in.
5.3 mm.

.625 in.
15.9 mm.

.698 in.
17.7 mm.
Min. ID

Notes

1. Needle to lock in place with mating holder

2. Stopper dimensions to allow for two positions as shown

POSITION 2
Collection of specimen

A

B

Fig. 5.10 *A,* Line drawing of assembled venipuncture set. *B,* Fully assembled venipuncture sets. (*A,* Courtesy Rick Davis; *B,* From Bonewit-West K. *Clinical Procedures for Medical Assistants,* 8th ed. St. Louis, Saunders, 2011.)

VEIN LOCATION EQUIPMENT

TOURNIQUETS

The purpose of the tourniquet is to increase resistance in the venous blood flow. When this happens, the veins become distended and can be more easily palpated or located. However, the tourniquet should not remain on the patient too long (the recommended maximum time is 1 minute to prevent hemoconcentration) (see Chapter 9) because this could adversely affect the test results and be uncomfortable or harmful to the patient. A variety of tourniquets are available, including blood pressure cuffs, rubber tubing, and rubber straps.

Although a blood pressure cuff is an ideal tourniquet because the pressure can be accurately regulated, it is not practical to use for routine venipunctures. However, when confronted with a difficult "stick," a blood pressure cuff is very helpful. The more commonly used tourniquet is the rubber strap, which is tied in a slip loop (see Chapter 6) above the venipuncture site. Some tourniquet straps are equipped with hook-and-loop Velcro fasteners, thereby eliminating the need for the slip loop. Some tourniquet straps have a buckle adjustment to allow ease of release and retightening if needed. See Fig. 5.11 for types of tourniquets. In most cases, tourniquets are latex free to prevent allergic reaction and are single use to prevent the spread of infection. In all cases, tourniquets must be cleaned properly if contaminated, a drawback of blood pressure cuffs and buckling tourniquets. If the tourniquet becomes contaminated, discarding it may be easier and more cost effective.

VEIN LOCATING DEVICE

Equipment is available that helps phlebotomists visualize veins. The Venoscope II (Venoscope, LLC, Lafayette, LA), the Neonatal Transilluminator (Venoscope, LLC, Lafayette, LA), the Transillumination Vein Locator (Promedic, McCordsville, IN), and the Vein Entry Indicator (Vascular Technologies, Ness-Ziona, Israel) are all devices that help visualize veins. They work by using light to visualize the location of veins beneath the skin surface (Fig. 5.12).

PERSONAL PROTECTIVE EQUIPMENT
GLOVES

With the implementation of the Occupational Safety and Health Administration (OSHA) regulations for bloodborne pathogens and the advent of Universal Precautions, now incorporated in Standard Precautions, gloves have become mandatory in blood collection and are a primary piece of personal protective equipment (PPE). They provide a protective barrier between the phlebotomist and any infectious agents that could enter the body through a cut or abrasion. Remember, just because cuts or abrasions cannot be seen does not mean they are not present. *There is no excuse for not using gloves during every phlebotomy procedure.* Failure to use gloves could result in disciplinary action depending on the policies of the facility.

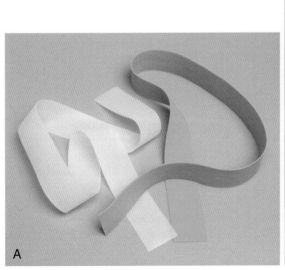
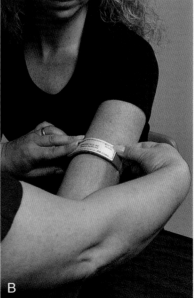

Fig. 5.11 In addition to the traditional latex tourniquets shown in *A*, *B* shows a hook-and-loop Velcro type of tourniquet.

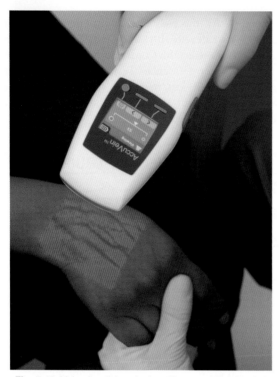

Fig. 5.12 *Vein-visualizing device. (Courtesy Rick Davis.)*

Gloves are made from a variety of materials, but the most commonly used materials are vinyl, latex, and nitrile. Vinyl gloves are probably the least desirable because they do not fit snugly and do not conform to the shape of the individual's hand. Latex gloves are the most commonly used because they fit nicely and conform to the individual's hand. Many phlebotomists prefer nitrile gloves, which are latex free. These have a fit similar to that of latex gloves but are more tear resistant and feel more comfortable on the hand. However, they are slightly more expensive. If a patient expresses a latex allergy, nonlatex gloves should be used.

Commonly, gloves are available with talcum powder lightly dusted inside them, which makes it easier for the wearer to put them on and take them off. Talc with calcium should be avoided because the calcium could cause altered test results. In addition, some individuals develop allergies to the powder, and occasionally the powder may interfere with some tests or be harmful to sensitive equipment. For these situations, powder-free gloves are available from a variety of vendors. Others

are allergic to latex and must use nonlatex gloves or a glove liner.

Gloves are available in dispenser boxes or are individually wrapped and sterilized, which is more costly. Generally, dispenser boxes are most commonly encountered in phlebotomy units. Phlebotomists should wash hands thoroughly after removing each pair of gloves to further prevent contamination or infection. Some phlebotomists may elect to use glove liners with powdered gloves, especially if they are sensitive to latex or the powder in the gloves. In summary, gloves should fit snugly and act as a "second skin." They should not be altered in any way, such as by removing a fingertip to allow direct contact, and hazardous access, between the phlebotomist and the patient.

OTHER PERSONAL PROTECTIVE EQUIPMENT

Safety goggles are recommended for use during some phlebotomy procedures; some places may use face shields in lieu of goggles. They both prevent the phlebotomist's eyes from being exposed to bloodborne pathogens from splashing or aerosol contaminants. Regular glasses are not acceptable substitutes for safety goggles.

Gowns and face masks (N-95 and/or surgical) are additional PPE that may be needed whenever a patient is in respiratory isolation. They may also be needed in a case of reverse isolation (to protect the phlebotomist). Additionally, since the advent of COVID-19, face masks may become a permanent addition for all phlebotomies. Only time will tell if face masks actually become a requirement for all blood-collecting procedures (same as gloves).

PHLEBOTOMY TRAYS

Phlebotomy trays are commercially available carriers that enable phlebotomists to conveniently carry all the equipment and supplies they may need to perform their job. These trays are generally carried, but some hospitals provide phlebotomists with push carts on which they may place their trays. The trays must allow the phlebotomist to carry an adequate supply of all the previously mentioned equipment. See Fig. 5.13 for a picture of a fully stocked phlebotomy tray.

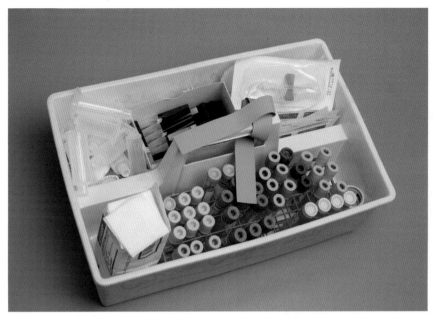

Fig. 5.13 Fully stocked phlebotomy tray. (Courtesy Rick Davis.)

PHLEBOTOMY CHAIRS

A final piece of equipment worth mentioning is the phlebotomy chair. These chairs are most often found in outpatient blood-collecting areas. There are several models available from manufacturers. However, they all provide a sturdy backrest, support for the arm, and a restraint system to keep the patient from falling out. They also generally have storage areas for tubes, needles, and so on. Fig. 5.14 shows an acceptable phlebotomy chair. Some phlebotomy chairs recline so that patients may lie down if they feel weak or faint.

TRAINING EQUIPMENT

All the equipment mentioned so far is used in both the actual practice of phlebotomy and in teaching phlebotomy students. However, some equipment is used specifically for training in most phlebotomy training programs. At one time, venipuncture training may have consisted of having students stick oranges or chicken legs; now, simulated arms and hands—complete with "blood"—are available from various manufacturers. Manikins are also available for teaching students how to hold infants for microcapillary collection.

OTHER COMMON SUPPLIES

Other common supplies that the phlebotomist needs are alcohol pads, gauze or cotton balls, surgical tape, pens, and adhesive bandages. Box 5.1 lists the common equipment that a phlebotomist may need.

SAFETY SUMMARY

- Ensure that consumable phlebotomy equipment is not expired.
- Ensure that collection tubes are filled properly if the blood/anticoagulant ratio is important.
- Wear gloves for all venipunctures or capillary punctures.
- Dispose of contaminated phlebotomy equipment properly.
- Follow all required local protocols.

SUMMARY

This chapter reviews the basic equipment used in routine phlebotomy. It is important for phlebotomists to keep their equipment organized, clean, and current.

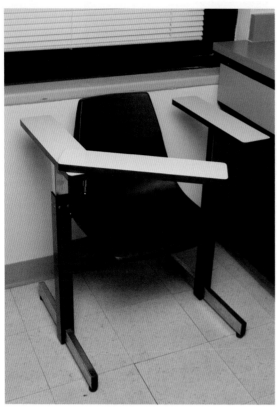

Fig. 5.14 Phlebotomy chair.

Also, as stressed in this chapter, attention to safety is paramount for both the phlebotomist and the patient.

BOX 5.1   Common Equipment a Phlebotomist Should Carry

- Needles (various sizes and microcapillary)
- Evacuated tubes (various sizes and colors)
- Microcapillary collection equipment
- Tube holders
- Tourniquets
- Alcohol swabs
- Gauze
- Adhesive bandages or tape
- Gloves
- Face masks
- Sharps containers
- Marking pens
- Clay sealer
- Goggles

CASE 5.1   Critical Thinking

During a routine venipuncture phlebotomists must remember many things about performing a proper procedure. They should not need to worry about the equipment. However, occasionally a phlebotomist is not successful when attempting a venipuncture. Discuss the possible ways that equipment may lead to an unsuccessful venipuncture.

■ REVIEW QUESTIONS

1. Identify the anticoagulant in a lavender-stoppered tube and explain how it prevents coagulation. _____

2. A small, sterile, disposable instrument used for skin puncture is the _____.

3. Explain the proper procedure for disposing of phlebotomy equipment after venipuncture. _____

4. What is the purpose of a tourniquet? _____

5. In an effort to reduce aerosol mist, a _____ is placed over the rubber stopper by some manufacturers.

6. Cells and serum are separated on the basis of _____ in tubes with gel separators.

7. _____ prevent aerosol from possibly exposing bloodborne pathogens to the phlebotomist via the eyes.

8. These alternatives to isopropyl alcohol are used to cleanse the skin when collecting blood culture tubes: _____

Proper Procedures for Venipuncture

John C. Flynn, Jr.

"Great dancers are not great because of their technique; they are great because of their passion."

—*Martha Graham (1894–1991)*

OBJECTIVES

At the conclusion of this chapter, the student should be able to:

- Greet and identify patients.
- Perform routine venipuncture with a needle and evacuated tube system.
- Perform blood collection using microcapillary blood collection equipment.
- Perform venipuncture using a butterfly collection needle.
- Name the proper order of draw for the various blood collection tubes.
- List several physiological and biological considerations that may influence laboratory results.

OUTLINE

KEY TERMS

analyte
basal state
circadian rhythm

diurnal variation
Luer adapter
supine

INTRODUCTION

The previous chapter discusses the equipment and anticoagulants used in common blood collection techniques. In this chapter, the actual techniques practiced in evacuated tube and microcapillary collections, beginning with greeting and identifying the patient and continuing through to labeling and transporting the specimen, are discussed and illustrated. (Syringe collection technique is discussed in a subsequent chapter.)

PATIENT GREETING AND IDENTIFICATION

The manner in which a phlebotomist greets a patient can often set the tone for the remainder of the phlebotomy procedure. Chapter 11 is devoted to interpersonal communication and professionalism, but it must be emphasized here that phlebotomists must always conduct themselves in a professional manner. Therefore, when greeting a patient, be courteous and respectful. Treat patients the way you would like to be treated. Additionally, if in a hospital and the patient's door is shut when you get to the room, knock and listen for a response before you enter. Of course, this may not always be feasible, depending on the patient and the surrounding circumstances. Also, there may be times when other people are with the patient, such as family, friends, clergy, or other health care professionals. Generally, if they are nonprofessionals, it is recommended that you ask that they step out for a minute while you collect the specimen. If other health care professionals are present, discuss with them whether they would like you to collect the specimen or return in a short while. Occasionally, the patient may not be present; this should be noted on the requisition and at the nurse's station. Familiarity with local protocol will guide you as to what you should do in this circumstance.

For patients in the hospital or similar settings, phlebotomists must identify themselves and tell the patient why they are there. One of the most important steps in venipuncture—possibly the most important—is proper patient identification. If the wrong patient's blood is collected, the consequences can be catastrophic, including possible patient death. Additionally, there may

be severe consequences for the phlebotomist and for the laboratory, clinic, and/or hospital in the form of lawsuits. Identification should be both visual and verbal. When you enter a patient's room, in addition to the test requisition, you will generally have certain information, such as the patient's name, identification number, and age or date of birth. Compare the information you have with the patient's physical appearance and the identification bracelet. For example, if your requisition lists the patient's name as Sarah Jones and you encounter a male patient, there may be a problem. Furthermore, do not use the information on the chart that is attached to the bed or on the nameplate on or above the bed. Patients may be transferred, and nameplates may not be accurate. The only dependable information is on the patient's wristband. Additionally, ask patients to state their name rather than having them respond to a question. For example, it is best to say, "Please tell me your full name," rather than, "Are you Mrs. Jones?" If the patient is incoherent or has difficulty hearing, they may answer "yes" no matter what is asked in an effort to be cooperative. Remember, caution is the name of the game; using a second and a third identifier to properly identify the patient may take a little extra time but may avoid potential trouble later. In the event that a wristband is lacking, a second person must identify the patient. This should also be documented; it is suggested the second person should verify the patient's identity by initialing the requisition. It is also good practice to ask some basic questions regarding allergies to latex, arm preference, and propensity to fainting.

When the patient is ambulatory, such as in an outpatient clinic, there may not be a wristband for identification purposes. You will still have a requisition with basic information, but the secondary identification may be a driver's license or some other form of identification, preferably with a photograph. The same procedures as mentioned previously must be followed for appropriate patient greeting. It is also good practice to note the physical disposition of the patient. Is the patient sweating, obese, acting nervous, or showing some other condition that may play a role in the success of the venipuncture? Asking the patient when they last ate is good practice, too, especially when collecting fasting or timed specimens. In all cases, the phlebotomist must be careful about discussing the patient's test requisition or any other conditions within earshot of other persons, whether they are professionals or laypeople. Such discussion, should it be overheard, could be a violation of the patient's Health Insurance Portability and Accountability Act (HIPAA) rights. HIPAA is discussed in Chapter 14.

ROUTINE VENIPUNCTURE

This section discusses the proper procedure (Procedure 6.1) for performing routine venipuncture. Remember that gloves must be worn at all times. After reviewing the photographs in Procedure 6.1, see the Venipuncture Competency Evaluation at the end of this chapter after the Review Questions. Also, Box 6.1 lists general considerations for all types of blood draws.

POSITIONING AND TOURNIQUET APPLICATION

Position the patient's arm in such a way that it is comfortable for both you and the patient, allowing clear access to the antecubital area. The arm should be supported by a firm surface such as an armrest on a phlebotomy chair or on the bed if the patient is lying down (i.e., in a supine position). It is courteous to ask the patient if they have an arm preference for the venipuncture, but the ultimate decision rests with the phlebotomist. Once the arm is positioned, place the tourniquet firmly around the upper arm approximately 4 inches above the antecubital area. The tourniquet needs to be tight enough to increase blood pressure in the veins but not so tight that it cuts off the circulation (see Fig. 6.1). Fig. 6.2 shows how the tourniquet should be tied. After some practice, you will learn how to adjust the tourniquet for proper snugness. Before working an actual patient, you will have practiced on laboratory partners or simulated arms to master the technique of tying a tourniquet. The tourniquet should not remain on the patient's arm for more than 1 minute. If this does occur for some reason, loosen the tourniquet, and wait 3 to 4 minutes before retying.

CHOOSING THE SITE

Try to locate the median cubital vein (generally the largest and best-anchored vein, near the center of the antecubital area) (see Fig. 6.3A). Other veins that may be acceptable are the cephalic and the basilic veins (see

Fig. 6.3B). Veins in the back of the hand may also be acceptable, but in these cases it is wise to use pediatric needles and evacuated tubes or a butterfly needle. (This is discussed later.) To enhance visualization of the veins, position the arm at a downward angle, using the force of gravity as an aid. Also, rubbing the forearm toward the antecubital area and instructing the patient to make a fist may enhance vein visualization. Palpating and feeling for the vein with the forefinger is also helpful; do not forget that you can look on both arms before a decision is made and that there will be times when you cannot see the vein but can feel it. A vein visualization device may be helpful as well. The prospective venipuncture site should be free of skin abrasions, lesions, and scar tissue.

ASSEMBLING THE EQUIPMENT

Assemble the needle, the barrel (also known as the *tube holder* or *adapter*), and the first tube you wish to use, as in Fig. 5.9 and Fig. 6.4. The needle should not be uncovered until you are ready to perform the venipuncture, nor should the tube be engaged onto the needle. Place any additional tubes to be used in a convenient location, keeping some spares handy. The gauze, alcohol pads, and bandages should be ready. (Note: It is preferable to assemble the equipment before applying the tourniquet.)

CLEANSING THE SITE

Cleanse the venipuncture site (see Fig. 6.5A, B) with 70% isopropyl alcohol by making outward concentric circles. *This area must be allowed to dry*, either by air drying or by using sterile gauze (however, typically, sterile gauze is not available to phlebotomists, so air drying is the preferred method). Do not blow on the area. Failure to adequately dry could result in red cell hemolysis in the collected sample and discomfort to the patient.

Once the site is cleansed, it must not be touched; if touched, it must be recleansed.

PERFORMING THE VENIPUNCTURE

With the bevel up (that is, with the bevel facing upward), quickly and smoothly insert the needle into the vein at approximately a 15-degree angle and engage the evacuated tube (see Fig. 6.6A, B).

PROCEDURE 6.1   Routine Venipuncture

Materials
- Tourniquet
- Phlebotomy chair
- Needle
- Gloves
- Tubes (appropriate colors)
- Alcohol wipe
- Bandage
- Pen or label for specimen
- Biohazard waste receptacle
- Face masks
  1. Position the patient's arm and apply the tourniquet (Figs. 6.1 and 6.2).

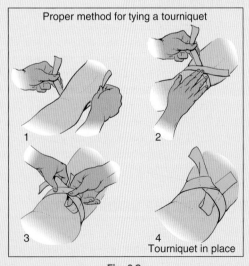

Fig. 6.1   (Courtesy Rick Davis.)

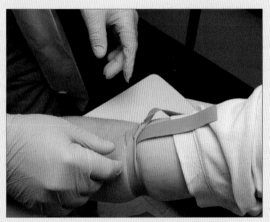

Proper method for tying a tourniquet

1

2

3

4
Tourniquet in place

Fig. 6.2

2. Choose the site (Fig. 6.3A, B). (You may need to apply the tourniquet to find an appropriate site and if necessary, release the tourniquet for a bit before reapplying and attempting the venipuncture if the 1-minute allowance is surpassed.)

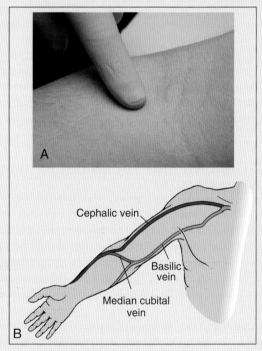

A

Cephalic vein

Basilic vein

Median cubital vein

B

Fig. 6.3   (A, Courtesy Rick Davis.)

3. Assemble the equipment, including the needle, barrel, and tube (Fig. 6.4). Have other tubes and equipment ready and nearby. (You may do this step before applying the tourniquet.)

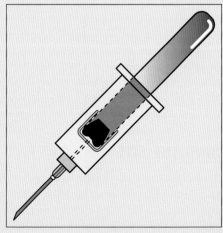

Fig. 6.4

PROCEDURE 6.1 Routine Venipuncture—cont'd

4. Cleanse the site using an alcohol sponge (Fig. 6.5A, B). Allow to dry.

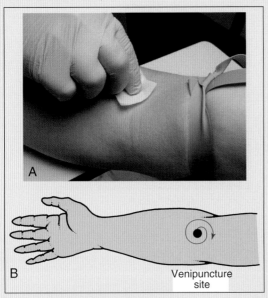

Venipuncture site

Fig. 6.5 (A, Courtesy Rick Davis.)

5. Perform the venipuncture (Fig. 6.6A, B).

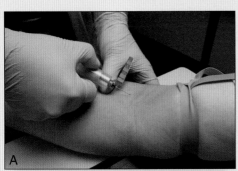

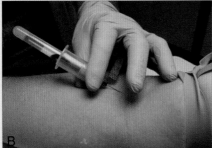

Fig. 6.6 (A–B, Courtesy Rick Davis.)

6. Release the tourniquet (Fig. 6.7).

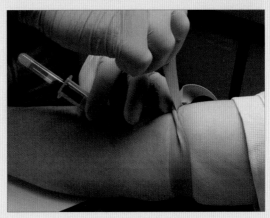

Fig. 6.7 (Courtesy Rick Davis.)

7. Remove the needle and apply pressure or a bandage as necessary (Fig. 6.8A, B). Snap the safety device into place (see Fig. 6.8C).

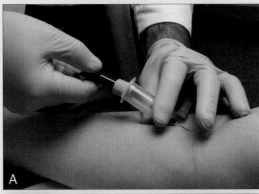

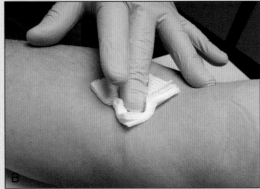

Fig. 6.8 (A–C, Courtesy Rick Davis.)

Continued

PROCEDURE 6.1   Routine Venipuncture—cont'd

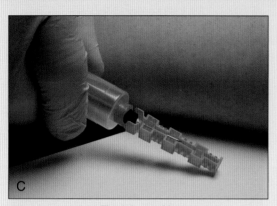

Fig. 6.8, cont'd

8. Dispose of the needle in an appropriate disposal container (Fig. 6.9A, B).

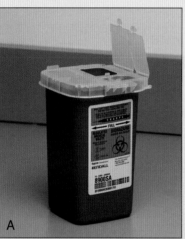

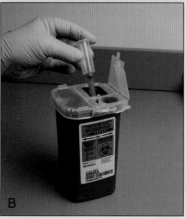

Fig. 6.9 (A–B, Courtesy Rick Davis.)

9. Label and prepare the specimen for transport (Fig. 6.10). Mix any specimens as necessary.

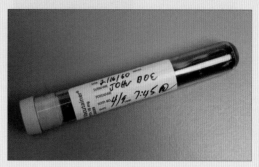

Fig. 6.10 (Courtesy Rick Davis.)

10. Properly dispose of gloves and other equipment, wash hands, and ensure the patient has no excessive bleeding.

BOX 6.1 General Considerations for Blood Collection

The following general considerations apply to blood collection either by venipuncture or by skin puncture:
1. Always act professionally and be considerate of the patient.
2. Never quarrel with a patient.
3. Use expendable equipment, such as needles, tube holders, lancets, and gauze, only once. Tourniquets may fall into this category as well, depending on local institutional policy.
4. Avoid performing venipuncture more than two times on a given patient.
5. Always wear gloves. The type of glove may depend on whether the patient has latex sensitivity.
6. Never recap needles, and always dispose of them properly.

Special Note: There is no right way or wrong way to hold the needle and adapter for venipuncture. Phlebotomy instructors may advocate one way over another because of familiarity and experience. The phlebotomy student must discover which way is most comfortable and which yields the best results. The key point is to prevent movement of the needle during tube exchange. Many advocate not switching hands, but again, rely on your instructor to guide you properly.

Be sure to stretch the skin surrounding the venipuncture site before inserting the needle; this will aid in anchoring the vein and will make needle insertion less painful. Anchor the vein by gently stretching the skin below the venipuncture site. Do not "straddle" the site with a thumb and finger; this increases the chance of inadvertently sticking yourself. Never tell patients that they will not feel the needle puncture or that it will not hurt. Be honest with the patient. If no blood is immediately forthcoming, slight manipulation of the needle may be helpful; you may have gone in too deep, not deep enough, or to one side of the vein. Avoid "probing," and do not attempt a venipuncture more than two times on a given patient. (See Chapter 9 for more discussion on what to do if you do not obtain blood.) If there are collection tubes that need to be mixed, you can do this while the other tubes are filling if easily manageable. Additionally, the patient should not be

instructed to pump the fist—this could lead to hemoconcentration.

RELEASING THE TOURNIQUET

Once good blood flow is established and before the final tube is filled, release the tourniquet (see Fig. 6.7). If the tourniquet was applied properly, you should be able to release it with a simple tug with minimal needle movement. Follow local protocol regarding whether the tourniquet is disposed or reused.

REMOVING THE NEEDLE

Once the last tube of blood is filled and you have removed it from the needle and tube holder, you may remove the needle (see Fig. 6.8A). Do this in a single, smooth, swift motion, and quickly apply clean gauze over the puncture site (see Fig. 6.8B). If the patient is able, instruct them to apply pressure and to keep the arm straight. If the patient is unable to do this, it is the phlebotomist's responsibility to apply pressure until the bleeding has stopped. Outpatients may use a bandage to cover the venipuncture site once bleeding has stopped or slowed significantly, but hospitals may have different policies about using bandages on inpatients. Be sure you are familiar with the policies at your institution.

NEEDLE DISPOSAL

Properly dispose of your needle in an approved disposal unit (see Fig. 6.9A, B). Do not lay it down, and do not recap it.

SPECIMEN LABELING AND TRANSPORTATION

Immediately label the specimen (the tubes should not be prelabeled) (see Fig. 6.10). Often, computer-generated labels are provided, but other times the phlebotomist must write the relevant information on the label. If any specimens require mixing and this could not be done during the collection process (e.g., blue- or purple-stoppered tubes or any anticoagulated tube), do so by gently inverting the tubes several times. Regarding labeling, remember that the patient's wristband is the primary source of information. In some hospitals, certain speci-mens (e.g., those for the blood bank) must be hand-labeled and initialed by the phlebotomist. Therefore be familiar with any special labeling requirements at your institution. Also, as a responsible phlebotomist, you must be aware of any special transportation requirements. Does the specimen need to be transported on ice (e.g., an ammonia test)? Does the specimen need to be maintained at 37°C (e.g., a cold agglutinin test)? Is the specimen a STAT (needing immediate analysis)? Be familiar with any special transportation requirements before collecting the blood specimen.

HAND WASHING AND DEPARTURE

Before moving on to the next patient, remove and properly discard your gloves, and then thoroughly wash your hands as discussed in Chapter 3. Thank the patient for their cooperation and ensure that the venipuncture site has been properly cared for and there is no exces-sive bleeding.

Occasionally, venipuncture must be performed on a young child or toddler. The equipment and procedure are basically the same as for an adult patient, but the child may need some restraint. See Chapter 9 for further discussion and an illustration of performing phlebotomy on a child.

MICROCAPILLARY BLOOD COLLECTION

Microcapillary blood collections are used primarily when the patient has no adequate veins for venipunc-ture, either because of age (very young or very old) or for some other reason, such as burns or dermatitis. Obviously, the amount of blood collected will be much smaller than that collected via venipuncture, which, in turn, means the physician must be very sure of the tests they want performed; there may be no excess blood available for additional tests. The technique for micro-capillary collection has some similarities to the veni-puncture technique described earlier. Gloves are used at all times, and the cleansing reagent and technique are similar. The site of the skin puncture is usually the finger but may also be the earlobe or the heel in the case of an infant (discussed further in Chapter 8). The third or fourth finger is preferred to the index or pinky finger. Procedure 6.2 illustrates the specifics.

After reviewing the procedure, see the Micro-capillary Blood Collection Competency Evaluation at the end of this chapter after the Review Questions.

VENIPUNCTURE USING A BUTTERFLY SET

A butterfly needle or winged infusion set may be used to access difficult veins (see Fig. 5.5). Butterflies are commonly used for pediatric or elderly patients, and a common site is the back of the hand. Butterfly needles can be used with either evacuated tube systems or with syringes. The evacuated tube system is more commonly used, especially by beginning phlebotomists. Occa-sionally, some phlebotomists will opt to use a butterfly set in place of an evacuated tube system for routine antecubital venipunctures.

The procedure is very similar to routine phlebotomy, including patient identification, site preparation, needle disposal, and precautions. A tourniquet is used, which is usually placed around the wrist if veins on the back of the hand are going to be used. The infusion needle is carefully threaded into the vein. It is very important to ensure that the needle is anchored; this is accomplished by taping or having a second person assist. However, a competent phlebotomist should be able to perform this procedure alone with a cooperative patient. A Luer adapter on the end of the infusion set can be threaded into the tube adapter, and then evacuated tubes can be filled. It is probably best to use pediatric tubes because full-size tubes may create too great a vacuum pull on the vein if the patient is elderly or an infant, thus leading to vein collapse. Extra precautions must be used when the needle is removed because the needle tends to dangle and can easily cause an accident. The safety device should be employed if one is present, and the needle and tubing should be disposed of properly as soon as possible. See Procedure 6.3 for a photographic series demonstrating the use of winged infusion sets. An additional consid-eration is that the air in the tubing in a butterfly set is significant enough to alter the blood/additive ratio in the first tube of blood collected. Therefore a tube without additives should be collected first, then the normal order of draw followed. If only additive tubes are requested, a "dummy" or throwaway tube should be collected first and discarded, followed by the normal order of draw.

ORDER OF DRAW

The order in which a phlebotomist fills tubes collected via evacuated systems is critical to ascertaining good test results. For example, tissue fluids may interfere with coagulation studies, and skin surface bacteria may lead to false positives in blood cultures. Additionally, additives from the tubes themselves may cause erroneous results if there should happen to be any carryover between collection tubes. For example, oxalate found in gray-stoppered tubes can interfere with red blood cell morphology. Therefore the order of draw in blood collection must be done in a way to minimize these potentially interfering factors.

PROCEDURE 6.2　Microcapillary Blood Collection

Materials
- Phlebotomy chair
- Microcapillary puncture device
- Microcollection tube
- Gloves
- Alcohol wipe
- Bandage or gauze
- Pen or label for specimen
- Biohazard waste receptacle

1. No tourniquet is applied, but instead the site is held firmly by the phlebotomist. Fig. 6.11A, B shows how to hold a finger to perform a skin puncture, which should be perpendicular to the lines of the fingerprint.

2. Site preparation (Fig. 6.12) is similar to venipuncture, but a microlance is used instead of a needle and tube (Fig. 6.13).

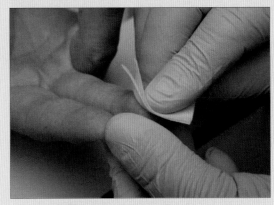

Fig. 6.12　(Courtesy Rick Davis.)

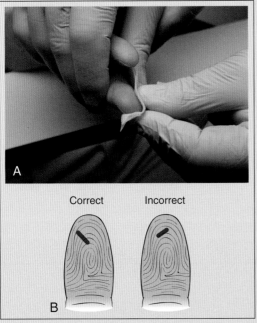

Correct　　Incorrect

B

Fig. 6.11　(A, Courtesy Rick Davis.)

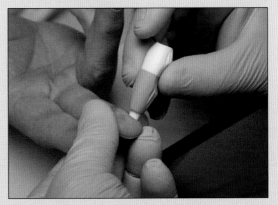

Fig. 6.13　(Courtesy Rick Davis.)

Continued

PROCEDURE 6.2 Microcapillary Blood Collection—cont'd

3. When doing a finger stick, make the puncture off the center of the finger (see Fig. 6.11*B*).
4. It is important to remember to wipe away the first drop of blood because the blood in this drop will be diluted with tissue fluid, which could alter the laboratory results (Fig. 6.14).

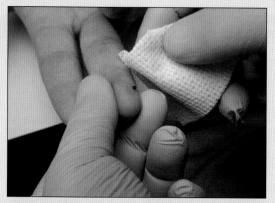

Fig. 6.14 (Courtesy Rick Davis.)

5. Some variation of a microcollection tube is used to collect the blood (Fig. 6.15). Be sure to mix the sample if appropriate.

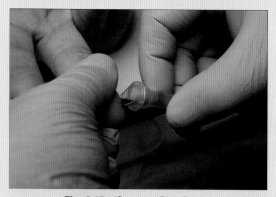

Fig. 6.15 (Courtesy Rick Davis.)

6. At the completion of the blood collection, either the phlebotomist or the patient must maintain pressure on the puncture site until bleeding has stopped (Fig. 6.16).

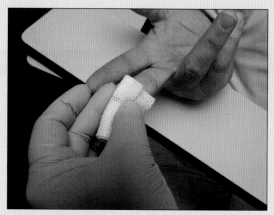

Fig. 6.16 (Courtesy Rick Davis.)

7. All used material is properly disposed of—the puncture device in puncture-proof container and the used gauze and gloves in an appropriate receptacle.
8. As in venipuncture, hands must be washed before going to the next patient.

The commonly accepted order of draw as recommended by the Clinical and Laboratory Standards Institute is as follows:

1. Blood culture tubes first, generally yellow tops (if not special blood collection bottles) to minimize the chance of bacterial contamination

PROCEDURE 6.3   **Winged Infusion Blood Collection**

Materials

- Phlebotomy chair
- Winged infusion set
- Collection tube
- Gloves
- Alcohol sponge
- Bandage or gauze
- Pen or label for specimen
- Biohazard waste receptacle

1. Apply the tourniquet, and locate a hand vein. (Fig. 6.17; note the location of the tourniquet in *A* and hand veins in *B*).

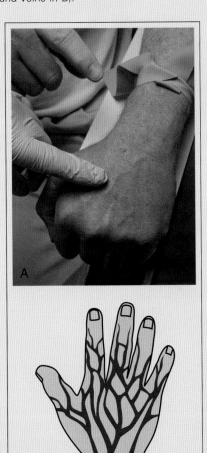

Fig. 6.17 (A, Courtesy Rick Davis.)

2. Cleanse the site using circular motion. Allow to air dry (Fig. 6.18).

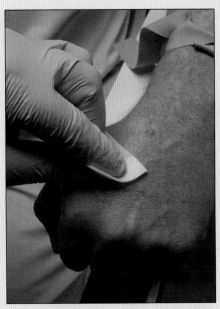

Fig. 6.18 (Courtesy Rick Davis.)

3. Perform the puncture; note the thumb stretching the skin and anchoring the site (Fig. 6.19).

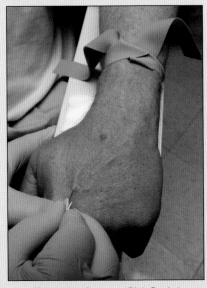

Fig. 6.19 (Courtesy Rick Davis.)

Continued

PROCEDURE 6.3   Winged Infusion Blood Collection—cont'd

4. Collect the blood (Fig. 6.20).

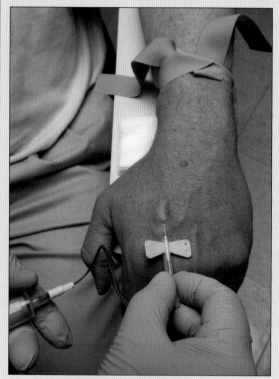

Fig. 6.20   (Courtesy Rick Davis.)

5. Remove needle and activate safety device. Apply pressure after collection (Fig. 6.21A, B).

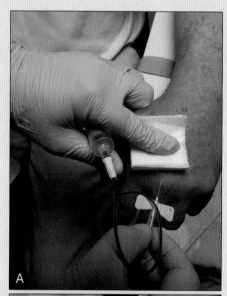

A

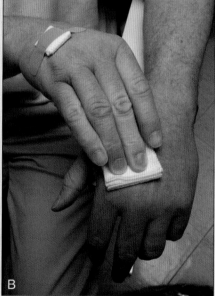

B

Fig. 6.21   (Courtesy Rick Davis.)

6. Properly dispose of all used material in the appropriate receptacle.

7. As in venipuncture, hands must be washed before going to the next patient.

2. Coagulation tubes (light blue)
3. Serum collection tubes: these could be with or without serum separators, such as red-top tubes with no additives for example
4. Additive tubes:
   a. Heparin, green top
   b. Lavender
   c. Pink
   d. Gray

Remember: Always follow the manufacturer's directions. Furthermore, local protocol may differ regarding the order of draw, especially with additive tubes, so be sure to follow your employer's standard operating procedure. Finally, if a coagulation tube (light blue) is the only one requested, collect a dummy or discard tube before this one and dispose of it in a biohazard disposal container. This eliminates the possibility of interference by tissue fluids during coagulation studies or excess air being introduced into the collection tube (if using a butterfly set) that can cause an improper blood/anticoagulant ratio. As always, check local protocol for order of draw and discard tubes.

PHYSIOLOGICAL AND BIOLOGICAL CONSIDERATIONS

Occasionally, laboratory testing of a blood sample results in a spurious result, which can be considered a mistake by a physician or nurse on the floor. Actually what has occurred is a variation from the basal state of the patient, which has influenced the analyte. In short, the basal state is the baseline condition of the patient before any treatment or medication. Any number of things can interfere with the basal state of a patient (e.g., diet, exercise, stress, trauma, or change in posture). These may also be referred to as *preanalytical conditions*. The time of day can also interfere with the baseline results one would expect to obtain on testing.

Diet is probably the most obvious factor that may affect testing. This is especially true when analyses for glucose or triglycerides are performed. The importance of collecting fasting or timed specimens is discussed more fully in Chapter 7, but it is important to note the time at which a specimen is collected and whether it is a fasting specimen.

The level of certain enzymes, such as creatine kinase (CK), in the blood may help diagnose heart damage. However, this same enzyme is also found in all other muscle tissue. If the patient has engaged in moderate to strenuous exercise in the 24 hours preceding the collection of the blood specimen, an elevated level of the enzyme, not related to a heart condition, may be found. (It should be noted that if an elevated CK level is encountered, a more specific test should be performed.) Exercise may also affect the levels of other enzymes, as well as various hemostatic factors. For the phlebotomist, it may be wise to note whether a patient has engaged in exercise in the 24 hours preceding blood collection. This information is usually more relevant in outpatients and can be determined through questioning.

Stress caused by the anticipation of having a blood specimen collected may alter the levels of certain constituents in the blood. For example, white blood cells may increase if the patient is overanxious about the phlebotomy. Therefore it is best—and easier—to collect the specimen when the patient is calm.

The *trauma* associated with an accident adversely affects the results of some tests. If the muscles are injured in a traumatic accident, CK is released into the blood system and may initially give a false indication of heart trouble.

A change in posture may not only change blood pressure, but it may also significantly alter the results obtained when testing for certain analytes such as proteins, lipids, iron, and enzymes. This is especially true when a patient has been in one position for a period and blood is collected shortly after they change position.

Finally, the time of day that a specimen is collected affects the results of testing. Serum cortisol, used to monitor adrenal function, is notably affected by circadian rhythm or diurnal variation, again illustrating the importance of noting the time at which a blood specimen is collected.

In addition to the physiological variations mentioned earlier, certain biological conditions may affect testing results. These include factors such as age, sex, race, and pregnancy. If appropriate, laboratories generally have different sets of normal values depending on what test is being performed. Table 6.1 shows how normal values for hemoglobin may vary. Often, the age, sex, and race are noted on requisition slips or computer-generated labels. If not, it will be very informative to the laboratory if the phlebotomist provides this information, in addition to noting whether the patient is pregnant.

The previous paragraphs mention only a few of the many blood constituents that may be affected by a

TABLE 6.1   Hemoglobin Values According to Age and Gender

	Normal Hemoglobin Value (g/dL)
Newborn	17–23
2-month-old child	9–14
Adult man	14–18
Adult woman	12–16

variety of physiological and biological conditions. For phlebotomists, any information that can be provided to the laboratory to help explain spurious results and avoid a "laboratory error" will be a great service in saving both time and money, as well as possibly saving the patient from a needless venipuncture.

SAFETY SUMMARY

- Properly identify the patient.
- Use the proper equipment for the venipuncture or microcapillary collection.
- Positively identify the vein selected for venipuncture.
- Thoroughly cleanse the venipuncture site.
- Do not probe if the initial phlebotomy misses the vein.
- Release the tourniquet before removing the needle.
- Ensure the patient is not bleeding after the venipuncture.
- Use the proper order of draw for the Vacutainer tubes.

SUMMARY

This chapter reviewed the proper procedure for conducting a routine venipuncture. This is the heart of the book and should be regarded by new phlebotomists as the most critical chapter in regard to procedures. The chapter also reviewed biological and physiological considerations when performing venipuncture. Subsequent chapters will review procedures in special circumstances.

CASE 6.1   Critical Thinking

You are just starting your phlebotomy collection rounds at 7 AM. You have been assigned the maternity ward, and you have a total of 22 patients from whom to collect. When you enter Room 345, you greet your patient properly and explain why you are there. She is your sixth patient. While you are putting on your gloves, you ask the patient to state her name. The patient replies, "I am Mary Jones." You look at your requisition slip and notice that the name the patient just gave you does not match your requisition. What should you do?

REVIEW QUESTIONS

1. Probably the most important aspect of phlebotomy is proper _____.
2. The cleanser of choice for routine venipuncture is _____.
3. The _____ should always be released before removing the needle from a vein.
4. You should always _____ before moving on to the next patient.
5. _____ may cause an elevation in blood enzymes.
6. Venipuncture needles are inserted at approximately a _____-degree angle.
7. A _____ needle is often used in elderly and pediatric patients.
8. If an anticoagulated tube is the only sample being collected, then a _____ tube should be the first tube collected using an evacuated system.

VENIPUNCTURE COMPETENCY EVALUATION

Student's Name _____ Date _____

Evaluated by _____

Result of Evaluation _____

Conditions for Testing:

The patient may be of any age.

The request is for multiple blood samples.

Equipment is readily available.

Student has undergone a training period for all previous labs.

Student has been given a copy of the exam before training period begins.

No references may be used or questions asked.

Scoring:

1. Steps 3, 15, 21, 27, 28, and 30 (in boldface) are critical. Exam is stopped if student omits such a step. Retest is required after additional training to be specified by the instructor.
2. More than two checks in the No column require a retest after additional training.

Criteria for Evaluation:

Competent (C): Student performs all steps as indicated and in the proper sequence. The numerical grade is 100.

Minimally Competent (MC): Student performs all critical steps as indicated. A maximum of two checks appears in the No column for the noncritical steps. The numerical grade is 80.

Incompetent (I): Instructor stops exam because a critical step is omitted; more than two checks appear in the No column; or steps are out of sequence. The numerical grade is 60.

COMPETENCY SCORE SHEET: EXPECTED OBSERVABLE PERFORMANCE

For venipuncture, the student:	YES	NO
1. Wears gloves and face mask		
2. Greets patient, puts patient at ease, explains the procedure		
3. Identifies patient: checks wristband, asks name, checks labels, and request forms		
4. Positions patient: supports patient's arm, patient appears comfortable		
5. Selects equipment to correspond with requested tests		
6. Places needle on holder		
7. Positions tube in holder without breaking vacuum		
8. Places sponges and other tubes within reach		
9. Reassures patient while positioning tourniquet; asks patient to clench fist		
10. Selects vein by palpation with index finger		
11. Cleanses area with alcohol sponge (student may repeat 8, 9, and 10)		
12. Removes needle cap		
13. Positions bevel up		
14. Fixes vein by placing thumb about 2 cm below site of entry and pulling skin downward to keep it taut		
15. Angles needle at approximately 15 degrees without contamination		
16. Inserts needle under skin and into lumen about 1 cm below prominent part of vein		
17. Pushes tube into holder without moving needle (order of draw)		
18. Obtains blood and allows tube to fill completely		

Continued

19. Removes tube and replaces with another tube without moving needle (may repeat 18)		
20. Asks patient to relax fist		
21. Removes tourniquet		
22. When last tube is filled, pulls tube back to line on holder to seal needle		
23. Covers site with gauze and removes needle slowly without changing angle, then activates safety device		
24. Applies pressure to gauze. Asks patient to hold gauze with pressure. Tells patient to keep arm straight		
25. Removes tube from holder and mixes tubes		
26. Activate safety device if not already activated		
27. Labels tubes		
28. Discards waste in proper containers		
29. Matches tubes to request slips		
30. Checks patient's arm to be sure hemostasis has occurred; asks patient if he or she is feeling all right; tells patient not to exercise arm immediately		
31. Places bandage on arm if needed		
32. Remove gloves and wash hands		
33. Leaves patient when appropriate		

MICROCAPILLARY BLOOD COLLECTION COMPETENCY EVALUATION

Student's Name _____ Date _____

Evaluated by _____

Result of Evaluation _____

Conditions for Testing:

The patient may be of any age.

The request is for multiple blood samples.

Equipment is readily available.

Student has undergone a 3-hour lab exercise training period.

Student has been given a copy of the exam before training period begins.

No references may be used or questions asked.

Scoring:

1. Steps 3, 15, 16, and 17 (in boldface) are critical. Exam is stopped if student omits such a step. Retest is required after additional training to be specified by the instructor.

2. More than two checks in the No column require a retest after additional training.

Criteria for Evaluation:

Competent (C): Student performs all steps as indicated and in the proper sequence. The numerical grade is 100.

Minimally Competent (MC): Student performs all critical steps as indicated. A maximum of two checks appear in the No column for the noncritical steps. The numerical grade is 80.

Incompetent (I): Instructor stops exam because a critical step is omitted; more than two checks appear in the No column; or steps are out of sequence. The numerical grade is 60.

COMPETENCY SCORE SHEET: EXPECTED OBSERVABLE PERFORMANCE

For capillary blood collection, the student:	YES	NO
1. Wears gloves and face mask		
2. Greets patient, puts patient at ease, explains the procedure		
3. **Properly identifies patient: checks wristband, asks name, checks labels, and request forms**		
4. Selects correct equipment and organizes all supplies before beginning		
5. Selects proper site		
6. Cleanses site with alcohol		
7. Dries site per local protocol		
8. Punctures ball of finger with one swift motion		
9. Wipes away first drop of blood		
10. Massages finger gently		
11. Holds capillary tube to blood source and allows to fill—does not touch tube to finger		
12. Wipes excess blood from outside capillary tube, seals it, or otherwise handles equipment according to previously specified instructions		
13. Collects all capillary blood samples in duplicate when specified		
14. Applies dry gauze to stop bleeding		
15. **Labels samples**		
16. **Checks patient's finger and applies bandage if needed**		
17. **Disposes of used equipment in appropriate manner**		
18. Remove gloves and wash hands		

7

Special Collection Procedures

John C. Flynn, Jr.

"Let each man pass his days in that wherein his skill is greatest."

—*Sextus Propertius (c. 50–c. 16 bc)*

OBJECTIVES

At the conclusion of this chapter, the student should be able to:

- Discuss the importance of the following tests:
  - Glucose tolerance test
  - Arterial blood gases
  - Cold agglutinin tests
  - Blood cultures
  - Therapeutic blood collections
  - Fibrin degradation tests

- Describe the procedure for syringe venipuncture.
- Compare and contrast routine venipuncture site preparation and blood culture collections site preparation.
- Perform peripheral blood smears.
- Discuss the steps in blood donor collection.
- Describe various peripheral venous access devices.

OUTLINE

KEY TERMS

aerobic
Allen test
anaerobic
diabetes mellitus
hypoglycemia

myasthenia gravis
phagocytosis
polycythemia vera
septicemia

INTRODUCTION

A skilled, well-trained, and experienced phlebotomist is a valuable asset to the clinical laboratory or any health care setting where venipuncture is performed. Often the phlebotomist is asked or required to do more than perform routine venipuncture or microcapillary collections. This chapter outlines other blood collection procedures or tests that phlebotomists may perform depending on the institution, laboratory, or clinic.

SYRINGE COLLECTIONS

At one time a syringe was the only option for blood collection. With the advent of the evacuated tube system, the use of a syringe to collect venous blood is no longer routine. With that being said, it will be an experienced phlebotomist that will typically be called upon to collect blood via a syringe. Generally, a syringe is used to collect blood from veins that may collapse when using an evacuated tube system because of the force of the vacuum (e.g., small or fragile veins often found in elderly patients and small children). See Fig. 7.1 for an illustration of a typical syringe.

As previously stated, an entry-level phlebotomist generally will not use a syringe for venipuncture. However, collecting blood via the syringe is straightforward. Preparation of the venipuncture site is the same as that for the evacuated tube system described in Chapter 6. Keep in mind that if the plunger is pulled back too hard, it will have the same effect as a strong vacuum collection tube—that is, it will collapse the vein. Once the needle is in the vein, blood will appear in the hub of the needle. The phlebotomist should pull back slowly and evenly on the plunger to fill the syringe. Because blood will begin to clot in the syringe, it is imperative that collected blood be added to the evacuated tubes immediately in the same order and to the same level as a routine venipuncture. Historically, the syringe needle was pushed through the stopper and

blood was "injected" into the tube, or the needle was removed from the syringe and the stopper removed from the tube and blood was ejected from the syringe into the tube in this manner. These methods have been abandoned because of safety issues and increased risk of causing hemolysis in the specimen. Now there are blood transfer devices (Fig. 7.2) that are used to transfer blood from the syringe into the evacuated tube. The phlebotomist should mix any anticoagulant tubes thoroughly after the blood has been added.

GLUCOSE TOLERANCE TEST

The glucose tolerance test (GTT) is done on individuals who are being screened for hyperglycemia, also known as **diabetes mellitus.** The test is also used to screen for **hypoglycemia.** The purpose of the test is to determine the patient's blood glucose level after the patient consumes a fixed amount of glucose (usually 100 g). The test takes from 3 to 5 hours. Although there is nothing unique about the actual collection process itself, the number of venipunctures performed in a relatively short period makes this test significant.

After a patient has fasted for at least 12 hours, a blood sample is collected using routine collection procedures. The blood may be collected in a plain tube (without any anticoagulant) or in a tube especially

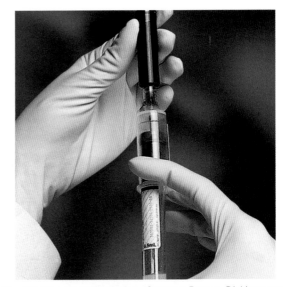

Fig. 7.2 Blood transfer device. (Courtesy Becton, Dickinson and Company, Franklin Lakes, New Jersey.)

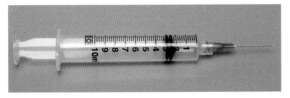

Fig. 7.1 A typical syringe. (Courtesy Rick Davis.)

designed to preserve glucose levels (such as a gray-stopper tube with sodium fluoride and potassium oxalate).

After the fasting sample is collected, the patient is directed to consume a dose of glucose determined by the patient's physician (100 g is common), often in liquid form. *It is critical to note the time of glucose consumption and of all subsequent venipunctures.* Blood is then collected at the half hour, 1 hour, 2 hours, 3 hours, 4 hours, and 5 hours after consuming the glucose. At each venipuncture, a urine specimen may also be collected. Again, it is very important to note the collection time on all specimens. The procedure may terminate in less than 5 hours depending on local protocol.

The laboratory analyzes the glucose levels in the blood specimens and plots them on a chart (Fig. 7.3). The results help the physician determine whether the patient is suffering from diabetes.

The phlebotomist plays a very crucial role in the administration of this test. Usually the patient receives a set of instructions about what to eat and a warning to avoid stressful exercise in the days leading up to the GTT. However, at times it is the phlebotomist who gives the patient instructions about dieting and fasting. The patient should eat a well-balanced diet for 3 days before the test. Generally, the patient is allowed water and is actually encouraged to drink water during the

fast and the test, but nothing else is allowed, including coffee and tea. Smoking is also discouraged. These instructions must be delivered in a clear and understandable manner. Patients should be encouraged to ask questions if they do not understand the instructions. If the phlebotomist does not perform this patient education function properly, much valuable time may be wasted.

Finally, the phlebotomist must be prepared to handle the situation when the patient becomes ill from consuming the glucose or lightheaded from fasting for several hours. Sometimes, nausea and vomiting occur early in the test, and it is a good idea to have towels and an emesis basin nearby. If the patient vomits within the first half hour, the test should be discontinued and will probably need to be rescheduled for another day. It is appropriate to notify the patient's physician and have them make the final decision. If the patient vomits or becomes faint later in the test, have them lie down and complete the testing. If repeated oral glucose administrations are unsuccessful, intravenously administered glucose is an option. The patient's physician will make this decision.

ARTERIAL PUNCTURES

Although they are very infrequently performed by phlebotomists, arterial punctures should be mentioned. Generally, a nurse or respiratory therapist collects an arterial blood specimen to assay blood gases such as O_2, CO_2, and pH present in the blood. This can be done using arterial blood only because venous blood is deoxygenated. The blood gas determination reveals, among other things, how well the lungs are functioning in terms of gas exchange and acid-base balance. It should be clearly explained to the patient that this procedure is not only procedurally different but more uncomfortable than venipuncture and more difficult to accomplish.

The obvious difference between the arterial puncture and the venipuncture is the blood vessel from which the specimen is collected. One artery that may be used is the brachial artery, which is located on the inside of the upper arm (Fig. 7.4). It can be found by feeling for a pulse using the middle finger and forefinger; the thumb is not used because its pulse may be confused with that of the artery. A more common site is the radial artery found in the wrist area, assuming a positive **Allen test**. Local protocol should be consulted to determine which site to use.

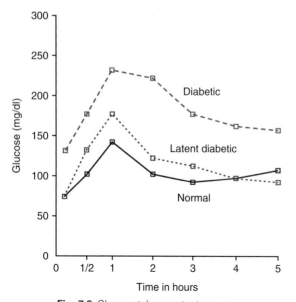

Fig. 7.3 Glucose tolerance test curves.

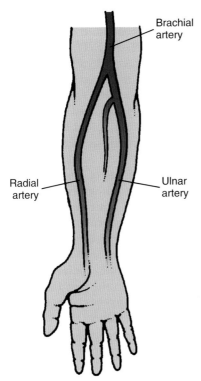

Brachial
artery

Radial
artery

Ulnar
artery

Fig. 7.4 The radial artery in the wrist area is the most common site for arterial puncture. The brachial artery may also be used.

The puncture site should be cleansed with a povidone-iodine (Betadine) solution. Do not use alcohol swabs because the alcohol may interfere with testing results. No tourniquet is needed because of the pressure that already exists within the arteries. A syringe may be used because generally only a small amount of blood (1 mL) is needed. The angle of entry is generally 30 to 45 degrees. The syringe safety cap should be engaged, placed in ice slurry, and transported to the laboratory as soon as possible after collection. The ice helps preserve the integrity of the constituents being assayed in the specimen. Ideally, the test should be run within 10 minutes after collection, which means that someone may have to transport the specimen to the laboratory.

The phlebotomist should maintain pressure on the site for at least 15 minutes after collection. It takes much longer for bleeding to stop in an artery than in a vein because of the arterial pressure. The patient should never be allowed to maintain pressure, and the patient's nurse should be made aware that an arterial puncture

was done so that they can periodically check the puncture site.

COLD AGGLUTININ TESTS

A cold agglutinin is an antibody that is made in response to a form of pneumonia called primary atypical pneumonia, which is caused by the bacteria *Mycoplasma pneumoniae*. Therefore the presence of a cold agglutinin is diagnostic. Occasionally the antibody can cause a form of autoimmune hemolytic anemia.

A critical part in the collection of a specimen that will be screened for cold agglutinins is maintaining the specimen at 37°C (normal body temperature) after collection. The specimen is collected in an empty evacuated tube (plain red stopper) after proper site preparation and delivered promptly to the laboratory, where it is placed in a 37°C incubator, at which temperature the blood must clot. If prompt delivery is not possible, the specimen may be placed in a temporary holding device such as a disposable warming device or cup of water that is 37°C. The water must not be warmer than 37°C because this may alter the test result. Conversely, should the specimen be allowed to cool, the cold agglutinin may appear stronger than it really is at 37°C, and the results may be invalid.

BLOOD CULTURES

In healthy individuals, blood is a sterile substance. When bacteria enter and remain in the bloodstream, it is referred to as *septicemia*. **Septicemia** is a serious condition and must be detected and treated as soon as possible; if not treated, the patient may die. Because blood circulates throughout the body, bacteria in the blood can be transported to other areas of the body, thereby spreading infection. The proper antibiotics must be administered intravenously to stop the infection as soon as possible.

To administer the proper antibiotics, the offending bacteria, as well as the antibiotic to which the bacteria are most susceptible, must be identified. To do this, a blood culture must be performed. The phlebotomist's role is to collect a specimen using special sterilization techniques.

One symptom of septicemia is a fever of unknown origin. Often such a fever will rise and fall on a regular basis. Therefore timing of the blood culture collection is crucial. It is often desirable to collect blood cultures before and after a fever spike. This maximizes the chances of collecting a specimen while the bacteria are present in the bloodstream.

After a vein is located, the site is specially prepared for venipuncture. All existing bacteria on the skin must be removed. Check with your local protocol because there are two acceptable preparation procedures. One uses a one-step chlorhexidine gluconate—isopropyl alcohol antiseptic. Others may still use a two-step method with isopropyl alcohol cleansing, followed by

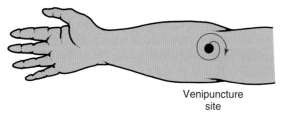

Venipuncture
site

Fig. 7.5 Proper method for swabbing a venipuncture site, moving in an outward spiral.

swabbing with an iodine or povidone solution applied in outward-moving concentric circles from the puncture site (Fig. 7.5). Please recall that this was also briefly reviewed in Chapter 5. ChloraPrep is a commercially available application to prepare the venipuncture site for a blood culture collection. This is allowed to air dry. The tourniquet is applied, and the venipuncture is performed. The site can be touched only with sterile gauze or with a finger that has been cleaned in the same way used for the site.

Although some aspects of blood culture collection vary from institution to institution, all techniques involve collecting blood either directly or indirectly into an **aerobic** and **anaerobic** culture system. Either a syringe or a specially designed evacuated tube is used. When a syringe is used, a safety transfer device is used to inoculate blood culture bottles to avoid possible contamination, and then the blood culture bottles are inoculated (anaerobic followed by aerobic) with the appropriate amount of blood.

The blood may also be collected into an evacuated tube made especially for blood cultures (Fig. 7.6, A).

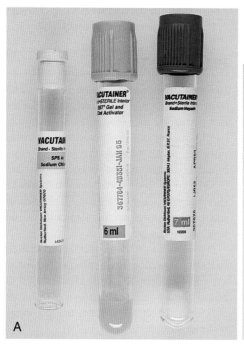

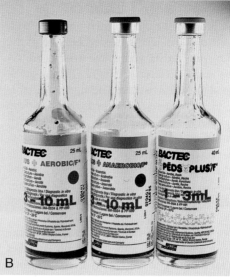

Fig. 7.6 Examples of culture systems used in collection of blood cultures. *A,* Specially designed Vacutainer tube for collecting a blood culture (direct method). *B,* Blood culture bottles (indirect method). (Courtesy Becton, Dickinson and Company, Franklin Lakes, New Jersey.)

This is usually a yellow-stoppered tube with sodium polyanethol sulfonate, which prevents coagulation and inhibits complement and **phagocytosis**. Then, in the laboratory, a syringe is used to remove blood from the evacuated tube and inoculate the blood culture bottles (see Fig. 7.6, *B*). However, no matter what collection method is used, care must be taken to maintain sterility by swabbing the septum of the culture bottles with iodine followed by alcohol.

After the blood is collected, any cleansing solution on the patient's arm should be removed using alcohol swabs. The culture bottles must be thoroughly mixed and labeled with pertinent information, including the time and site of collection. This is important because blood cultures are collected rather frequently and the policy at some hospitals is to alternate arms at each blood culture collection.

BLOOD DONATION COLLECTIONS

Phlebotomists may be employed in a blood donation center, where they collect blood that will ultimately be used for transfusion. These centers may be American Red Cross centers, community blood centers, or hospital blood banks and collection centers.

Phlebotomists who collect blood from volunteer donors must be very competent in the skill of venipuncture and must possess good interpersonal skills. Because relatively few individuals (less than 5% of the population) provide donor blood for the entire country, it is critical that every phase of the donation process be performed smoothly and professionally. The health care system cannot afford the loss of these volunteer donors, and an unpleasant experience may discourage them from volunteering again.

This type of blood collection varies from routine venipuncture in several ways; two very important ones are the amount of blood that is collected (usually 450 mL) and the nature of the "patient." Individuals who donate blood must undergo a thorough medical history and screening. The history should include frequency of donation, present and past medications, exposure to transfusion-transmitted disease such as hepatitis B and human immunodeficiency virus (HIV), recent vaccinations, foreign travel, and cancer history. The medical screening includes blood pressure, temperature, hemoglobin or hematocrit levels, weight,

pulse, and assessment of skin lesions and general appearance. Donors also complete a donor self-exclusion form, which allows them to confidentially ensure that their blood will not be used for transfusion if they have any misgivings. The American Association of Blood Banks' *Technical Manual* contains a more thorough discussion of donor criteria. Once the donor passes the medical history and screening, the actual phlebotomy can be performed. The antecubital area of the arm is the preferred site and must be thoroughly cleaned and disinfected. (See the procedure discussed earlier for blood culture preparation.) The step-by-step procedure for performing blood donor phlebotomy is listed in Procedure 7.1.

THERAPEUTIC BLOOD COLLECTIONS

As mentioned in Chapter 1, in ancient times, therapeutic phlebotomy was the only treatment used for many different conditions. Today the treatment is used judiciously. Blood is collected as an aid to treatment of some diseases, such as hemochromatosis, **polycythemia vera,** and **myasthenia gravis.** It is rarely the definitive treatment but instead serves as symptomatic treatment until the underlying cause can be identified and treated.

Therapeutic phlebotomies are very similar to donor blood collection, but the underlying purpose is different. Whereas donated blood is destined to be used for transfusion, blood collected for a therapeutic reason is generally discarded or occasionally is used for research purposes. Therefore no additional pilot tubes of blood need be collected for additional testing nor is the "donor" screening as rigorous. In addition, the amount of blood collected may be different; an amount less than 450 mL may be appropriate depending on the patient's age and condition. However, site preparation is the same, and the same precautions must be observed when performing therapeutic phlebotomies.

TESTS FOR FIBRIN DEGRADATION PRODUCTS

Fibrin degradation products (FDPs) are the result of the splitting or disintegration of fibrin or fibrinogen by plasmin, a coagulation enzyme. Increased levels of

PROCEDURE 7.1   Blood Donor Phlebotomy

Materials
- Gloves
- Site preparation material
- Blood bag with clamp
- Needle
- Tourniquet or sphygmomanometer (blood pressure cuff)
- Sterile gauze
- Tape
- Pilot tubes

1. Once the donor is comfortably situated—generally on a bed or special donor chair—locate the vein.
2. Prepare the site.
3. Prepare the blood collection bag and scale. Be sure there is a clamp between the bag and the needle.
4. Apply the tourniquet or blood pressure cuff (inflated to 40 to 60 mm Hg), and give the donor something to squeeze. These techniques will help distend the vein.
5. Perform the venipuncture and place the needle approximately half an inch into the vein.
6. Release the clamp; if there is a steady flow of blood into the bag, tape the needle to the arm. Cover the area with sterile gauze.
7. Release the tourniquet or blood pressure cuff, but instruct the donor to slowly clench their fist. Monitor the donor for any adverse reactions. (These are infrequent; see Chapter 9.)

8. When the appropriate volume of blood (405 to 450 mL) is collected, instruct the donor to stop clenching the fist, and clamp or tie a knot in the tubing.
9. Collect pilot tubes—samples of donor blood that will be tested before the unit is released for transfusion—before removing the needle from the donor's arm.
10. Strip the tubing and thoroughly mix the blood, then allow the tubing to refill. At this time the tubing may be segmented.
11. Place the units in storage as specified by the collection room nurse or technologist.
12. Do not allow the patient to arise or leave the area until bleeding has stopped and at least 10 minutes have elapsed. Because the donor has lost a significant amount of blood, be sure to instruct them to increase fluid intake over the next 24 hours, avoid alcohol until after a meal, avoid smoking for at least 30 minutes, refrain from strenuous exercise for a few hours, apply pressure if bleeding resumes, and sit down if dizziness occurs. Patients may have to return to the blood bank or see their own doctor if symptoms continue.
13. Finally, *always be polite and professional, and thank the donor for donating.* The donor should leave with a positive feeling so that they will be inclined to donate blood again.

FDPs are generally associated with such conditions as myocardial infarctions, pulmonary emboli, certain complications of pregnancy, and disseminated intravascular coagulation.

A popular test for detecting FDPs is the Thrombo-Wellcotest (Burroughs Wellcome, Triangle Park, NC). For the phlebotomist, this test involves performing a routine venipuncture using a tube provided with the test kit. The tube holds 2 mL of blood and contains a special enzyme inhibitor plus thrombin. It is important to avoid traumatic venipunctures that might result in hemolysis, and the sample must be gently but thoroughly mixed after collection. Additionally, it must be allowed to stand for 15 minutes before any centrifugation. D-dimer testing may be an alternative to FDPs. (D-dimer tests measure a fraction of the FDP.) Be sure to check with your institution to see which test is the preferred protocol.

Once the sample is collected, assays are performed in the laboratory to semiquantitate the FDPs. This information is important to the clinician in making the proper diagnosis. Occasionally, urine specimens may be tested for FDPs.

PERIPHERAL BLOOD SMEARS

Peripheral blood smears are important to the clinician for a number of reasons. Examination of the blood smear may reveal abnormal red cell morphological findings characteristic of certain disease states such as sickle cell anemia (Fig. 7.7). The variety and proportion of white blood cells may also be ascertained;

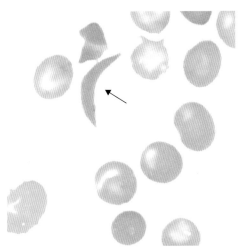

Fig. 7.7 Blood smear from a patient with sickle cell anemia. (From Carr JH, Rodak BF. *Clinical Hematology Atlas,* 3rd ed. St. Louis, Saunders, 2009.)

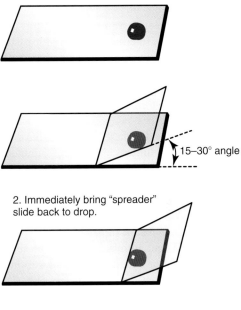

1. Place slide on flat surface; apply drop of blood.

15–30° angle

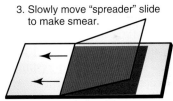

2. Immediately bring "spreader" slide back to drop.

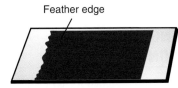

3. Slowly move "spreader" slide to make smear.

Feather edge

Fig. 7.8 "Wedge" method, the suggested method for making blood smears.

information of this nature may also help in the diagnosis of disease. For example, infectious mononucleosis is characterized by an increased number of atypical lymphocytes.

Although the process is becoming increasingly semiautomated, phlebotomists may still be called on to make a blood smear. This may be done either at the patient's bedside using standard microscope slides and capillary blood or in the laboratory using well-mixed, recently collected (within 1 hour) anticoagulated (with ethylenediaminetetra-acetate) blood.

The "wedge" method is probably the most common manual method (Fig. 7.8). The following important points should be remembered:

- Keep the smear slide on a flat surface.
- Make the smear immediately after placing the blood on the slide.
- Make the smear in a smooth fashion to avoid ridges and bubbles.
- Allow the smear to air dry; never blow on it.

A straight-edge smear is preferable to a bullet-shaped smear because of better distribution of leukocytes.

It takes a great deal of practice to become proficient at making smears, and therefore it may be desirable to assign slide-making to certain members of the phlebotomy team. Improperly made blood smears can contain an uneven number of blood cells and yield inaccurate results.

PERIPHERAL VENOUS ACCESS

Following is a brief discussion on peripheral venous access and related devices. Generally, a nurse or someone with specialized training withdraws blood through a venous access device, but it is beneficial for beginning phlebotomists to be familiar with the apparatus and precautions associated with them when performing routine venipuncture.

Central venous catheters are surgically inserted with the client in the operating room. First, a tunnel is made through subcutaneous tissue, usually between the clavicle and the nipple. Next, the catheter tip is inserted through the cephalic, internal, or external jugular vein, or a similar large vein, and threaded into the right atrium or the superior vena cava. The catheter tip cannot rest in the right atrium as that would create a risk of cardiac arrhythmias. Accurate placement must be verified by chest x-ray examination before the catheter can be used. These catheters have single, double, or triple lumens, allowing simultaneous administration of several infusions. The subcutaneous tunnel allows the catheter to remain in place longer because it creates space between the end of the catheter and the actual vein. The risk of infection is lower.

A *percutaneously placed catheter* is inserted directly through the skin and into a large vein of the neck, usually the internal or external jugular or subclavian.

Peripherally inserted central catheters (PICC lines) are inserted through large veins of the antecubital fossa and threaded into the tip of the right atrium. These lines can be in place for up to 6 months.

A *midline catheter* (MLC) may be placed between the antecubital fossa and the head of the clavicle. MLCs are shorter than PICC lines, with the tip resting in the larger vessels of the upper arm. The arm in which a PICC or MLC is in place should be avoided for taking blood pressures or drawing blood.

BLOOD DRAWING AND FLUID ADMINISTRATION

Vascular access devices are designed for repeated access to the venous or arterial systems. These catheters may be used to obtain blood samples. It is the nurse's responsibility to draw the blood from a central venous catheter. If a central venous line has more than one lumen, blood specimens should be obtained from the proximal lumen.

Some catheters have three ports: The proximal lumen is the port closest to the site of insertion, the medical lumen is the port in the middle, and the distal lumen is the port farthest away from the insertion site.

You should determine how many tubes of blood are required; in some situations, several tests can be run from one blood tube sample. For example, potassium, calcium, and magnesium test results can all be obtained from one full tube of blood versus three separate tubes. Repeatedly withdrawing more blood than necessary can place the client at risk for anemia.

If an intravenous (IV) solution is to be infused, follow the blood-drawing procedure by connecting the ordered fluids. It is best to schedule blood sampling with fluid administration to limit the number of entries into the vascular system.

Routine venipuncture should be avoided, if possible, from the arm that has an IV port in place. If there is no alternative, blood may be drawn from below the IV port, but *never above it.* Drawing blood above an IV port may result in the specimen being diluted with IV fluid, and there are safety issues in play for the patient. A nurse must stop the IV infusion before beginning the phlebotomy.

SAFETY SUMMARY

- Thoroughly cleanse phlebotomy or skin puncture site.
- Avoid phlebotomy on patient's side with mastectomy.
- Blood donors must meet all criteria.
- Blood culture collection requires special site preparation.
- For timed tests, the timing must be closely monitored and recorded.
- All glucose must be consumed for glucose tolerance tests.

SUMMARY

This chapter reviewed some of the special collection procedures with the desire to give the entry-level phlebotomist some knowledge and understanding of these procedures. As with any textbook that reviews a given topic, there is always more information and more procedures than presented. As you become more experienced as a phlebotomist, you will encounter these less common procedures. Furthermore, you will undergo special training wherever you work. Always be sure to review the protocol of your institution for proper procedures and techniques.

CASE 7.1   **Critical Thinking**

You are collecting blood from a patient undergoing a glucose tolerance test (GTT). After the 2-hour collection, you notice that the container with the glucose solution is in the trash can and is still about half full. There have been no other GTTs performed on this day. What should you do if anything?

CASE 7.2   **Critical Thinking**

The supervisor of the phlebotomy unit has received a call from the microbiology laboratory. They are reporting that a recent specimen is demonstrating the presence of a very common skin bacteria. How could this happen, and what should be done in the future?

REVIEW QUESTIONS

1. Arterial puncture is the method of choice for _____.
2. The volume of blood usually collected during blood donation is _____.
3. Bacteria in the blood are referred to as _____.
4. The _____ is used to test patients for diabetes mellitus and hypoglycemia.
5. What is the importance of fibrin degradation products (FDPs)?
6. Sodium polyanethol sulfonate is an additive in _____-stoppered tubes.
7. Why are special site preparation steps taken when blood is being collected for culturing?
8. Name the types of peripheral venous access devices and where they are located.
9. Antibiotics are administered _____ to fight septicemia.
10. With the advent of COVID, this type of personal protective equipment (PPE) may be become mandatory at all times in health care settings.

BIBLIOGRAPHY

Burtis C, Bruns D, eds. *Tietz Fundamentals of Clinical Chemistry and Molecular Diagnostics.* 7th ed. St. Louis: Saunders; 2014.

Clemente CD, ed. *Gray's Anatomy of the Human Body.* 30th ed. Philadelphia: Lea & Febiger; 1986.

Cohn C, et al. *Technical Manual.* 20th ed. Arlington, VA: American Association of Blood Banks; 2020.

Dougherty L. *Central Venous Access Devices: Care and Management (Essential Clinical Skills for Nurses).* Malden, MA: Blackwell Publishing; 2006.

Rodak BF, Fritsma GA, Keohane E, eds. *Hematology: Clinical Principles and Applications.* 4th ed. St. Louis: Saunders; 2012.

Slockbower JM, Blumenfeld TA. *Collection and Handling of Laboratory Specimens.* Philadelphia: JB Lippincott; 1983.

8

Neonatal and Geriatric Procedures and Considerations

John C. Flynn, Jr.

*"Resolve to be tender with the young, compassionate with the aged,
sympathetic with the striving, and tolerant with the weak and the wrong.
Sometime in your life you will have been all of these."*

—*Dr. Robert H. Goddard (1882—1945)*

OBJECTIVES

At the conclusion of this chapter, the student should be able to:

- Name common tests performed on newborn infants.
- Describe the procedure for collecting blood from newborns.
- Define *iatrogenic anemia.*
- Describe the scope of the geriatric population in relation to the total U.S. population.

- Discuss the major medical considerations associated with aging when performing phlebotomy.
- Describe the phlebotomy considerations relevant to the major medical conditions associated with aging.
- Explain why arthritis may make phlebotomy more difficult.

OUTLINE

KEY TERMS

arthritis
cataract
dementia
elasticity
galactose

hemolytic disease of the newborn
iatrogenic anemia
osteomyelitis
phenylalanine

INTRODUCTION

Generally speaking, most of the venipunctures a phlebotomist will be asked to perform in a general hospital setting will be on individuals that can easily understand instructions and comprehend what will happen during the blood collection procedure. However, every phlebotomist at some point in their career will be required to collect blood from an infant or an older adult patient. There are certain procedures and considerations that a phlebotomist must be aware of when working with these populations. This chapter discusses some of these issues.

NEONATAL BLOOD COLLECTION

With the increasing sophistication of medical testing and care, premature infants have a better chance of survival today than they did as recently as the late 1900s. Infants as small as 2 pounds or less and more than 10 weeks premature are surviving. To monitor the progress of care and treatment, blood must be collected for analysis. Common neonatal tests include screening for increased bilirubin, sickle cell disease, cystic fibrosis, human immunodeficiency virus (HIV), phenylketonuria (PKU), galactosemia, and hypothyroidism; screenings for the latter three conditions are required by law in the United States on all newborns. Bilirubin is a screen for **hemolytic disease of the newborn**, and PKU screens the infant for the ability to metabolize **phenylalanine**. Inability to metabolize phenylalanine can result in brain damage and mental retardation. Galactosemia is an inherited condition in which the infant is unable to use (metabolize) the simple sugar **galactose**, which is found in milk. Should newborns ingest galactose, they may become ill and die if not treated. The infant must have all galactose removed from their diet and can safely be fed soy milk. Screening for hypothyroidism detects if the thyroid gland is underperforming, which can result in a general slowing of many functions such as heart rate and can produce low temperature and low blood pressure. It can also lead to fatigue, weakness, and joint pain, so it is important to detect this condition as early as possible.

Collecting blood from infants involves using a variation of the microcollection techniques previously discussed in Chapter 6. The site of collection is generally the infant's foot, specifically the heel. Care must be exercised when performing the skin puncture to avoid damaging the heel bone, which can cause **osteomyelitis** in the newborn. Fig. 8.1A illustrates the safe areas in which to perform the puncture. Commercial automatic, spring-loaded retractable puncture devices specifically for infants are available and recommended for use. The recommended depth of a heel puncture is 2 mm or less.

When preparing to perform the blood collection, take only the equipment necessary into the bassinet area to avoid needlessly exposing a generally immune-weakened infant to additional bacteria. You will usually be required to wear at least a gown and face mask in addition to gloves. Try not to disturb the infant any more than necessary, and if you must change the infant's position, do so only with permission of the nurse because of the many tubes and lines that are often attached to premature infants. Prepare the puncture site as described in Chapter 6, and hold the heel firmly as shown in Fig. 8.1B. Perform the skin puncture (see Fig. 8.1C) and wipe away the first drop of blood to avoid dilution of the blood with tissue fluid. Collect blood into the appropriate container, being careful not to apply too much pressure to the heel; this could adversely affect the results of testing and may hurt the infant. When you are finished, apply pressure until bleeding has stopped. Do not apply a bandage, and do not leave anything in the bassinet. (Bandage application could damage the skin of the infant and cause needless pain when removed for a later collection.) Label the collected specimens appropriately and deliver them to the laboratory. The collection for the PKU and hypothyroidism involves blotting of the infant's blood on specially prepared testing paper (see Fig. 8.1D). The surface of the heel cannot touch the testing paper. As with all procedures, carefully read instructions and follow local protocol.

Because of the small total blood volume of newborns (Fig. 8.2), a log should be kept of the total blood removed from infants. Often anemia becomes a problem because of the amount of blood collected from a given newborn. This is called **iatrogenic anemia**. Therefore accurate records must be maintained. Each hospital will have established guidelines for the amount of blood that can be collected from neonates. The infant's body weight will determine the allowed amount to be collected.

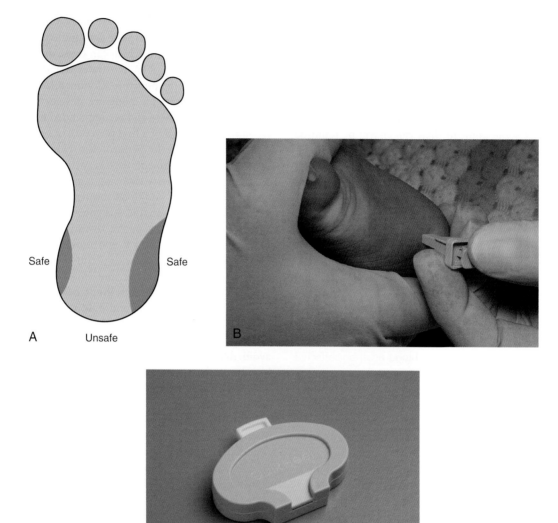

Fig. 8.1 *A,* Safe areas on an infant's foot for microcapillary collection. *B,* A properly held heel for skin puncture. *C,* An infant blood incision device. *D,* A neonatal phenylketonuria screening card. (B from Chester GA: *Modern Medical Assisting.* Philadelphia, Saunders, 1998; C, Courtesy Rick Davis.)

GERIATRIC COLLECTION CONSIDERATIONS

The Geriatric or Older Adult Population

The geriatric segment of the population is the fastest growing of all segments. One dilemma with categorizing the older adult population is determining the age at which it begins. Traditionally, 65 has been the age considered "elderly" but, as is discussed later, age-related changes happen much sooner and need to be considered in phlebotomy. According to the U.S. Census Bureau, the number of people aged 65 and older composed about 16% of the population in 2010 but will rise to nearly 1 in 5 (21%) by 2030. This equates to

Client keep top copy

2376607

Neo ● Gen
SCREENING

(412) 220-2300

2376607

S&S® 903™ LOT # W-011 (Rev. 12/02)

BABY'S LAST NAME		FIRST		HOSPITAL OF BIRTH	BIRTHDATE	BIRTHTIME	BABY'S MED. REC. NO.	DRAWN BY
						SEX M		BABY'S RACE
DRAW DATE	TIME AM PM	CHECK HERE IF BABY IS LESS THAN 24 HRS. OLD				F	AM PM	☐ WHITE ☐ ASIAN ☐ BLACK ☐ AMER. IND. ☐ OTHER
MOTHER'S LAST NAME		FIRST		GESTATION	BIRTHWEIGHT	BIRTH		HISPANIC? ☐ YES ☐ NO
				(WEEKS)	(GRAMS)	☐ SINGLE ☐ A ☐ B ☐ C	☐ OTHER	
ADDRESS				TRANSFUSED?		SPECIMEN	IF REPEAT	
				☐ SM. VOL.		☐ INITIAL	☐ REQUESTED	
CITY, STATE, ZIP				☐ EXCHANGE DATE ___		☐ REPEAT	☐ ROUTINE	(PREVIOUS CARD #)
PHONE (MOTHER)				BABY'S PHYSICIAN			SUBMITTER	
MOTHER'S SOCIAL SECURITY NUMBER				PHONE (PHYSICIAN)				ADDRESS IF OTHER THAN BIRTH FACILITY

A D D R E S S   A R E A   O G A   A P H

Fig. 8.1 cont'd

Instructions

Screening Instructions
The sample should be drawn by a health professional experienced in this type of collection.
Specimens should be obtained between 24 and 48 hours of age, as close to 48 hours as possible.

Sample Collection
• Sterilize the heel area with alcohol, air dry, and puncture with a sterile disposable lancet.
• Apply blood to the front side of the filter paper only.
• Completely fill each of the four circles on the filter paper with a single, free-flowing drop of blood.
• Make sure the blood soaks through to the back of the filter paper.
• Do not layer successive drops.
• The use of capillary tubes is not recommended. Do not use devices that contain EDTA.

Drying the Sample
• Air dry on a clean, flat surface for 3 to 4 hours away from heat and light.
• Do not stack, or allow the blood spots on the filter paper to touch other surfaces while drying.
• Place in the glassine (wax paper) envelope when dry.

Mailing to the Screening Laboratory
Place the glassine envelope containing the filter paper in the postage-paid envelope, and mail to the laboratory as soon as possible to ensure accurate and timely processing. Refrigerate sample if you are unable to mail it immediately. If urgent screening results are needed, we recommend shipping the sample by overnight courier.

DO NOT TOUCH BLOOD COLLECTION AREA. IT MAY CONTAMINATE RESULTS.

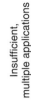

COLLECT SAMPLE FROM SHADED AREA

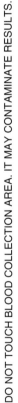

RIGHT   ACCEPTABLE
Circle filled and evenly saturated

WRONG   UNACCEPTABLE
Layering

Insufficient, multiple applications

Serum rings present

Fig. 8.1 cont'd

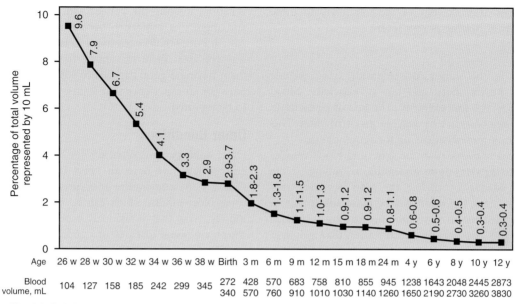

Fig. 8.2 Relationship of 10 mL book sample to total volume and age of patient. (Blood volumes for calculations: Prematures, 115 mL/kg; Newborns, 80-110 mL/kg; Infants/children, 75-100 mL/kg.)

nearly 85 million people. Additionally, the group 85 years and older is the fastest growing segment as a percentage of the population.

We all age, and we will all experience the effects of aging. The age at which we first experience those effects and the intensity of the effects may vary, but rest assured that we will all experience them. The following section briefly describes some of the changes associated with aging.

PHLEBOTOMY CONSIDERATIONS FOR SELECTED MEDICAL CONDITIONS

Vision

Some people as early as their 30s have reported minor vision problems, such as not being able to read without holding the material further away or with the aid of reading glasses. They may also need more light than in the past and may notice that their eyes take longer to adjust to sudden changes in light. This is all because the muscles around the eye cannot adjust the lens adequately or as quickly. Some people have clouding of the eyes (actually the lens) or **cataract** formation, thus making it even more difficult to see. Thus, the blood collection area of any hospital or clinic must be well lit. It is also advisable to have any written instructions available in large-print format to assist with vision problems.

Hearing

With age often comes a loss of hearing, particularly of high-pitched sounds. This is because of the loss of auditory hair cells or nerve damage. Patients may also report having trouble distinguishing or filtering out "background noise" even when able to hear the person speaking to them.

If you suspect your patient is having difficulty hearing, do not shout. This may make the situation worse. Instead, be sure you are speaking directly to your patient, preferably in front of them. Ask if the patient understands what you are saying (although the patient may agree just to agree) and look for nonverbal signs that the patient understands you, such as starting to roll up their sleeve if this is something you would expect after giving instructions. Also, having printed instructions available may be the solution with those whose loss of hearing is very severe.

Skin

Changes in the skin associated with aging include wrinkles, brown spots, and loss of **elasticity**. Blood vessels may also lose elasticity. The loss of elasticity in the skin demonstrates by sagging and wrinkling. This may make it more challenging for venipuncture.

The loss of elasticity in the skin (and blood vessels) may make the veins more susceptible to "rolling" so the need to adequately anchor the vein becomes very important. Also, the veins may be more susceptible to excessive bleeding so postvenipuncture care is critical. Older adults may bruise much easier than younger patients. It is important to use smaller-gauge needles and less traumatic equipment such as syringes and butterflies to collect blood specimens from older adult patients. If there is a history of excessive bruising, evacuated tubes should not be used. This will help preserve the veins for more venipunctures in the future.

Mental and Emotional

Dementia, whether caused by Alzheimer disease or not, is a condition that the phlebotomist must be able to recognize. Although less severe than dementia, other conditions in older adults like increased forgetfulness, difficulty focusing attention, and taking longer to recall knowledge may be problematic. Also, some patients may not accept the fact that they are aging and now must make adjustments in their lifestyle and what they can expect of themselves. This could manifest itself by depression or aggression. In any event, a phlebotomist must be acutely aware of the mental or emotional state of the patient.

Many older adult patients do not have much contact with visitors, so many will want to visit with you while you are collecting blood. Be prepared to carry on a conversation while you work. Being friendly will make the phlebotomy experience more pleasant for both of you. As noted previously, some older adult patients suffer from dementia, so they may not be as cooperative as you would like. They may try to pull away, remove the needle, or even push you away. You may have to ask a nurse or other health care professional to help with the collection by trying to soothe or gently restrain the individual. Although not necessarily making the venipuncture any more complicated when taken in isolation, treating the patient with the utmost respect and dignity is critical. (This should be true for any patient but perhaps even more so for older adults.) The way you treat them may make the difference between them having a good experience with you as a phlebotomist or an experience that is unsettling and may need to be repeated.

Other Conditions

Older adult patients often do not eat or hydrate properly, which may have an effect on blood collection. Changes in temperature may present a challenge to some older adults, which can be because of a loss of muscle mass that individuals experience as they age. There are some diseases or conditions that are more prevalent in older adults. Of special note is **arthritis**. Patients suffering from this often have joint stiffness and it may be uncomfortable for them to straighten their arms or grasp with their hands. Phlebotomists must be aware if a patient is suffering from arthritis and thus not ask the patient to move in any way that may aggravate their condition. See Table 8.1 for a summary of medical conditions associated with older adults. One last item of note is that many older adults also use assistive devices such as wheelchairs and walkers. A phlebotomist may need to assist an older adult patient

TABLE 8.1	Common Geriatric Conditions	
Condition	**Manifestation**	**Consideration**
Vision	Unable to read fine print, need more light	Well-lit areas, large print available
Hearing	May not completely understand instructions	Speak clearly and directly, do not raise voice
Skin	Loose or sagging	Must anchor vein securely
Mental/ Emotional	Depressed, uncooperative	Use utmost respect and treat with dignity
Arthritis	Joint stiffness	Avoid asking patient to use stiff joints, avoid painful areas

into the phlebotomy chair or collect the blood while the patient stays seated in their wheelchair.

SAFETY SUMMARY

- Perform phlebotomy or skin puncture in well-lit areas.
- Never leave any equipment in a bassinet.
- Perform skin puncture on infants only in the safe area of the foot.
- Ensure any instructions or communications are understood by the patient.
- Anchor veins securely and safely.
- Be aware of any joint stiffness or pain.

SUMMARY

As discussed previously, there are many similarities between "routine" venipuncture and the same procedure performed on infants and older adults. In fact, there are more similarities than dissimilarities. However, it is also imperative that the phlebotomist take into consideration the special circumstances faced when collecting blood from these special populations. As

always, the ultimate goal is successful collection of blood while maintaining the safety and comfort of the patient.

CASE 8.1   Critical Thinking

It is the first time you are asked to go to the neonatal unit to collect blood on a premature infant. Your orders say to collect blood for a hemoglobin and hematocrit assay and a bilirubin assay. When you are done, you notice a notebook labeled "log of blood collected" where the amount of blood you just collected is recorded. What purpose does this log serve?

CASE 8.2   Critical Thinking

While preparing to collect blood from a 78-year-old man, you gather your tubes, needle, and other equipment while you are asking him his name and requesting that he roll up his sleeve. When you have collected your equipment, you realize that he did not state his name nor begin to roll up his sleeve. What should you do now?

■ REVIEW QUESTIONS

1. These tests are required by law of all newborns: _____

2. Damage to the heel bone of an infant is called _____.

3. In addition to gloves, what other piece of personal protective equipment will you be required to wear when collecting blood from a newborn? _____

4. Why is the first drop of blood not collected? _____

5. Why is a bandage not used on infants? _____

6. What percent of the population will be considered geriatric in 2030? _____

7. Name the changes associated with aging that may make phlebotomy more challenging? _____

8. Why does the loss of skin elasticity make a venipuncture more challenging? _____

9. What equipment should you use when you draw blood from an older adult patient? _____

10. What determines the amount of blood that can be collected from an infant? _____

Considerations and Complications of Phlebotomy

John C. Flynn, Jr.

"If history repeats itself, and the unexpected always happens, how incapable must Man be of learning from experience."

—*George Bernard Shaw (1856–1950)*

OBJECTIVES

At the conclusion of this chapter, the student should be able to:

- List situations when phlebotomists may encounter an uncooperative or absent patient and know how to address each situation.
- List and address common considerations of phlebotomy.
- List and address common complications of venipuncture.
- Describe less common complications of venipuncture.
- Describe various technical problems associated with phlebotomy practice.
- Discuss how to avoid unacceptable specimens.

OUTLINE

KEY TERMS

coagulation factors
convulsions
edema
expired
hematoma
hemolysis

hemorrhage
hypovolemia
mastectomy
short draw
syncope

INTRODUCTION

If phlebotomy is done correctly and consistently, unexpected outcomes or complications can be avoided. However, even when all procedures and techniques are performed correctly, complications can still occur. This chapter discusses common considerations and various complications that can be encountered when performing or attempting to perform phlebotomy. These include uncooperative or absent patients, medical and physiological complications, and technical problems.

THE UNCOOPERATIVE OR ABSENT PATIENT

Every phlebotomist has encountered an uncooperative patient. The patient may be uncooperative for a variety of reasons, such as age (young or old), which may preclude them from understanding the procedure; mental dysfunction; or an objection to having the phlebotomy done for some other reason.

When a patient is too old or young to understand what is going on and will probably resist or struggle, do not attempt to perform the venipuncture alone. Get help from the patient's nurse; a fellow phlebotomist; or a parent, relative, or guardian. If phlebotomy is a regular routine for the patient, the parent, relative, or guardian may be accustomed to being asked for assistance. Take precautions to ensure the safety of the individual but do not compromise your own safety. For example, a common and safe way to hold a child is

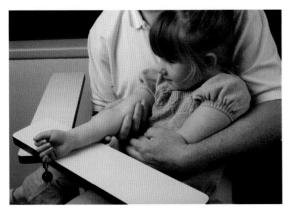

Fig. 9.1 A suggested way to restrain a child for phlebotomy. (Courtesy Rick Davis.)

shown in Fig. 9.1. However, you as the phlebotomist must instruct the patient's parent or guardian in the proper techniques for restraining the patient. Do not assume they know how to do it.

Occasionally phlebotomists are required to collect blood from a patient who is mentally disturbed, mentally impaired, or suffering from substance abuse. In such a case, the patient may not understand the procedure and may react violently. You must do what you can to reassure the patient and secure cooperation. However, if there is any doubt about how the patient will react, do not attempt to collect the specimen until you have secured some assistance, even if the patient is in restraints. Also, it may take more than one person to assist in restraining the patient while blood is being collected.

Sometimes a patient may be of sound mind and yet still refuse to have the procedure performed. At these times, you must use your skills of persuasion to convince the patient to allow you to collect the blood sample. Point out that the physician needs the blood test results to properly manage the patient's illness and prescribe the proper medication. The patient's nurse may try to convince the patient to cooperate as well. Never attempt to force, either physically or with threats, a patient in this situation. Remember, a patient has the legally protected right to refuse a blood draw (see Chapter 14). Ultimately, if the patient refuses to allow the blood collection, this must be noted on the requisition form, which is returned to the laboratory and reported to the patient's physician; the patient's nurse must also be informed.

Another situation that often confronts a phlebotomist is that of an absent patient—that is, the patient is not where they are supposed to be. The patient may have been moved to another room or transported to surgery or the radiology department or simply sitting in a patient lounge area. They may have been discharged or perhaps may have **expired**. Generally, the phlebotomist can find out where the patient is by asking the nurse in charge. If the patient has simply been moved to another room, collect the blood specimen, noting the room change on the requisition form and on the tube of blood. If the patient is inaccessible (e.g., in the radiology department or the operating room), inform the patient's nurse and note on the requisition form why the blood was not collected.

A sleeping or unconscious patient is yet another situation that calls for the phlebotomist to adapt to an unusual situation. If gentle rousing does not waken a patient, check with the care nurse on duty who may explain that the patient is in a coma, is under sedation, or is a heavy sleeper, for example, and give some guidance to the phlebotomist. Do not attempt the phlebotomy until you know exactly what the circumstances are.

MEDICAL AND PHYSIOLOGICAL CONSIDERATIONS

Common Considerations

Syncope

Syncope, more commonly referred to as *fainting*, results from insufficient blood flow to the brain. This can be caused by fatigue, a sudden decrease in blood volume, cardiac arrhythmia, hypoglycemia, or hyperventilation. However, in individuals who are having their blood collected, fainting is primarily from psychological causes. Merely the sight of blood or needles is enough to cause some people to faint.

To prevent fainting or to deal effectively with it, the phlebotomist must always be aware of the condition of the patient. Observe the patient before and during the phlebotomy. Are they acting nervous or hyperventilating? Try to engage the patient in conversation to keep their mind off the procedure. After performing the venipuncture, ask the patient how they feel. Also, always be sure the phlebotomy is being done with the patient in a well-supported position. Always be sure that you follow your facility's policy and procedure for patients who suffer episodes of syncope.

The volume of blood collected during routine phlebotomy is not enough in itself to cause fainting from **hypovolemia**; however, in blood donation, hypovolemia may cause fainting. As stated in Chapter 7, blood donation results in approximately a 450-mL loss of blood from the donor. This loss may be enough to cause syncope if the patient attempts to get out of the donor chair or off the table too quickly. For this reason, the donor is not allowed to leave the chair for at least 10 minutes after the collection. This amount of time, along with the consumption of some liquids, gives the body a chance to adjust to the decreased total blood volume.

If a patient is sitting in a phlebotomy chair and faints before the venipuncture, guide the patient's head between their knees (Fig. 9.2).

A cold compress placed on the back of the neck is also helpful. Once the patient recovers, have them lie

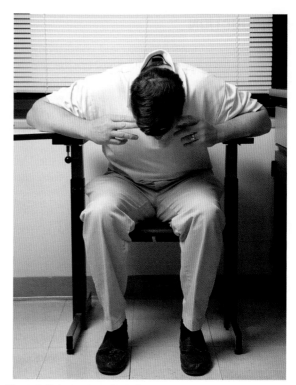

Fig. 9.2 If the patient feels faint, place the head between the knees. (Courtesy Rick Davis.)

down for the phlebotomy to be performed. A cool drink of water may also help the patient feel better if the fainting happens before venipuncture. (Note that water is recommended because some other beverage may affect the results of the blood test to be performed.) Patients who are lying down very seldom feel faint. If the patient feels faint after the phlebotomy has been started, remove the tourniquet, carefully remove the needle, and, while applying pressure, support the patient and call for help. Never leave the patient!

Hematoma

Perhaps the most common complication from phlebotomy is the **hematoma**. This occurs when the needle is improperly placed in the vein, allowing blood to escape from the vein and collect under the skin (Fig. 9.3). The primary indication of a hematoma is swelling around the venipuncture site when the needle is being inserted. By adjusting the depth of the needle, it may be possible to stop the hematoma from enlarging. Otherwise, remove the needle and apply

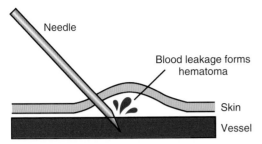

Fig. 9.3 A hematoma occurs when an improperly placed needle causes blood to escape from the vein.

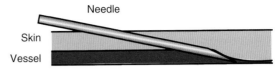

Fig. 9.4 One possible cause of a short draw or failure to obtain blood. The vacuum causes the vessel to collapse.

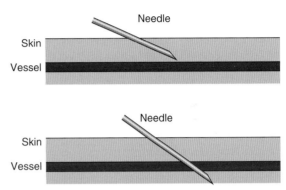

Fig. 9.5 Possible explanations for not collecting blood. In the *top* picture, the needle is not inserted deep enough. In the *bottom* picture, the needle is inserted too deep.

firm pressure to the site. This may help the blood disperse somewhat. It is usually good practice and common courtesy to inform the patient that a day or two later they may notice a bruise at the venipuncture site. It is nothing to be alarmed about and will disappear in a few days.

If removal of the needle is required and not enough blood was collected, another venipuncture must be performed. This venipuncture should be at an alternate site.

Hematomas may occur after the phlebotomy is completed, even if the procedure is done correctly. This is why it is very important to maintain pressure on the venipuncture site until bleeding has stopped.

Short Draw or No Blood Collected

When insufficient blood is collected in a given tube or for a given test, this is often referred to as a **short draw**. Occasionally, the phlebotomist will enter the vein and the blood flow will be slow, stop after a short time, or will not flow at all. There are some general technical errors that can occur; these are discussed later. There are also some occasions when the needle is in the vein but blood flow is reduced. In such cases, the needle bevel may be against the vessel wall, thus preventing the flow of blood. Slight manipulation of the needle will generally remedy this problem. In other cases, the suction of the tube vacuum may be too great, causing the vessel to collapse (Fig. 9.4). In these cases, smaller tubes or a syringe may be used to collect the blood. Additionally, when using a syringe, collapsed veins may also occur if the syringe plunger is withdrawn too quickly.

Another cause of insufficient blood collection may occur when the needle is not inserted far enough. The needle may be below the skin surface but above the vein. Gently inserting the needle into the vein should result in blood flow. Conversely, the needle may have

been inserted through the vein; thus no blood is collected. Slowly withdrawing the needle back into the vein may correct this problem (Fig. 9.5).

Finally, it should be noted that anticoagulated tubes—that is, blue-stoppered, lavender-stoppered, and so on—must be filled to the proper level. Short draws in these tubes will alter the anticoagulant-to-blood ratio, producing spurious results.

Nonanticoagulated tubes and/or serum tubes—that is, for example, red and speckled-stoppered—may be used if a short draw occurs and the blood collected is of sufficient quantity to perform the requested tests. The phlebotomist should check with local protocol and procedures if uncertain how to proceed.

Other Complications
Petechiae

Petechiae are small red dots that appear on the skin as the result of capillary **hemorrhage**. In such cases, the capillaries bleed excessively because of a coagulation problem, generally one related to platelets. As stated in Chapters 2 and 7, the function of platelets is to stop bleeding from blood vessel walls. If you notice petechiae, you should realize that it may take a little longer than normal for the patient to stop bleeding from the

---

venipuncture site. Petechiae can also be the result of tying the tourniquet too tight and leaving it on too long. For this reason, the tourniquet should not be on for longer than 1 minute.

Edema

Edema results when excessive fluid collects in the tissues of a patient, causing swelling. Venipuncture should be avoided in these areas because (1) it is often difficult to locate a vein, and (2) the specimen may be diluted with tissue fluid, which could adversely affect the testing results.

Excessive Bleeding

A phlebotomist must not leave a patient until bleeding has stopped after venipuncture. Normally this is a few minutes. However, occasionally patients on anticoagulant therapy may take much longer. Even the patient's use of aspirin may result in prolonged bleeding because aspirin interferes with platelet function. It is the phlebotomist's responsibility to be certain that bleeding has stopped before the phlebotomist leaves the patient or the patient leaves the phlebotomy area in the case of an outpatient.

Intravenous Lines

As reviewed in Chapter 7, phlebotomy should be avoided from an area adjacent to or above an intravenous (IV) line. Use the arm without the IV or some other site. If a phlebotomy must be collected from the arm with the IV, draw the blood from below the IV. If blood is drawn above the IV, the IV should be stopped and a note sent to the laboratory indicating that the blood was collected above an IV. Be sure to check your institution's guidelines for collecting blood from an arm with an IV.

Obesity

Locating and palpating a vein may be difficult in an obese patient because the veins are generally deeper and cannot be seen. However, with practice and patience, you will learn to locate these veins and perform the phlebotomy with minimal difficulty. A blood pressure cuff may be used for vein location or some other vein locating devise.

Allergies

Occasionally patients may indicate that they are allergic to a sterilizing solution or to the adhesive on bandages.

When a patient expresses these concerns, the phlebotomist should find an alternative. Additionally, the patient may be allergic to latex or the powder used in latex gloves. In these cases, the phlebotomist must use a nonlatex tourniquet and gloves or powder-free gloves if that is appropriate.

Nausea

It is not unusual for patients to feel nauseated before or immediately after venipuncture. The cause is generally psychosomatic, and it may be advisable to have an emesis basin nearby. This also demonstrates the importance of being very aware of the patient and how they are feeling.

Unintentional Arterial Puncture

Unintentional arterial puncture is extremely rare if proper venipuncture procedures are followed. It is more likely to happen as a result of excessive probing, especially when attempting to puncture the basilic vein, and is a good reason to use the basilic vein only as a last resort. Arterial puncture can be recognized by the brightness of the blood (because it is fully oxygenated) and the "pulsing" of the blood into the collection tube. The phlebotomy should be stopped immediately, and it is imperative that firm pressure be applied for at least 5 minutes. Bleeding from a punctured artery after phlebotomy is much more likely than from a vein and can result in hematoma and potentially nerve damage.

Damaged or Scarred Veins

Occasionally you will encounter a patient who has had so many venipunctures that scar tissue has developed around the area that you plan to use for phlebotomy. For example, it is not unusual for IV drug users to have a lot of scar tissue. A situation in which the patient has a lot of scar tissue requires an alternative site for venipuncture, and if none can be located (which is unusual), a microcapillary procedure should be considered. Veins may also be damaged or occluded (blocked) to the degree that even if the venipuncture is successful, little blood is collected. Again, an alternate site must be located.

Burned Areas

Burned areas must be completely avoided because they are very susceptible to infection. The phlebotomist must take extra precautions when performing venipuncture on patients with burns. Gowns, in addition to face masks and gloves, are required because the patient is at risk for contracting an infection from the phlebotomist (see Chapter 3).

An alternate site for venipuncture must be chosen or a microcollection technique used.

Convulsions

Although **convulsions** resulting from phlebotomy are rare, nonetheless a phlebotomist must be prepared to deal with them. It is a good practice to ask patients if they have had any previous adverse reactions to phlebotomy. Although many things can cause convulsions, simple hysteria causes most convulsions in phlebotomy patients. The most important objective is to not allow patients to harm themselves. If the needle is in the arm, quickly remove the needle and the tourniquet if the latter is still on the arm. Move anything that could harm the patient and try to protect the patient's head from striking an object that could cause injury. Do not forget to call for help and notify a physician. If the patient is in a phlebotomy chair and starts to fall out, help guide them to the floor. *Do not panic, and never leave the patient alone!* Be sure to record the date, time, and circumstances under which the convulsion occurred. Once the patient recovers, assess the situation to determine whether the phlebotomy can be performed or repeated, if required, or whether the patient should return at a later time. Finally, the supervisor of the phlebotomy team or unit must be notified.

Mastectomy

Venipuncture should be avoided in the arm on the same side on which a **mastectomy** was performed. This is because the patient may be susceptible to infection on that side of the body because of the removal of lymph nodes with the breast. In the case of a double mastectomy, the patient's physician or nurse should be consulted.

Nerve Injury

Occasionally, even when proper technique and equipment are used, a patient may sustain nerve injury. This is usually signified by a "shooting" pain in the forearm. As pointed out in Chapter 2, nerves may overlie the vein identified for phlebotomy. If a patient complains of this type of pain, the phlebotomy should be discontinued immediately, and the patient should be cared for according to local protocol. Of course, excessive probing, going significantly through the vein, or sudden movement by the patient during phlebotomy may increase the chance of nerve injury.

Reflux or Backflow of Anticoagulant

Although rare, this occurs when anticoagulant is introduced into the patient's vein. The way to avoid this is to have the patient's arm in a downward position when phlebotomy is attempted and perform the venipuncture in an upward motion.

TECHNICAL PROBLEMS

The technical problems discussed in this section include situations that result in no blood being collected because of either faulty equipment or simply missing the vein. Occasionally everything is done properly, but when the tube is pushed onto the needle, no blood is forthcoming. This could be the result of a faulty collection tube that does not contain any vacuum or because the phlebotomist unknowingly pushed the tube onto the needle during the process of preparing to perform the venipuncture, thus releasing the vacuum. It is always a good practice to carry extra collection tubes and keep them within easy reach whenever performing a phlebotomy.

Another technical problem that occasionally occurs is having the needle unscrew from the barrel during the phlebotomy. If this occurs, do not attempt to correct the problem; simply discontinue the phlebotomy, and repeat the procedure. Make sure that the needle is properly seated in the hub of the barrel so that the problem does not happen again, and be sure the needle cover is pulled and not twisted when being removed.

All phlebotomists, at some point in their career, will miss the target vein completely. When this occurs, it may be possible to simply redirect the needle slightly and obtain blood. The needle may be to one side of the vein or perhaps did not enter the patient deeply enough. *However, avoid probing!* And never remove the needle from the arm and reinsert it. You must completely start over. The more experience you get as a phlebotomist, the less often you will miss, and when you do, it will be easier for you to redirect the needle without having to repeat the entire venipuncture procedure.

UNACCEPTABLE SPECIMENS

This section outlines some of the common reasons for unacceptable specimens that are rejected by the clinical laboratory.

Hemolysis

Hemolysis occurs when red blood cells are destroyed, thus releasing a red-tinted substance called hemoglobin. Hemolysis may not be evident at the time of collection but becomes evident in the laboratory when the specimens are centrifuged to separate the cells from the serum or plasma. The serum or plasma will have a pink or red tint. The greater the hemolysis, the more color will be present and the more laboratory test results may be affected. Depending on the test being performed, a hemolyzed specimen may not be acceptable. For example, hemolysis may interfere with testing done in the blood bank as it could be a false positive. In other areas, the hemolysis or hemoglobin itself may not be a problem, but other constituents released when the cells were destroyed may interfere with testing or give falsely high or low values. See Table 9.1 for some common tests and the effect hemolysis may have on them.

Hemolysis may be a result of a physiological condition, such as autoimmune hemolytic anemia or a transfusion reaction that causes hemoglobin to be present in the patient's plasma. More often, it is a result of the venipuncture procedure itself or the handling of the specimen after collection. See Box 9.1 for a list of items that may result in a specimen being hemolyzed.

If the phlebotomist follows standard procedures and is conscientious, most cases of phlebotomy-induced hemolysis can be avoided. This, in turn, will save time, money, and, most importantly, the need to perform a repeat phlebotomy on the patient.

Hemoconcentration

Hemoconcentration occurs when the tourniquet is on the patient's arm too long. It results in a "backing up" or concentration of blood at the venipuncture site. As the blood backs up, specimens collected from the area will have falsely elevated red and white cell counts. This may only be detected if prior laboratory results are available for comparison. If prior laboratory results are available and if there is a significant change in the cell counts without adequate explanation, the latest specimen may be rejected and a new specimen requested.

Clots

Clot formation occurs when **coagulation factors** are activated. Normally, if no anticoagulants are present in the collection tube, these factors are activated almost immediately. When a clot forms in an anticoagulated specimen, generally the specimen will be rejected and a new one will have to be collected. When a clot begins to

TABLE 9.1 **The Effects of Hemolysis on Common Tests**	
Test	**Effect**
Chemistry	
Potassium	Increased value
Magnesium	Increased value
Aldolase	Increased value
Lactate dehydrogenase	Increased value
Blood Bank	
Antibody screen	May invalidate test; specimen rejected
Hematology	
Prothrombin time	Increased value if severe
Activated partial thromboplastin time	Increased value if severe

BOX 9.1   **Causes of Hemolysis**
Technical
• Vigorously shaking the tube of blood
• Using a needle that is too small
• Drawing too hard on the syringe plunger
• Expelling blood too quickly through the syringe into the collection tubes
• Allowing the specimen to overheat
• Drawing blood via an intravenous line
• Incomplete drying of alcohol
Physiological
• Transfusion reaction
• Autoimmune hemolytic anemia
• Paroxysmal nocturnal hemoglobinuria
• Disseminated intravascular coagulation

form in an anticoagulated tube, it may indicate that the blood and anticoagulant are not in proper balance or that the correct procedure was not followed for mixing the specimen. If too little blood is collected, or if too much blood is added to an anticoagulant tube—as, for example, via a syringe—a clot may form. Therefore whenever using an evacuated tube system, always fill the tube with the amount of blood indicated.

Clots may also be present when blood is collected into a syringe and not expelled soon enough into an anticoagulant tube. For this reason, blood must be transferred as quickly as possible from the syringe into the appropriate tubes. Finally, clots may form because the anticoagulant itself is not active or is not present in the proper quantity. The phlebotomist may not be aware of this, and therefore it is important to check the expiration date on the tubes. As long as they are in date, everything should be acceptable.

Short Draw

A short draw, as discussed earlier, is a specimen that does not contain enough blood. Depending on the tests being performed, a short draw may result in specimen rejection. A short draw may occur when the needle comes out of the vein, the vein collapses, or the vacuum was not sufficient to fill the tube. If the vein collapses, you will probably have to redraw the specimen from a different site or possibly use a syringe. If the needle comes out of the vein (but remains in the patient) and you can reinsert it, you will avoid a short draw. Otherwise the venipuncture may need to be repeated. Possibly the vacuum was not strong enough (because of a manufacturing error or an expired tube); in this case, the extra tubes you should be carrying will enable you to collect the specimen without needing to repeat the venipuncture on the patient.

MISLABELED SPECIMENS

Mislabeled specimens or clerical discrepancies occur when the name or some other important identifying information on the requisition form does not match the name on the tube of blood. Depending on the institution and the laboratory department, there will be variations in how clerical discrepancies are handled. For example, a specimen with a slightly misspelled patient name may be acceptable for hematological analysis if the patient's hospital number, room number, and so on are correct. However, for transfusion units or blood banks, which have the strictest requirements, the slightest deviation in name or hospital number may require collection of a new specimen. The reason should be obvious: A transfusion based on the results of an incorrectly labeled specimen could be fatal! It must be noted that mislabeling is a much less frequent problem now that specimen labels are preprinted. However, specimen tubes should never be prelabeled and only labeled after the patient is positively identified and the specimen is collected.

SAFETY SUMMARY

- Never force a patient to undergo phlebotomy.
- Watch for signs of syncope before, during, and after collecting blood.
- Be aware of hematoma development during venipuncture and act accordingly.
- Always fill anticoagulated tubes to the proper volume.
- Recognize unintentional arterial punctures and terminate immediately and take proper precautions.
- Be sure the patient has sufficiently stopped bleeding before leaving.
- Never probe to find a vein during an unsuccessful venipuncture.
- Do not leave a tourniquet on beyond 1 minute; this may result in hemoconcentration.
- Always positively identify the patient and accurately label all specimens.

SUMMARY

This chapter reviewed many considerations and complications associated with phlebotomy. It is important for the phlebotomist to be familiar with how to handle and address situations that may arise before, during, and after venipuncture. It is very important to always keep in mind the patient's safety and comfort first and foremost. By remembering this rule, the new phlebotomist has a very good chance of success in this profession.

CASE 9.1   Critical Thinking

Joseph was preparing to collect a fasting specimen on Albert. Just before Joseph was going to perform the venipuncture, Albert said he was feeling light-headed. Joseph did not continue with the phlebotomy but asked for a nearby technician, Jane, to get a cold compress. Joseph had Jane hold the compress on the back of

Albert's neck. When he was feeling a little better, Joseph helped Albert to a nearby bed, gave him some apple juice, and continued with a successful phlebotomy.

Please discuss Joseph's handling of this situation.

REVIEW QUESTIONS

1. Small red dots on the skin indicating a possible coagulation problem are _____.
2. Low blood volume is referred to as _____.
3. _____ is a condition in which fluid collects in the tissues and results in swelling.
4. _____ is the destruction of red blood cells that results in the release of hemoglobin.
5. Blood that escapes from a blood vessel and collects under the skin may result in a _____.

6. Blood donors are not allowed to leave the donor chair for 10 minutes because of the possibility of _____.
7. In women, venipuncture should be avoided in the arm on the side of a _____.
8. Aspirin may cause prolonged bleeding because it interferes with _____.

BIBLIOGRAPHY

1. Rifai N, Horvath AR, Wittwer CT. *Tietz Fundamentals of Clinical Chemistry and Molecular Diagnostics*. St. Louis: Saunders; 2018, 8th ed.

Dorland's Illustrated Medical Dictionary. 32nd ed. Philadelphia: Saunders; 2012.

Roback J, Combs MR, Grossman B, Hillyer C. *Technical Manual*. 16th ed. Arlington, VA: American Association of Blood Banks; 2008.

The Versatile Phlebotomist and Point-of-Care Testing

Kristy Matulevich*

"I'd like to be a bigger and more knowledgeable person ten years from now than I am today. I think that for all of us as we grow older, we must discipline ourselves to continue expanding, broadening, learning, keeping our minds active and open."

—*Clint Eastwood (1930-)*

OBJECTIVES

At the conclusion of this chapter, the student should be able to:

- Explain cross-training and how it applies to phlebotomists.
- Discuss the importance of cardiopulmonary resuscitation (CPR) training for phlebotomists.
- Describe how to assess patient vital signs (temperature, heart rate, respiration, and blood pressure).
- Explain the procedure of an electrocardiogram (ECG) test and results interpretation.

- Describe the skills necessary to work at a blood donor center.
- Discuss the Clinical Laboratory Improvements Amendments (CLIA '88) in relation to waived testing.
- Define point-of-care testing (POCT) and list its advantages.
- Describe the importance of quality control in POCT.
- Identify POCT used in clinical practice and their applications.

OUTLINE

* The author gratefully acknowledges the original contributions of Joyce E. Hill, on which portions of this chapter are based, and Debra Eckman and David Delvecchio.

KEY TERMS

alveoli
calibration
cross-training: training performed to become proficient in more than one skill
electrocardiography (ECG)
glucometer

hypothalamus
point-of-care testing (POCT)
quality control
respiration
waived testing

INTRODUCTION

In today's fast-paced and competitive health care environment, many institutions have implemented **cross-training** requirements for their employees. The idea is that employees with direct patient care who are competent in performing multiple skills can improve efficiency and effectiveness in the patient care process. Medical facilities cross-train phlebotomists to perform additional duties besides collecting blood for laboratory testing. However, some hospitals have eliminated the phlebotomist's position and instead employ patient care technicians who not only draw blood but also perform other duties such as assisting in patient care (bathing, feeding, and toileting), taking vital signs, performing electrocardiograms (ECGs), and performing point-of-care testing (POCT). Phlebotomists can also cross-train to perform clinical lab assistant duties, which include processing laboratory specimens, performing data entry, transporting specimens, and maintaining processing equipment. The ability to be successful in these positions where multiskilling is necessary requires workers to not only have effective technical skills but also have well-developed self-regulation skills, such as time management, organization, communication, and social perceptiveness. Because the health care field is ever changing with new test procedures and novel technologies, it's important for the phlebotomist to commit to lifelong learning and maintain versatility in their skill sets. These skills can include, but are not limited to, those listed in Box 10.1.

BOX 10.1   Skills for Cross-Training Phlebotomists

Administering cardiopulmonary resuscitation (CPR)
Assessing vital signs
Performing electrocardiograms (ECG)
Providing direct patient care
Conducting donor center/clerical duties
Performing CLIA '88 waived point-of-care testing

CROSS-TRAINING SKILLS
CARDIOPULMONARY RESUSCITATION

Phlebotomists can be employed at a myriad of medical facilities including hospitals, medical clinics, physician offices, and outpatient and blood donation draw centers. In addition, some phlebotomists travel to patients' homes as part of a medical facility's laboratory outreach program or as a contractor for insurance companies. Regardless of where a phlebotomist is employed, a crucial credential to possess is cardiopulmonary resuscitation (CPR) certification. CPR is a technique that provides artificial respiration and circulation to someone who has stopped breathing or has no heartbeat.[1] Often, a phlebotomist is positioned in a situation where they are one-on-one with the patient. If a medical emergency should arise while the phlebotomist is performing their duties, this lifesaving technique can provide the critical need of supplying oxygen-rich blood to the patient's brain and vital organs until emergency medical responders arrive.

Both the American Red Cross (ARC) and the American Heart Association (AHA) offer a Basic Life Support (BLS) course designed for health care professionals that teaches people how to perform CPR. Courses are also offered that provide instruction on basic first aid and automated external defibrillator (AED) certification.[2] These courses are made available at a large number of training centers and medical facilities across the country. CPR certification requires that a refresher course be taken every 2 years to maintain the credential. Many educational programs for phlebotomists incorporate CPR certification training within the curriculum because it is not only medically valuable but also provides the phlebotomist with a marketable skill.

VITAL SIGNS

Another skill that phlebotomists are often cross-trained to perform is assessing and recording patients' vital signs. These signs include patient temperature, heart rate, respiration rate, and blood pressure. Depending on where the phlebotomist is employed, these skills are usually learned through on-the-job training. It is essential that vital signs are measured and recorded accurately because they provide the clinician with valuable information to help diagnose and treat a patient.

Temperature

The measurement of a patient's body temperature allows the provider to assess whether or not they have a fever. A fever is a rise in body temperature as a reaction mechanism of the immune system, usually because of a disease-causing stimulus. An elevated temperature prompts the body's immune response to defend against foreign invaders such as bacteria or viruses.

The **hypothalamus** gland in the brain controls the body's balance of heat production and heat loss. The body temperature of a healthy person fluctuates throughout the day depending on a number of factors, including age, sex, and activity level. Normal body temperature is usually stated as 97.0° to 99.0° Fahrenheit (F) or 36.0° to 37.2° Centigrade (C); however, the temperature depends on the site of measurement, which should be noted. The five areas of the body used to measure temperature are the oral cavity (mouth), rectum, an auxiliary area (armpit or groin), ear (tympanic), and temporal artery (forehead). Many health care facilities continue to take temperatures orally by placing a digital thermometer under the patient's tongue, but with the advent of the noncontact infrared thermometer, which measures thermal radiation emanating from the body, more facilities are employing this touchless method.

Oral and rectal temperature measurements provide the most accurate readings because these areas have a rich supply of blood flow and the ability to be a closed cavity. The average oral temperature for a healthy person is 98.6°F (37°C). A rectal temperature is 0.5° to 1.0°F (0.3° to 0.6°C) higher than an oral reading and a tympanic, auxiliary, or forehead temperature is 0.5° to 1.0°F (0.3° to 0.6°C) lower than an oral reading. It is imperative that whichever method is used to take a patient's temperature the manufacturers' instructions are carefully followed to obtain the most accurate results. See Fig. 10.1 for an illustration of temperature-recording devices.

Heart Rate

The heart rate, or pulse, is defined as the number of times a patient's heart beats per minute. It can be measured by taking the index and middle fingers and compressing the area over an artery and counting the number of beats in 60 seconds. The most common sites to measure heart rate are the radial (wrist), brachial (middle of arm), and carotid (neck) arteries. To assess circulation in different areas of the body, additional sites may be used to obtain a heart rate reading (Fig. 10.2). Heart rates can vary according to the patient's age, sex, fitness and activity level, disease state, body position, medications, and emotional state, and if they smoke. See Table 10.1 for the normal resting heart rate by age group.[3]

When taking a patient's heart rate, the rhythm and volume of the beat should be noted. Rhythm refers to the intervals between heart beats, with a normal rhythm having the same time interval between beats. Arrhythmias (abnormal rhythms) are characterized by irregular or unequal intervals between beats and should be noted for the clinical provider. The volume of the heart rate, which should also be noted, refers to how strong of a beat is felt. It should feel strong and full rather than weak and thready (disappears with slight pressure).

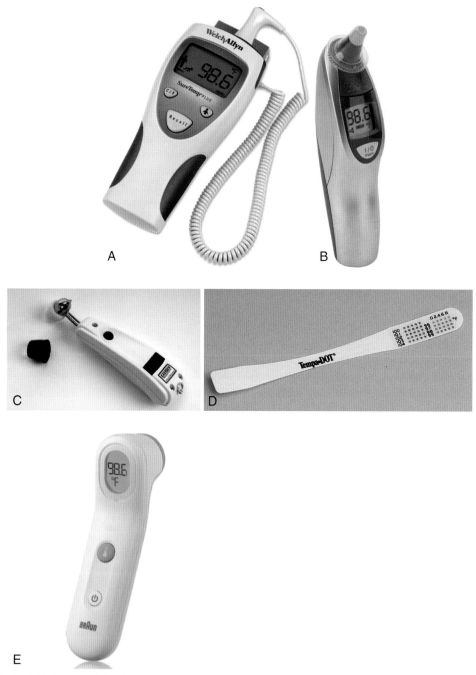

Fig. 10.1 Various models of thermometers. *A,* Digital thermometer. *B,* Tympanic thermometer. *C,* Temporal artery thermometer. *D,* 3M Tempa-DOT disposable strip thermometer, *E,* Noncontact Infrared Thermometer. (A—B Courtesy Welch Allyn, D from Braun, Kronberg, Germany.)

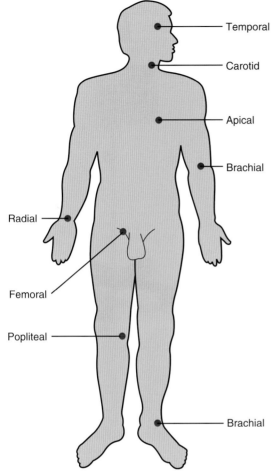

Fig. 10.2 Heart rate sites.

TABLE 10.1	Normal Resting Heart Rate by Age	
Age		**Normal Resting Heart Rate (beats/min)**
Newborns ages 0–1 month		70–190
Infants 1–11 months old		80–160
Children 1–2 years old		80–130
Children 3–4 years old		80–120
Children 5–6 years old		75–115
Children 7–9 years old		70–110
Children 10 years and older and adults (including seniors)		60–100
Athletes in top condition		40–60

TABLE 10.2	Normal Resting Respiration Rates by Age	
Age		**Normal Resting Respiration Rate (breaths/min)**
Newborn to 12 months		30–60
1–2 years old		24–40
3–5 years old		22–34
6–12 years old		18–30
13–17 years old		12–20
Adult less than 65 years old		12–20
Adults 65–80 years old		12–28
Adults over age 80		10–30

Respiration

The act of **respiration** entails the exchanging of gasses by inhaling and exhaling. External respiration is the exchange of oxygen and carbon dioxide taking place in the lungs between the **alveoli** and the blood. Internal respiration is the exchange of oxygen and carbon dioxide between the body cells and blood. The measurement of the respiration rate is vital because it is sensitive to the detection of various adverse or pathological conditions. There are a variety of factors that affect the respiration rate in healthy patients including age, physical activity and emotional stress levels, body temperature, and medications.[4]

Characteristics of respiration include rate, rhythm, and depth. Respiratory rate is the number of respirations per minute. Table 10.2 lists the normal resting respiratory rate by age.[5] To measure the respiration rate, the number of times a patient's chest or abdomen rises over the course of 1 minute is counted, and this number is recorded. The ratio of respirations to pulse rate is typically 1 to 4. The breathing pattern, or rhythm, is noted for irregularities and the depth of respiration, which can be described as normal, deep, or shallow, is also evaluated.

Blood Pressure

The pressure of the blood against the walls of the arteries is known as the blood pressure (BP) and is

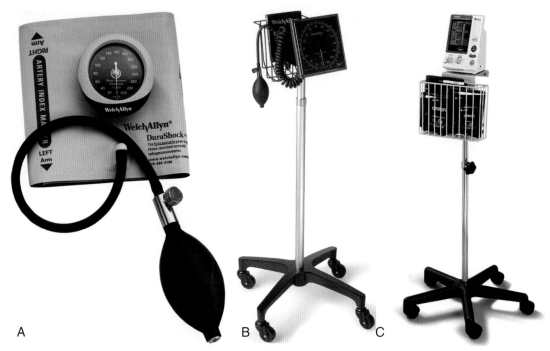

A

B

C

Fig. 10.3 Blood-pressure equipment. *A,* Aneroid dial system with an inflatable cuff. *B,* Aneroid floor model with a large, slanted face, *C,* Digital floor model device. (A—B Courtesy Welch Allyn; C from OMRON Healthcare, Inc.)

measured in millimeters of mercury (mm Hg). There are two components to this measurement: the systolic and the diastolic pressures. The systolic pressure is the force exerted on the arterial walls by the blood during the heart's ventricular contractions and is noted as the first number. Diastolic pressure, the second number, represents the force exerted on the artery walls while the heart is resting between beats. The average BP of a healthy adult is 120/80 mm Hg. Many factors can influence a BP reading, including patient age, sex, activity level, dehydration, anemia, medications, and if the person is a smoker.

Measuring BP is important because it plays a critical role in determining the risk factor for heart disease and stroke. High BP, or hypertension, if uncontrolled, leads to an increase in serious health issues and even death. Hypotension, or low BP, is also a dangerous condition that needs to be controlled and monitored. There are two common methods of measuring BP, typically performed on the bare upper arm. The manual method uses a stethoscope to amplify the sounds of the

heartbeat while a sphygmomanometer measures the pressure of blood in an artery. It is imperative that an appropriate-size cuff be used for the most accurate readings. An alternate method that is commonly employed in health care facilities is the use of a digital BP cuff. This device automatically inflates and deflates as sensors in the cuff measure the pressure in the artery; no stethoscope is needed. Fig. 10.3 displays the two methods of BP measuring devices.

ELECTROCARDIOGRAM

A valuable test to determine heart health is the ECG, which is a graphic recording of the heart's electrical signals. It measures the electrical impulses, or waves, produced by the heart during the process of contraction and relaxation and the time it takes for these impulses to travel through the heart during each heartbeat.[6] To understand the measurement obtained from an ECG, one must be familiar with the electrical activity of the heart.

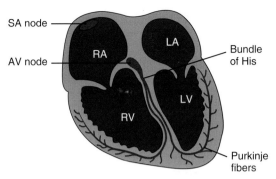

Fig. 10.4 Figure depicting the electrical components of the heart. *LA,* Left atrium; *LV,* left ventricle; *RA,* right atrium; *RV,* right ventricle. (IA Courtesy Nipro Diagnostics, Inc. Fort Lauderdale, Florida. Courtesy Stanbio Laboratory, L.P., an EKF Diagnostics Company. C From Young AP, Proctor D: *Kinn's The Medical Assistant,* 11th ed. St. Louis, Saunders, 2011.)

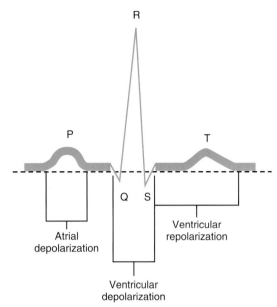

Fig. 10.5 Normal electrocardiogram cycle highlighting waves.

The heart contains specialized masses of tissue that form the conduction system. The sinoatrial (SA) node, located in the upper part of the right atrium, is referred to as the body's "pacemaker" because it sends out an electrical impulse that begins and regulates the heartbeat. As each electrical impulse is dispersed, it causes the heart's atria to contract or depolarize. From the atria, the electrical impulse travels to the atrioventricular (AV) node and then to the Bundle of His. The electrical signal slows down slightly, which allows the ventricles to fill with blood. The AV node then sends another signal that travels along the ventricular walls, via the Purkinje fibers, causing them to contract and pump blood out of the heart. Then the ventricles relax briefly, and a new impulse is sent by the AV node, starting the next heartbeat cycle (Fig. 10.4).

This cardiac cycle represents one complete heartbeat consisting of a contraction (systole) and relaxation (diastole) of the atria and ventricles. Each cycle takes approximately 0.8 seconds for an average of 75 heartbeats per minute. The normal ECG cycle consists of waves that have been labeled P, QRS, and T (Fig. 10.5).

The flat, horizontal line that separates the various waves is known as the baseline. The baseline is divided into segments and intervals so interpretation and analysis can be performed by the health care provider. A segment is the portion of the ECG recording between two waves. An interval is either the length of a wave or the length of a wave with a segment.

The PR interval represents the time it takes from the start of the atrial contraction to the start of the ventricular contraction. The ST segment represents the time period from the end of the ventricular depolarization to the beginning of ventricular recovery (repolarization). The QT interval represents the time from the beginning of ventricular depolarization to the end of ventricular repolarization. The baseline occurring after a T wave represents the period the heart is resting or in its polarized state (Fig. 10.6). Rarely, the U wave, depending on its size, is seen after the T wave. It is thought to represent repolarization of the Purkinje fibers.

The test procedure starts with the phlebotomist, who is cross-trained, placing small electrodes on a patient's arms, legs, and chest. These electrodes are connected to wires attached to an ECG machine at the patient's bedside. When the machine is turned on, it starts recording the electrical signals of the patient's heart. An ECG provides the clinician interpreting the results with important data about a patient's heart. By observing and measuring the time intervals of the ECG, the clinician can determine whether the length of time it takes for the electrical waves to pass through the heart is slow, normal, fast, or irregular. Secondly, the measurement of the heart's electrical activity can help

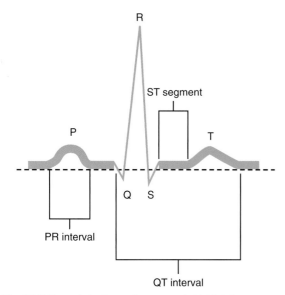

Fig. 10.6 Normal electrocardiogram cycle highlighting segment and interval.

identify if there is any structural abnormality or heart damage such as a myocardial infarction (heart attack) or arrhythmia.

DIRECT PATIENT CARE

The role of a patient care technician includes performing the duties of a phlebotomist in addition to those that a medical assistant performs under the direction of a nurse or physician. These duties can include feeding, bathing, and toileting the patient and other skills depending on the clinical facility. Because the phlebotomist has extensive patient contact, the aspects of this cross-training flow naturally, and can be learned through on-the-job training. In this role, it is vital that the phlebotomist employ excellent communication skills, empathy, and intuition, because a great deal of interaction is required with not only the patient but also appropriate medical providers.

BLOOD DONOR CENTER SKILLS

A blood donor center is a place where donors are screened, and blood is collected for the purpose of transfusion to a patient in need. These centers can be stand-alone buildings, sites located within other medical facilities, or sites (temporary or permanent) situated

at various community locations where blood drives take place. Employment involving blood donation requires the phlebotomist to possess not only venipuncture procedure competency but also skills such as professional interactions with donors, the ability to provide simple first aid, proficient specimen processing, and efficient clerical duties.

A prospective blood donor's screening process starts upon their arrival at the site. The phlebotomist may be required to ask questions to first gather relevant demographic information and obtain the donor's consent to proceed with the donation process. After this, the phlebotomist conducts a verbal medical history inquiry including questions pertaining to illnesses, medications taken, travel history, recent surgeries, tattoos or body piercings, and sexual history. The answers to these questions enable the blood center personnel to determine whether or not the prospective donor is an acceptable candidate for blood donation.

Once it is determined that a donor is able to give blood, the phlebotomist conducts a brief physical examination, which includes evaluating their general health status and assessing their vital signs. Next the donor's hemoglobin level is determined using the copper sulfate method to ensure adequacy using a small amount of blood obtained from a finger stick. The donor's body weight is also measured to make sure they meet the minimum donation requirement.

If it is determined that the prospective donor is an acceptable candidate, they will need to complete an informed consent document. This form notifies the donor that their blood will be tested for infectious diseases and that they will be notified of any positive test results. Before the blood donation, the prospective donor should understand the entire procedure of blood donation and have the opportunity to ask questions and refuse consent. Blood donation centers have strict policies and procedures that must be followed throughout the entire process, starting with screening the donor to collecting and processing the donated blood and blood products. Often, specific training is required for phlebotomists employed at blood donor centers.

CLIA '88 WAIVED TESTING

Legislation was enacted in 1988 by the United States Congress known as the Clinical Laboratory Improvements Amendments (CLIA '88), which included regulations designed to improve the quality of clinical laboratory testing. CLIA '88 was enacted in response to concerns about laboratory testing errors and established specifications for quality assurance (QA) and quality control (QC) in the laboratory. Any clinical laboratory in the United States that performs human diagnostic testing must be CLIA certified by the Centers for Medicare and Medicaid Services (CMS). Along with CMS, the Food and Drug Administration (FDA) and the Centers for Disease Control and Prevention (CDC) oversee the administration of CLIA certificates.

CLIA '88 legislation was enacted to ensure that regardless of where patient testing is performed (e.g., a hospital laboratory, an outpatient clinic, a physician's office), the results are reliable, accurate, and completed in an appropriate time frame.[7] The FDA established several categories of laboratory testing based on the complexity level of the test procedure: **waived testing**, moderate complexity testing, high-complexity testing, and provider-performed microscopy.[8] There are personnel standards for each level of testing, but phlebotomists who have been properly trained can perform waived testing.

Waived tests are simple to perform, and the category includes tests cleared by the FDA that can be performed at home. When the manufacturer's instructions are followed, waived tests carry little risk of causing harm to patients due to an erroneous result. However, incorrect results may lead to unintended negative consequences for patients and therefore care must be taken to precisely follow the testing instructions and interpretation. Box 10.2 is a list of CLIA waived tests. For a complete list of approved tests, methods, and instruments, visit http://www.cms.gov/CLIA/10_Categorization_of_Tests.asp.

POINT-OF-CARE TESTING

POCT is defined as laboratory tests performed near where the patient is located. This could mean testing samples from a patient at their hospital bedside, in a physician's office examination room or clinic, at a blood donation center, or at a community health fair table, just to name a few. This type of testing is also known as decentralized testing because it is done outside the confines of a core clinical laboratory. POCT may be classified as waived or nonwaived.

> ### BOX 10.2 CLIA '88 Waived Tests
>
> Dipstick or tablet reagent urinalysis
> Urinalysis by approved chemistry analyzers
> Urine pregnancy tests by visual color comparison
> Fecal occult blood and gastric pH and occult blood
> Blood glucose devices approved by the Food and Drug Administration (FDA) for home use
> Hemoglobin
> Drug screening
> Cholesterol monitoring
> Chemistry panel
> Glucose
> PT/INR
> Influenza A and B
> *Streptococcus* Group A
> Respiratory Syncytial Virus (RSV)
> SARS-CoV-2 (COVID-19) (under Emergency Use Authorization)

Diagnostic laboratory tests are vital to providers in diagnosing, treating, and monitoring patient's medical conditions. According to the CDC, it is estimated that 70% of today's medical decisions are based on laboratory test results.[9] Because it is performed near the patient, POCT provides the advantages of being convenient for the patient, having a quick turnaround time, and using a smaller volume of sample, all of which contribute to test results that can lead to improved patient care.[10] However, often, the cost of POCT is higher compared with the same test performed in a centralized laboratory.

Testing devices and instrumentation developed for POCT are designed to be low maintenance, require minimal quality control steps, and use bar code technology to minimize the chance of human error. The POCT menu of analytes depends on the clinical facility, but can include blood gases and electrolytes, cholesterol, coagulation tests, drugs of abuse, Group A strep, glucose, respiratory viruses, hemoglobin and hematocrit, occult blood, urinalysis, and urine pregnancy testing. Some devices can connect to the testing facility's wireless internet so the results can be automatically uploaded into the patient's electronic medical record (EMR).

Phlebotomists who are performing versatile patient care duties must be conscientious, adequately trained, and deemed competent to perform POCT on patients. Strict care must be taken to perform all required quality control and correct testing procedures to obtain accurate results. Phlebotomists must also use critical thought processes to troubleshoot spurious results, be aware of critical values, and be able to effectively communicate with the patient care team. Fig. 10.7 shows various types of POCT equipment.

Quality Control

One of the most essential aspects of providing accurate patient results is **quality control** testing. Regardless of whether the POCT apparatus is a small test cartridge, a handheld device, or a tabletop analyzer, quality control must be tested every day that patient samples are run to ensure that the testing device is working properly. Many facilities designate one employee to oversee personnel training and competency and to verify that quality control is being appropriately performed and documented. It is of critical importance that phlebotomists are aware of the importance of quality control procedures because patient results and outcomes depend on the accurate functioning of POCT instruments.

Quality control material used for testing should be of the same specimen type as the patient sample and usually two levels are run before patient testing: a positive and negative control (qualitative results) or a low and high quality control level (quantitative results). All control values are documented and evaluated by the testing personnel. Some POCT devices use an internal control and require **calibration** for each testing device.

Mathematical calculations are done using quantitative quality control results to obtain the acceptable numerical ranges. The acceptable range is two standard deviations from the average of the data points (mean). If controls fall outside the acceptable limits, then corrective action must be taken and documented. This corrective action may include retesting the quality control material or possibly recalibrating the point-of-care analyzer using manufacturer's calibration material. All steps taken to troubleshoot and resolve quality control issues must be documented. Patient samples cannot be tested until the control values fall within the acceptable range.

Blood Coagulation

One test available through POCT is the monitoring of blood coagulation, which involves the body's ability to form blood clots. The most common tests being performed in this manner are the prothrombin time (PT) assay, including the international normalized ratio (INR) and activated partial thromboplastin time (aPTT). These tests can monitor patients who are on anticoagulant medications, such as warfarin, and can also detect factor deficiencies and other coagulopathies that can put patients at risk for bleeding. Most often, results are obtained through simple capillary puncture and are available within 5 minutes of testing.

Blood coagulation monitoring is of utmost importance in a cardiac-catheter laboratory, the operating room (OR), emergency room (ER), and critical care units. When this type of testing is performed in an outpatient setting, such as at a physician's office or during the patient's home visit, it allows for immediate adjustment of the patient's medication, improves patient compliance, and minimizes laboratory-to-laboratory variability. The CoaguChek System (Roche Diagnostics, Indianapolis, IN) is a commonly used POCT instrument for this purpose.

Blood Gases and Electrolytes

Blood gas analysis involves the measuring of analytes crucial to maintaining homeostasis, or steady-state conditions, in the body. Blood gas analysis involves measuring the pH, partial pressure of oxygen (PaO_2), partial pressure of carbon dioxide ($PaCO_2$), bicarbonate (HCO_3), oxygen saturation (O_2 Sat), and oxygen content (O_2 CT). Imbalances in these analytes can indicate the presence of various medical conditions related to the body's acid-base balance. POCT analyzers can be used to perform blood gas analysis and can often provide electrolyte test results as well. These tests include sodium, potassium, and chloride, which can aid in diagnosing and monitoring patient conditions.

Because these POCT instruments perform more than one test, there may be more complex quality control, maintenance, and testing procedures required. Also, blood gases are often performed on arterial blood samples, which requires additional phlebotomy training for the collection procedure. The iStat system (Abbott Laboratories, Abbott Park, IL) and Nova Biomedical Stat Profile pHOx (Nova Biomedical, Waltham, MA) analyzers are widely used for point-of-care blood gas and electrolyte testing.

Cholesterol

A point-of-care analyzer is also available to test cholesterol levels, which include total cholesterol, triglycerides, high-density lipoproteins, and low-density

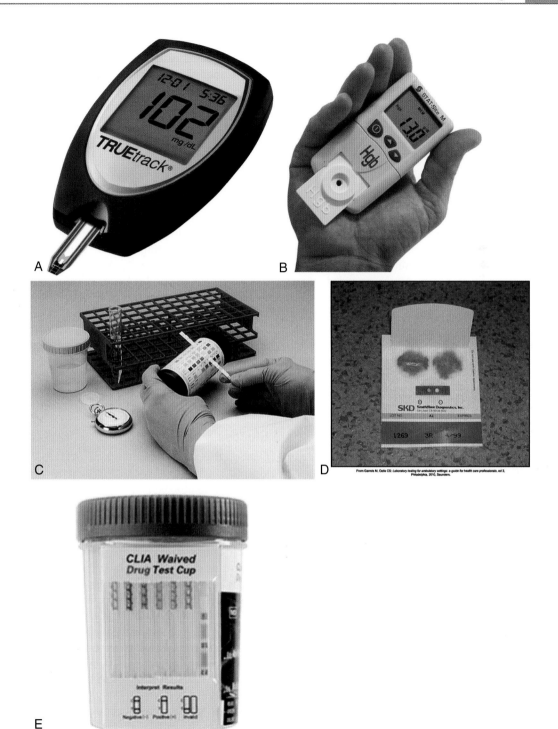

Fig. 10.7 **Point-of-care equipment.** *A,* Blood Glucose Monitor. *B,* Hemoglobin tester. *C,* Urine reagent strips, *D,* Fecal occult blood test card, *E,* Urine drug test cup. (D From Linné & Ringsrud's Clinical Laboratory Science, *Concepts, Procedures and Clinical Applications,* 8th ed. Elsevier, found in Chapter 9, Fig. 9.4, page 224. E from Healgen Scientific, LLC.)

lipoproteins. This information can provide patients with their risk of atherosclerosis, which can lead to heart disease. The CLIA-waived Cholestech LDX™ Analyzer (Abbott Laboratories, Abbott Park, IL) uses a capillary specimen obtained from a fingerstick to provide quick results. The testing is often seen as part of a health fair sponsored by a local hospital, clinic, or community college.

Drugs of Abuse Screening

The testing of patient samples for drugs of abuse occurs in many clinical settings, including the ER, outpatient testing facilities, and physician's offices. POCT devices provide rapid results, often within a few minutes, so immediate action or treatment can be provided. Most point-of-care devices analyze a small amount of a random urine sample; however, other sample types, such as hair, saliva, and nails, can be used for testing in forensic settings. One type of POCT device is a self-contained plastic cup that is integrated with a visual testing panel for multiple drug metabolites.[11] These tests provide qualitative preliminary results, which can be confirmed using more sophisticated testing methods. Collection protocols must be strictly followed to ensure specimen integrity.

Fecal Occult Blood

Fecal occult blood (FOBT) is a POCT that screens patient fecal samples for occult, or hidden, blood. A positive screening test indicates the presence of blood in the large intestine, which can lead a clinician to early detection of colorectal cancer. The test procedure entails placing a thin film of a patient's stool sample in two small boxes of special filter paper on one side of a test card. The sample is allowed to dry, and a chemical developer is added to the flip side of the card in the area the sample was applied. A reaction will take place and turn the test card blue if blood is present because of the reagent reacting with hemoglobin in the sample. The color developer is also added to a control area on the card containing a positive and negative performance area. The positive area should show a blue color when added, and the negative area should show no color for a valid patient test result.

To prevent false-positive reactions, patients must refrain from foods such as certain fruits, vegetables, and red meat before sample collection. For patients with gastrointestinal disease, early detection and treatment is vital for optimal patient outcomes. The test can also be used to monitor patients for gastrointestinal bleeding and other inflammatory conditions. One test card widely available for a rapid qualitative screening method is Hemoccult II SENSA [elite] (Beckman Coulter, Brea, CA).

Gastroccult

POCT can be used to detect occult blood and also determine whether the pH level is abnormal in gastric aspirate or vomitus. Various conditions can be detected and monitored by employing the gastroccult test in multiple clinical settings including the ER, intensive care units (ICUs), and ORs. Measuring the pH of the sample can be helpful for evaluating the use of antacid therapy. The test procedure is similar to the FOBT in that the patient sample is applied to certain areas on the test card area. A color developer is then added to one area to detect if hemoglobin is present, and the pH comparator is used to determine the pH of the gastric sample. Quality control is performed in a similar fashion as in the FOBT for hemoglobin testing, and for the pH testing a colorless, buffered reference is used.

Glucose

One of the most common uses of POCT is blood glucose monitoring. Such determination allows the doctor to monitor patients diagnosed with the disease diabetes mellitus (DM) and choose appropriate treatment. DM is a chronic metabolic disease in which the pancreas cannot produce enough insulin, or the body is not able to use the insulin that is produced. Insulin is a chemical released into the bloodstream by the pancreas in response to increased blood glucose, especially after meals. Insulin allows the glucose from the bloodstream to be absorbed by the body's cells, where it is converted into energy. If this process does not or cannot occur, then glucose in the bloodstream can rise to dangerously high levels, which can lead to strain on major body organs, especially the kidneys and heart, causing shock or even death.

Because of the strict control of glucose levels necessary in patients with DM, the use of a small glucose POCT analyzer, called a **glucometer**, has become commonplace in the patient's home, in doctor's offices, and at the hospital bedside. These glucose monitors are known by many different names

---

BOX 10.3 Various Point-of-Care Glucose Testing Devices

Precision Xceed Pro Blood Glucose and beta-Ketone Monitoring System (Abbott Diabetes Care)
Assure Platinum (Arkray)
Accu-Chek (Roche Diagnostics)
One Touch (Life Scan)
Glucose 201 DM Analyzer (HemoCue)
StatStrip Hospital Glucose Monitoring System (Nova Biomedical)
Glucometer Elite (Bayer)

(Box 10.3). These monitors require whole blood samples collected by skin puncture from the finger of an adult or the heel of an infant. As with any equipment used to perform testing, adherence to quality control procedures and manufacturer's instructions is of vital importance. Careful recording of results must include date, time, and phlebotomist's initials.

New technological advances have enabled continuous glucose monitoring devices to be developed and used to track patients' glucose levels throughout the day and night. These devices work via the insertion of a tiny sensor under the patient's skin that measures glucose readings. Results can be transmitted electronically for monitoring patient therapy.

Group A Strep

Group A *Streptococcus* (*Streptococcus pyogenes*) is a bacterium that causes strep throat. When patients present with symptoms including a sore throat and fever, a throat swab can be obtained and tested using a waived kit for Group A *Streptococcus*, which can help determine whether the cause is a bacterial or viral infection. To collect the specimen, a sterile swab is rubbed along the back of a patient's mouth along the pharyngeal wall. Usually two swabs are obtained; one is used for the rapid test and the other is used for a throat culture and sent to a clinical laboratory microbiology department. The throat culture, which can take several days, is subsequently performed if the results of the Group A *Streptococcus* POCT is negative to confirm that there are no *Streptococcus pyogenes* organisms present.

Numerous types of rapid screening kits are available that test for the specific proteins of the Group A *Streptococcus* organism, and it is important to follow the manufacturer's steps for accurate results and interpretation. Positive and negative controls are run simultaneously with the patient's test, and the result is typically a color reaction on a test cartridge or strip. Usually, the result is obtained within 15 to 30 minutes, which is helpful for the provider when prescribing appropriate treatment. If left untreated, strep throat can cause various patient complications including rheumatic fever and glomerulonephritis.

Hemoglobin and Hematocrit

Hemoglobin and hematocrit are tests that have been available as a POCT for quite some time. Most doctor's offices have a hemoglobinometer available to quickly screen for anemia. Anemia is a medical condition in which a person lacks a sufficient amount of healthy red blood cells, consisting of hemoglobin, which transport oxygen throughout the body. This condition can result in the patient developing weakness and shortness of breath. There are various causes of anemia, and treatments vary from medications to diet modifications to requiring a blood transfusion.

The ER is another location where hemoglobin and hematocrit levels may be tested. Also, blood donor centers screen potential donors for an acceptable hemoglobin level prior to donation. Hematocrit centrifuges have long been in use in ORs to monitor a patient's blood loss during surgical procedures.

Pregnancy Tests

This POCT is designed to detect very small amounts of human chorionic gonadotropin (hCG), a glycoprotein hormone that rapidly increases during the early stages of fetal growth and development. In a normal pregnancy, detectable amounts of beta hCG can be found in both the serum and urine a few days after a fertilized egg attaches to the uterine wall lining. The beta hCG (a subunit of the glycoprotein) can be detected using a POCT around 12 days after a missed period. For urine testing, the first morning sample is optimal, since the urine is most concentrated; however, serum testing is more sensitive because of a lack of this variation in beta hCG level.

The test procedure involves adding several drops of either serum or urine to a sample area on a test cartridge and timing the reaction. The test cartridge contains antibodies that will react with the beta hCG molecules, and a color reaction is seen to indicate the test is positive. Most test kits employ an internal control that shows a color reaction to ensure the cartridge is working properly, and the sample has been added. The test results are qualitative, meaning only a positive or negative reaction is reported.

The POCT is widely used in medical facilities to determine whether a patient is pregnant. The ER setting uses this test to screen for pregnancy if a patient needs radiological studies performed because these can have detrimental effects on a fetus. Often providers will follow up a positive screening test for hCG with a blood test run in the core laboratory as a confirmatory test, which gives a quantitative result.

Respiratory Viruses

Phlebotomists can be trained to collect nasal and nasopharyngeal swab specimens for respiratory virus testing. These waived test kits and platforms can detect and differentiate influenza A and influenza B, respiratory syncytial virus (RSV), and SARS-CoV-2 (the novel coronavirus that causes COVID-19) viral infections by using immunoassay tests or molecular methods to detect viral proteins.[12] Results of the tests can be obtained in as little as 15 minutes so proper care can be provided to the patient.

Each test kit or device has been authorized to use only a specific specimen type and it is crucial that proper specimen collection and handling occur and adherence to manufacturer's instructions for use are followed to ensure accurate test results. If applicable, both external and internal control must be performed during the testing process and care should be taken, such as regular disinfection and changing of gloves, to avoid cross-contamination of materials.

Urinalysis

One of the most frequent tests a cross-trained phlebotomist may perform in a point-of-care setting is urinalysis. This waived test consists of observing the physical characteristics and performing a chemical analysis of the patient's urine sample. A third component of the urinalysis test, a microscopic examination of

the sediment, if required, is performed in a clinical laboratory. Urinalysis is a screening test often performed because the sample is easy to obtain from the patient, and the results can provide valuable information to the physician about the patient's medical condition related to diabetes, kidney function, and urinary tract infections.

When performing urinalysis, the specimen to be tested should be a freshly voided sample that is well mixed and at room temperature. The urinalysis includes first recording the color and clarity of the urine sample. Next the phlebotomist dips a multiple-reagent test strip into the urine and either manually observes the chemical reactions or places the test strip on a tabletop point-of-care analyzer, which measures and records the reactions. These test strips are thin plastic strips containing individual test pads. When the urine sample is added to the test pad, a chemical reaction takes place, resulting in color changes to the pads. Manual reading of the results consists of comparing the color of the test pads to a comparator chart on the side of the urine test strip bottle. If the phlebotomist is manually performing the chemical analysis, adequate lighting for reading is required, and the manufacturer's directions must be precisely followed because the timing of the reactions is essential to recording accurate results. The use of an automated urinalysis analyzer will standardize the testing process by removing the variables of timing and color differentiation of the test pads.

The test strips must be stored properly to avoid deterioration, which can lead to inaccurate results. The multiple-reagent test strips must be kept away from light and moisture, and the container should be tightly capped. Quality control must be performed on each day of patient testing using a normal and abnormal level of controls for both manual and automated testing.

SUMMARY

A phlebotomist who is cross-trained to perform additional duties, such as reading vital signs and POCT, is well equipped to provide essential medical care to patients in a fast-paced and ever-changing health care environment. By keeping an open mind with regard to obtaining a versatile skill set, committing to life-long learning, and developing their self-regulation qualities, phlebotomists can continue to be valuable assets to the patient care team.

CASE 10.1 Critical Thinking

You are required to obtain glucose readings on five patients before 8 AM. Before testing
 your patients, you test the quality-control samples, and the results are outside the acceptable
 range.
 Should you proceed with patient testing? Why or why not?

REVIEW QUESTIONS

1. The five major areas in which a patient's temperature may be taken are _____, _____, _____, _____, and _____.
2. Involuntary breathing is controlled by the _____.
3. The primary purpose of point-of-care testing is _____.
4. A graphic recording of the heart's electrical activity is an _____.
5. The average resting heart rate _____ as people mature.
6. _____ is a combination of artificial respiration and circulation.
7. A sphygmomanometer and a _____ are needed to ascertain blood pressure.
8. True or False: Blood donation centers have strict policies and procedures that must be followed throughout the entire process starting with screening the donor to collecting and processing the donated blood and blood products. CORRECT ANSWER IS "true"
9. This category of testing, established by CLIA '88, which includes tests that are simple to perform, cleared by the FDA, and can be performed at home are called _____ tests. CORRECT ANSWER IS "waived"
10. Two advantages of POCT testing are _____ and _____. CORRECT ANSWERS CAN BE "convenient for the patient, having a quick turnaround time, and using a smaller volume of sample"
11. Name three common POCT procedures: _____, _____, and _____.
12. What is the importance of quality control? _____
13. What roles can a phlebotomist fulfill? _____

REFERENCES

1. Cardiopulmonary resuscitation (CPR). *First aid. Mayo Clinic.* Published February 12, 2022. Accessed August 2, 2022. https://www.mayoclinic.org/first-aid/first-aid-cpr/basics/art-20056600.
2. Red Cross training & certification, and store. Red Cross. Accessed August 2, 2022. https://www.redcross.org/take-a-class/cpr?utm_source=RCO&utm_medium=For_Individuals_Find_Classes_and_Certification&utm_content=CPR.
3. Hipp D. Normal heart rate by age. Forbes. Published May 3, 2022. Accessed August 2, 2022. https://www.forbes.com/health/healthy-aging/normal-heart-rate-by-age/.
4. Nicolò A, Massaroni C, Schena E, Sacchetti M. The importance of respiratory rate monitoring: From healthcare to sport and exercise. *Sensors (Basel).* 2020; 20(21):6396. https://doi.org/10.3390/s20216396.
5. Meadows A. What is a Normal Respiratory Rate for Sleep? Sleep Foundation. Published July 8, 2021. Accessed August 1, 2022. https://www.sleepfoundation.org/sleep-apnea/sleep-respiratory-rate.

6. The Electrocardiogram explained - What is an ECG? Heart Sense. Published September 28, 2014. Accessed August 2, 2022. https://heartsense.in/electrocardiogram-explained/.

7. Clinical laboratory improvement amendments (CLIA). U.S. Food and Drug Administration. Accessed August 2, 2022. https://www.fda.gov/medical-devices/ivd-regulatory-assistance/clinical-laboratory-improvement-amendments-clia.

8. Waived tests. Cdc.gov. Published September 3, 2021. Accessed August 2, 2022. https://www.cdc.gov/labquality/waived-tests.html.

9. Strengthening clinical laboratories. Cdc.gov. Published November 15, 2018. Accessed August 2, 2022. https://www.cdc.gov/csels/dls/strengthening-clinical-labs.html.

10. Turgeon ML. *Linne & Ringsrud's Clinical Laboratory Science: Concepts, Procedures, and Clinical Applications.* 8th ed. Mosby; 2019.

11. Wiencek JR, Colby JM, Nichols JH. Rapid assessment of drugs of abuse. Makowski GS. *Adv Clin Chem.* 2017;80: 193–225. https://doi.org/10.1016/bs.acc.2016.11.003.

12. CDC. Guidance for SARS-CoV-2 rapid testing performed in Point-of-Care settings. Centers for Disease Control and Prevention. Published July 28, 2022. Accessed August 2, 2022. https://www.cdc.gov/coronavirus/2019-ncov/lab/point-of-care-testing.html.

11

Interpersonal Communication and Professionalism

John C. Flynn, Jr.

> *"When people talk, listen completely. Most people never listen."*
> —*Ernest Hemingway (1899–1961)*

OBJECTIVES

At the conclusion of this chapter, the student should be able to:

- Discuss why communicating clearly is important.
- Name several attributes of professionalism.
- Discuss the Patient Care Partnership.
- Identify several organizations that certify phlebotomists.
- Discuss the importance of continuing education.

OUTLINE

KEY TERMS

empathy
HIPAA
jargon

stereotyping
subordinates

INTRODUCTION

The purpose of this chapter is to discuss the importance and the role of interpersonal communication and professionalism in the daily life of a phlebotomist or, for that matter, any health care professional. The two topics are included in the same chapter because they are intricately related. The chapter concludes with a brief discussion of continuing education (CE), a topic that is very important to all professionals.

EFFECTIVE COMMUNICATION

What is effective communication? Does it always imply either written or oral communication? Is one better than the other? Does how you say something matter? *STAT!* This is a word that is used every day in the clinical setting, but the word has different meanings for different individuals in the health care setting. To some, it means "drop everything and do it now"; to others, it means "do it when you can get to it"; and to still others, it may mean something else entirely. This example of the use (and abuse) of the word STAT illustrates a problem with effective communication that is confronted by phlebotomists.

Communicating is something that laboratory personnel, including phlebotomists, do every day during the course of their jobs. However, the backgrounds of the people with whom they must communicate are diverse, as illustrated in Chapter 1 (see Fig. 1.3).

In some situations, *communication*, which is a noun, is often thought of as a commodity or substance, as illustrated by the phrase "we must have more communication"; however, communication can be more accurately described as a process, not a commodity. For example, if a plant is lacking water, the situation can be corrected by adding more water. However, if there is a lack of communication, adding more communication does not necessarily correct the problem; in fact, it can make matters worse. In other words, the trouble with communication problems is not always the *quantity* of communication but instead the *quality* of the communication. Additionally, the context of any communication matters too. Going back to the example of STAT, an emergency room (ER) nurse running into a blood bank with a sample from a gunshot wound victim asking for four units of blood for transfusion STAT may be more critical than a morning round glucose test on an inpatient that is labeled STAT.

A LIFE SKILL

There are certain activities common to all people that can be regarded as life skills. These include maintaining one's health and family relationships, self-evaluation, self-reflection, and decision making.

Communication is also a life skill, and yet what training do most people receive in communication? Most have had some grade school and secondary school training in grammar, composition, and public speaking; there are even collegiate programs of "communication." However, most people receive no training in interpersonal communications, which is what phlebotomists and all laboratory workers must use daily. It is assumed that if a person is certified or has a degree, then they must be able to communicate. In other words, being able to communicate effectively is often taken for granted. For many people, after meeting with any number of individuals—be they lawyers, doctors, or accountants—it will be demonstrated that effective verbal communication is not guaranteed by virtue of certification or degree.

Laboratory and health care workers must realize that there are several levels of communication, all of which must be used properly to do their job well. First is what may be called *intrapersonal* communication. This often takes the form of meditation or self-reflection. "How could I have handled that situation better?" or "What could I have done differently to be more effective?" are examples of self-reflective thoughts. It also includes the ability to think and plan in advance how to react in a given situation. Second, there is *one-way* communication. Examples of this are the important but sometimes annoying memos or notes received from supervisors, subordinates, or peers. The information on these notes (i.e., the communication), if not written properly, is open to improper interpretation. Finally, there is *interpersonal* (two-way) communication, which is how phlebotomists and laboratorians communicate most often with patients, with each other, and with other health care professionals. Additionally, it is very useful for phlebotomists to show empathy, which is the ability to see and understand other persons' perspectives—in other words, understanding what it is like "being in someone else's shoes."

KEYS TO SUCCESSFUL COMMUNICATION

Before interpersonal communication can be successful, certain fundamental conditions must be present. First, both parties must be attentive and willing to engage in the communication process. For example, have you ever tried to talk about something with a friend, supervisor, patient, or coworker and at some point, noticed that the person had tuned you out? Or rather than listening to you, the person constantly looked at their watch or a clock or gazed out a window? These experiences can be frustrating and counterproductive. Therefore in addition to being a good communicator, the importance of being a good listener cannot be overlooked. In fact, good listeners will repeat back to the original speaker what they heard to demonstrate that the message was understood.

Second, both parties must act as senders and receivers of messages. Once an individual receives a message (by being a good listener), they must then become a sender and let the other party know that the message was received and understood or that more information is needed. This is very important. If a message is received and not clearly understood, it is imperative that clarification or further instruction be requested. Again, repeating back the message is a good way to demonstrate understanding. The two participants are interdependent; for the communication process to be complete, they must interact.

Finally, and most importantly in the health care setting, communication must be based on mutual understanding. This implies that a given phrase or term, such as STAT or "type and hold," means the same thing to both parties. We all have had the experience of being misunderstood because the person we were talking with interpreted something differently from the way we intended. At times this could actually be dangerous. Laboratory personnel must be careful when using jargon, which, although used daily in the laboratory, may not be understood outside the laboratory setting.

OBSTACLES TO SUCCESSFUL COMMUNICATION

Unfortunately, all people encounter obstacles or barriers to effective communication. One of these is distrust. Distrust can lead to defensive interpersonal communication, especially when the recipient perceives the communication as an attempt to control, reprimand, or manipulate or thinks that the person "only talks to me when there is a problem to address." Additionally, if the sender has a superior attitude, this will trigger a defensive response. Distrust can be overcome if questions or directives are communicated in a nonthreatening way that makes the issue a mutual problem. In this manner,

respect and equality are communicated to recipients, giving them the feeling that their help and judgment are valued and truly part of the health care team. Lastly, it is vital to focus on the issue at hand, even if it is an uncomfortable topic, and not the person. Thus how something is communicated must not be overshadowed by the way it is communicated.

Another common barrier that hinders effective communication is a reference gap. This is analogous to a generational, cultural, gender, or racial gap, in which background and environments affect the way people think, act, perceive the world or environment, and, in this case, communicate. As for their training and background, phlebotomists have a different frame of reference from others with whom they must communicate, including laboratory personnel in other departments, nurses, physicians, social workers, and patients. For example, you may wonder why a test is ordered STAT. Your frame of reference is different from that of the physician; the physician obviously knows something about the patient that you do not know. Similarly, when you are asked by a physician why a STAT request is not done, you may have to explain that all tests from their service are ordered STAT (an abuse of the STAT designation) or that an emergency has arisen, thereby communicating to the physician your frame of reference.

Often, participants of health care teams take part in group discussions or decision making. Disagreement with an idea that you have put forth should not be interpreted as personal dislike. (Again, keep in mind context and how the issue is communicated.) This is unhealthy, another barrier to effective communication, and it must be realized that everyone involved in the process is seeking the best solution, whether the decision regards a patient or where to put a new piece of equipment. The facilitator of the group discussion should set the parameters for the discussion, including respect for each other and the notion that there are no bad ideas! Furthermore, remember that in a group process, the ultimate decision is usually the best one.

Hearing loss, language limitations, and cultural differences (gaps) may also become a barrier to effective communication. These types of barriers are most often seen when trying to communicate with patients but could be a problem between professionals as well. Therefore, as mentioned earlier, it is critical that all communication be clear and easily understood.

One final issue to be addressed is the use, or often the misuse, of body language. After the spoken word, our eyes are the most potent communicator we possess. For example, rolling eyes say one thing, and tear-filled eyes another; surprise, disappointment, and anger are all expressions and feelings we can communicate with our eyes. Reluctance to make eye contact also sends a message to the recipient. Therefore communication must be both verbal and nonverbal. This is especially important for a phlebotomist, who must interact with patients. Establishing eye contact with the patient will go a long way toward establishing trust. However, keep in mind that in some cultures, eye contact is not the norm.

Therefore be sure to make eye contact if appropriate when speaking or listening to patients. Avoid constant monitoring of the time by either looking at your wristwatch or checking a wall clock. Avoid deep sighs or fidgeting with a pencil, sorting supplies, reading, or tapping your toe, all of which signal boredom or impatience. Avoid assuming a defensive posture such as crossing your arms. Your aim is to put the patient at ease, which is best accomplished by acting confident, maintaining eye contact when speaking or listening to a patient or colleague, and appearing relaxed.

COMMUNICATION BREAKDOWN

In most instances, communication between the phlebotomist and others goes rather smoothly. Communication works well, for example, when a physician or nurse calls for testing results to determine whether blood is ready for the next day's operation's schedule or to inquire about what color tube is needed for a given test. In these relaxed situations, communication is open and friendly. Communication often breaks down during times of increased stress, the very times when it is most critical that communication be smooth and effective. A classic example is when an emergency is occurring either in the emergency department or in the operating room and there is a strain in the communication chain between these places and the laboratory. Someone may ask for the results of a test that was never ordered or question why blood is not ready for a trauma victim when the phlebotomist was never informed that there was a trauma patient or that they needed to collect a specimen. However, with patience and self-control and staying focused on the message, the communication process will work even during times of stress.

GENERAL GUIDELINES FOR EFFECTIVE COMMUNICATION

The following guidelines are primarily for oral communication but can easily be adapted to written communication. First, communication should be open and honest. This applies whether you are a subordinate, peer, or supervisor, and the key is respect and courtesy for the individual with whom you are communicating. Glibness, deceptiveness, and sarcasm have no place during communication if you wish to be taken seriously.

Second, avoid generalizations, assumptions, and stereotyping. We have all been guilty of this at some time, whether it was regarding someone in the health care field or of another race or cultural group. Talk to the *individual* because that is what they deserve.

Third, consider your environment or frame of reference. Explain where you are "coming from," including the pressures and time constraints you are under. It is equally important to consider the environment of the individual with whom you are communicating. As a rule of thumb, listen to *what* is said, not *how* it is said.

Next, communicate with a humanistic approach. In addition to the guidelines presented here, one should be sensitive, empathetic, or sympathetic to another's concerns or problems. Often, all a frustrated patient or coworker desires is to have someone listen.

Lastly, indicate you have listened carefully or if you have been the "transmitter," ask if your communication was understood (received), and ask if there are any questions.

These guidelines, which are the hallmarks of professional behavior, are summarized in Box 11.1.

Unfortunately, in some situations, these guidelines cannot be observed. You may be under pressure or

---

BOX 11.1 General Guidelines for Effective Communication

- Be open and honest.
- Avoid generalizations.
- Consider environments.
- Use a humanistic approach.
- Be a good listener and ask the other party if they understand or have any questions.

short of time, but you must keep in mind that you are dealing with another individual who may not be aware of your circumstance or situation. In other words, they do not understand where you are "coming from." When the immediate situation improves, contact the person with whom you may have been curt or impatient, explain the situation that led to your abruptness, and thank the person for their cooperation, understanding, and patience. This way we are not forgetting our obligation to a fellow health care provider to be courteous, responsible, professional, and, above all else, human.

PROFESSIONALISM

Historically, there were three professions—law, medicine, and theology (also known as the three "robed" professions)—and three types of professionals—lawyers, doctors, and clergymen. In the 19th and 20th centuries, the number of professional fields greatly expanded to include businesspeople, accountants, computer programmers, social workers, and people in all areas of health care, to name a few.

Strictly speaking, a profession is an area or field that has (1) a distinct field of knowledge requiring specialized training or education; (2) a full-time occupation, often defined and regulated by a peer organization; (3) an occupation that has a service orientation; and (4) a high degree of autonomy. Today an increasing number of occupations are considered professions. Phlebotomy became a profession when it moved from being a task or procedure of clinical laboratory personnel (Medical Laboratory Scientist and Medical Laboratory Technician/Clinical Laboratory Technician) to being performed by specialists, who are referred to today as *phlebotomists*.

Regardless of the definition of a profession, anyone can act professionally while conducting business or employment duties. In one regard, professionalism can be thought of as a state of mind. In this sense, acting as a professional encompasses how you look, act, communicate, and present yourself. For a phlebotomist, being well dressed and well groomed is one key to looking and acting professional, but looking good is only part of the picture. How you communicate with superiors, peers, and patients and their families is obviously very important to acting professionally. How you conduct yourself and handle adversity will further

> **BOX 11.2 Patient's Bill of Rights/ Partnership**
>
> - The patient has the right to high-quality hospital care.
> - The patient can expect a clean and safe environment.
> - The patient will be involved in their own care.
> - The patient's privacy will be protected.
> - The patient can expect help when leaving the hospital.
> - The patient can expect help with billing claims and procedures.

define whether you act professionally. Obviously, if you throw fits or temper tantrums, act defensively, and so forth, you are not acting as a professional.

One aspect of most professions is the incorporation of a pledge or code of ethics into their training. For example, physicians have the Hippocratic Oath. A profession's oath or creed does not have to be a formal one, but it should include a set of standards to abide by. As discussed in Chapter 1, the American Society for Clinical Laboratory Science (ASCLS) has published a pledge that can also be applied to phlebotomists; in summary, this pledge states that:
- Confidentiality will be maintained.
- Phlebotomists will "maintain and promote standards of excellence."
- Conduct will always be of a high standard.

Ethical or professional conduct in general also includes respect for patients and their rights, as outlined in the Patient Care Partnership. This replaced the American Hospital Association's Patient Bill of Rights in 2003 but ensures essentially the same thing. The Patient Care Partnership is available in an easy-to-read brochure from local hospitals or http://www.aha.org/aha/issues/Communicating-With-Patients/pt-care-partnership.html. Box 11.2 summarizes the key points of the Partnership.

Finally, another characteristic of a profession is the certification or credentialing of its members. Certification indicates that the individual has mastered the body of knowledge associated with the given profession. In addition, it gives employers some assurance that a potential employee has baseline skills and can more quickly become a productive member of the health care team. Box 11.3 lists the various organizations that offer certification examinations for phlebotomists, the

> ### BOX 11.3   Phlebotomy Certification Examination Options
>
> American Society for Clinical Pathologists (ASCP)*
> Phlebotomy Technician—PBT (ASCP)
> www.ascp.org
> (This is probably the most popular examination.)
> American Society of Phlebotomy Technicians (ASPT)
> Certified Phlebotomy Technician—CPT(ASPT)
> www.aspt.org
> National Phlebotomy Association (NPA)
> Certified Phlebotomy Technician—CPT(NPA)
> www.nationalphlebotomy.org
> National Healthcareer Association (NHA)
> Certified Phlebotomy Technician—CPT(NHA)
> www.nhanow.com
> American Medical Technologists
> Registered Phlebotomy Technician—RPT(AMT)
> americanmedtech.org/Phlebotomy-Technician

certification title, associated initials, and the organization's website.

CONTINUING EDUCATION

Once phlebotomists are credentialed and certified, they should not rest on their laurels. As defined earlier, a profession includes a distinct field of knowledge. Knowledge is not stagnant, and what is regarded as today's truth may be tomorrow's fiction. New theories, equipment, and methods are being discovered and tested every day on topics such as losing weight, treating patients and illness, and coping with stress. This is also true in phlebotomy; over the years, some examples of changes include the use of evacuated tubes instead of syringes, keeping the arm straight rather than bent after collecting a blood specimen, using blood transfer devices, and increasing use of plastic versus glass collection tubes.

Once you are credentialed and working, how do you learn about new techniques and changes in the field? Some learn by attending workshops, having in-service programs at their place of employment, or even hearing from sales representatives. This type of learning is known as *continuing education (CE)*.

CE is a very important aspect of professionalism. Physicians, lawyers, teachers, and those in many other professional groups participate in CE and are often required to accumulate a minimum number of CE credits in a given time period. (Generally, it takes 8 to 10 hours of contact time, depending on the organization, to earn one continuing education unit [CEU].) Once you are certified, some organizations, such as the ASCLS and the American Society of Phlebotomy Technicians, require accumulation of CEUs to maintain certification. Many other certification and credentialing organizations do not require CE, but they all strongly encourage it. In addition, the Joint Commission on Accreditation of Healthcare Organizations requires in-service training. Some CE applies to most professions. An example is the Health Insurance Portability and Accountability Act of 1996 (HIPAA). This is an act that outlines the steps and measures to be taken to ensure that confidential medical information is kept confidential; obviously, this is important to many groups.

Most of the previously mentioned organizations provide educational experiences for individuals to earn CEUs, such as workshops at local and national meetings, videoconferences/webinars, audio conferences, and self-instructional units. Other non-credentialing organizations, such as the American Association of Blood Banks and the American Association of Clinical Chemistry, offer CE that is recognized by the credentialing organizations. Still other organizations, such as the National Laboratory Training Network, American Society of Clinical Pathologists, and Area Health Education Center, provide continuing educational opportunities for laboratory personnel. The Mayo Medical Laboratories also offer workshops for phlebotomists.

As you can see, there is ample opportunity for phlebotomists to acquire CE. As a professional, you should want to continue your education and keep abreast of changes and new technologies in your field. In addition, not only should you attend your organization's CE offerings, but also you should become active in your organization. Volunteer to assist at workshops by organizing and scheduling speakers, rooms, or refreshments. Attend CE (you may not have a choice) and become active in the organization of your choice.

Finally, as discussed in Chapter 10, multi-skilling and cross-training are common. Some feel that phlebotomy-only technicians will soon be obsolete. Although this has yet to be borne out, there will always be a need for the well-trained, professional, and proficient phlebotomist.

SUMMARY

This chapter covered several topics under the general topic of professionalism. It is important to remember that often the phlebotomist is the "face" of the laboratory and the health care provider patients may encounter more than any other provider. Therefore it is critical to always act, speak, look, and perform as a professional.

CASE 11.1 Critical Thinking

You are returning to work after a day off. While you were off, a colleague, who usually collects blood only from outpatients, used your phlebotomy tray and left it in disarray. Luckily you came in a few minutes earlier than normal so you could restock and straighten out your tray before starting morning collections. When you get back to the laboratory, the colleague that used your tray the day before is collecting blood from an outpatient. You want to address the issue of using your tray. How should you approach the subject with your colleague?

CASE 11.2 Critical Thinking

When you are returning from afternoon rounds on the fourth floor, you overhear a doctor and nurse discussing a patient while you and some visitors are with them in the elevator. One statement you overhear is, "I can't wait until Mr. Jones gets discharged; he is such a needy patient!" What is wrong with this exchange and what should you do about it?

▮ REVIEW QUESTIONS

1. Activities such as maintaining one's health, self-evaluation, and decision making are examples of _____.

2. The ability to "walk in someone else's shoes" is known as _____.

3. When our background and environment are different from those with whom we communicate, this can be called a _____.

4. An occupation with a high degree of autonomy, service orientation, and specialized training is known as a _____.

5. _____ is an activity that is provided by most employers and professional organizations.

6. What are the key features of the Patient Care Partnership?

7. Why is continuing education important for a phlebotomist?

8. When communicating with a patient, what is the most important thing to keep in mind during this exchange?

BIBLIOGRAPHY

Adler RB, Rodman G, du Pre A. *Understanding Human Communication.* 14th. New York: Oxford University Press; 2019.

Donnelly E, Pavord E. *Communication and Interpersonal Skills (Health & Social Care).* 2nd. New York: Lantern Publishing; 2015.

Harwood J. *Understanding Communication and Aging: Developing Knowledge and Awareness.* 2nd Revised. San Diego: Cognella Academic; 2017.

Pease B, Pease A. *The Definitive Book of Body Language.* New York: Bantam; 2006.

12

Phlebotomy Department Management

Jeanne Gable

"Management—the art of juggling resources, people, and time."

Anonymous

OBJECTIVES

At the conclusion of this chapter, the student should be able to:
- Describe the role of the phlebotomy department.
- List key elements for a new-hire training and orientation program.
- Describe the layout of an outpatient draw station.

- Explain the need for an inpatient collection schedule.
- Explain the need for a Quality Improvement Program.
- Describe the responsibilities of managing a phlebotomy department.

OUTLINE

KEY TERMS

ambulatory
collection schedule
expenditures
operational plan

product review committee
quality assurance
quality control
revenues

INTRODUCTION

The purpose of this chapter is to give phlebotomy students a very brief introduction to managing a phlebotomy department. It is not intended to provide all the information needed for prospective managers nor the details behind the key functions of a manager such as budgeting. Several topics are also included in other chapters such as quality control (see Chapter 13) and equipment (see Chapter 5), but this chapter pulls them together as relevant to a manager. It is hoped that after reviewing this chapter a new phlebotomist will have an understanding of what goes on "behind the scenes."

ORGANIZATION

The phlebotomy department is the foundation of the clinical laboratory. The most skilled technician using the best equipment can produce reliable and valuable test results only if the specimens are from the correct patient and are properly collected, labeled, handled, and transported. Phlebotomists are also the face of the laboratory. Courtesy and professional treatment by the phlebotomy staff are critical to a positive patient experience. The phlebotomy department acts as a liaison among the laboratory and hospital departments, physicians, patients, and the public. Public opinion of the laboratory, hospital, clinic, and other medical services is often based on the treatment received from the phlebotomy department.

The phlebotomist's role is generally determined by the size of the facility. In large facilities the phlebotomist's role may only be specimen collection. In small to midsize facilities, the phlebotomist may also be involved with specimen processing for in-house and reference laboratory testing.

The manager of this department should possess all of the standard managerial training and skills. The manager monitors activity in the laboratory, schedules staff, ensures adequate inventory of supplies and equipment and is a link with the laboratory employees and other professionals in the laboratory, clinic, or hospital. They make decisions that will effectively and efficiently carry out phlebotomy duties while being committed to excellence in patient satisfaction. This individual should have special expertise in relating to people: communicating, listening, and adapting. Organizational skill is critical. Some technical skill, training, and understanding of laboratory tests have always been managerial assets especially if the department is responsible for processing specimens. Furthermore, budgeting and financial expertise is extremely important in these days of changing medical care payment systems.

TRAINING AND PROFESSIONAL ATTRIBUTES

Phlebotomy plays a major role in the diagnosis and treatment of diseases. Phlebotomy procedures must be performed by qualified and trained professionals. It is highly recommended that employed individuals have completed a phlebotomy program. These programs teach the technical aspects of phlebotomy and include safe practices and how to communicate with patients and medical staff. Some hospitals offer their own in-house training programs for phlebotomy. Look for a phlebotomist who is certified, if possible. Certification is proof of the technician's knowledge and skills.

Develop and institute an orientation and instruction program for new employees. The orientation provides an introduction to the department. Additionally, job performance expectations and the specific requirements related to their role and within the laboratory are formalized. The length of the orientation, content, and corresponding instruction will vary based on the job duties and the amount of previous experience. For instance, if the phlebotomist's only role is to collect specimens, the orientation may be only 1 to 2 weeks.

Additional duties such as receiving and ordering tests in a computer system or preparing and processing specimens will add additional time. Essential items that need to be covered in any orientation period are (1) safety policies; (2) organizational policies; (3) specimen collection and processing procedures; (4) infection control and prevention policies; and (5) computer training and use. The program should be longer, if necessary, to familiarize the employee with the methods, procedures, and general operating protocol of the department. A standard operating procedure manual should be provided, and employees should understand that uniformity is necessary. If less experienced phlebotomists are employed, the orientation and training period must be longer and more in depth.

A competency program to evaluate proficiency and performance should be in place. This program should consist of observing employees in their different settings to demonstrate they meet performance standards and expectations in the workplace. In addition to direct observation, a quiz may be given to determine competency in procedures that may be performed infrequently, and therefore, not easy to observe. The phlebotomist should expect an initial competency assessment and thereafter on an annual basis.

In addition to formal education and training, phlebotomists should possess the following professional attributes:
1. Professional appearance and behavior
2. Ability to relate well to people by showing concern and being courteous
3. Patience
4. Able to prioritize tasks
5. Ability to remain calm during emergencies
6. Flexibility
7. Willingness to adhere to the rules of the department
8. Accountability and responsibility
9. Ability to communicate effectively

PERSONAL PROTECTIVE EQUIPMENT

Personal protective equipment (PPE) is worn by phlebotomists and other health care workers to protect them from contact with infectious substances. PPE is mandated by the Occupational Safety and Health Administration (OSHA) for all health care professionals, including phlebotomists. The PPE used by phlebotomists may include face masks, nitrile gloves, eye goggles, face shields, laboratory coats, PPE gowns, coveralls, and respirators.

PPE provides a barrier against infection to protect the mucous membranes, airways, skin, and clothing of an individual. The prevalence of contagious respiratory infections has made it necessary to wear a surgical mask at all times within the health care setting. The masks are worn to protect health care workers from droplets generated by sneezing or coughing. Gloves must be clean, nonsterile, and worn at all times when collecting or handling blood and other body fluids, handling contaminated items, and touching nonintact skin or mucous membranes.

In certain situations, enhanced PPE precautions must be followed. This includes wearing an N95 mask, a face shield or goggles, and a disposable gown. Face shields and goggles are worn to protect the eyes, nose, and mouth from body fluid splashes. Disposable gowns protect from contamination and help prevent cross-infections. It is very important that adequate supplies of PPE are stocked, and all PPE is used and disposed of correctly according to hospital policies and procedures to protect the phlebotomist and prevent the spread of infections.

PLANNING

When planning a phlebotomy department, the following should be considered:
1. Number of patients to be served
2. Source of patients (such as hospital inpatients, outpatients, off-site locations)
3. Type of patients (such as age and whether the patient is in the hospital or ambulatory)
4. Location of the laboratory or laboratories to which specimens will be sent
5. Type of specimens the department will be collecting (blood, urine, specimen cultures from various sources, blood requiring special pretreatment or posttreatment, or other bodily excrements)
6. Responsibility associated with transporting specimens
7. Availability and type of computer system and how involved the department will be in its use—that is, who will be responsible for registering patients, billing, and ordering the laboratory studies

8. Responsibilities of the phlebotomist, including specimen processing for in-house and reference laboratory testing
9. Receipt and storage of stock supplies

The information necessary for these considerations can be obtained from the following sources:
1. Hospital administrators
2. Hospital statistics
3. Local or hospital-based physicians
4. Laboratory directors and department managers

OUTPATIENT COLLECTIONS LOCATION AND FACILITIES

The location and physical layout of the phlebotomy unit are important. The unit should be easily accessible to ambulatory patients from the central registration area and the outside entrance. The phlebotomy unit should have a reception area that is readily visible to people entering the unit. Test requisitions of ambulatory patients are reviewed in this area here, and all necessary patient information should be obtained and recorded. A computer system with the ability to order the laboratory tests and print labels is essential for this work. Ambulatory traffic through the unit is directed from this area. All telephone calls are received here and directed to the proper location.

The actual venipuncture area should be private and should contain a comfortable chair for the patient with an area on which to place either arm comfortably. The armrest areas should be at a comfortable height for the phlebotomist; most phlebotomy chairs have adjustable arms. The area should also be equipped with a wheelchair draw station and an infant draw station. Each area should be equipped with a help button or some other system of requesting assistance if needed. There should be adequate supplies neatly stored, as well as a sink, biohazard disposal, eye wash station, and sharps containers in each area. A location should be provided in each area to hang patients' coats.

The ideal phlebotomy drawing station has a place where the patient can lie down if needed, such as a bed with rails or a reclining phlebotomy chair. If each individual area cannot be equipped with a place for the patient to lie down, there must be at least one centrally located private space for (1) patients undergoing a blood test that requires rest before the specimen is collected or (2) patients who have a history of or experience adverse reactions to venipuncture, such as syncope or dizziness. All venipuncture drawing stations should promote patient dignity and privacy through the use of screens or curtains at the entrance of the station and sound insulation between stations to allow private discussions and minimize noise from carrying.

Licensed medical personnel should be available in the event the patient has an adverse reaction such as seizure or fainting. Adverse reactions should always be documented following the facility's policies.

Restrooms should be adequate, meet the requirements of the Americans with Disabilities Act, and be located in close proximity to the venipuncture areas. Each restroom must be equipped with some type of emergency call system. Convenient and secure shelf space should be provided for containers and other equipment used before and after collecting the specimen.

It is often advantageous to have the patient collect a urine specimen while waiting for the phlebotomist to perform the venipuncture procedure. The urine container should be properly labeled when it is given to the patient; this includes labeling the cup and not the container lid. To prevent embarrassment, provide a place where the patient may leave the labeled specimen before returning to the waiting room. This should be convenient to the restrooms and venipuncture areas.

INPATIENT COLLECTIONS
COLLECTION SCHEDULES

A collection schedule must be developed for the institution. There are no two hospitals that function exactly alike. The number of patients and the time projected to complete the procedure per patient are not the same in each facility. The expected draw per hour and turnaround time factor into what time collections begin and end. Adult acute hospital patient needs differ from a cancer center, which differs from a pediatric hospital. The physical layout of each facility may impact the collection schedule, especially if there is no pneumatic tube system and the phlebotomists must transport specimens back to the laboratory. The schedule may need to be varied on days when special procedures are being performed.

A specified time for early morning specimen collection (that is, morning rounds or sweep) is required in all hospitals. During this time, routine, fasting, and presurgical specimens are collected by the phlebotomists. Turnaround time of inpatient blood collection is very important. If results are not back in time for physician rounds, there may be delays in patient management and increased length of stays. The collection schedule and the number of employees involved varies, depending on the following:

1. The number of patients who require blood draws
2. When the clinicians need the results
3. Types of patients (infants, children, geriatric, and intensive care patients usually take longer and are more difficult)

The morning collection usually starts between 4:00 AM and 7:00 AM. Phlebotomy carts should be stocked and ready for the morning shift when phlebotomists arrive, and any devices should be fully charged. The phlebotomists should be prepared to immediately start drawing patients.

Several other collection times are typically scheduled throughout the day to help with the organization of the work. Three to four other scheduled collection times (or phlebotomy rounds or sweeps) are recommended: midmorning, midafternoon, and early and late evening. The times chosen for scheduled rounds are determined by the routines of the other departments involved in patient care and the laboratory performing the test. The collection time schedule should be strictly adhered to by all departments involved. Many intradepartmental phone calls and STAT ordered tests can be prevented when there is a set collection time.

PROCESSING REQUESTS

The task of processing requests depends on the computer software system used to create, access, and receive them in the laboratory. The processing procedure in your department should be such that the requests are promptly sorted and allocated to ensure timely and proper attention. In most hospitals, orders are entered into a computer system. Collection lists are then created for the phlebotomy rounds. Each collection has an order cut-off time, which is the latest time orders may be placed for that specific round. If an order is placed after the stated cut-off, the laboratory will not have knowledge of the request, and it will default to the next

collection round. If the cut-off is missed, and the round has not yet begun, a preprinted laboratory label or manual requisition may be placed on the phlebotomy clipboard before the phlebotomist arrives to the unit, depending on protocol. This is less likely as many hospital laboratories are moving toward assigning inpatient phlebotomists a handheld device that can be taken into the patient's room. A scanning device can be used to verify a patient's identity, view collection instructions and tube types, and print labels. With the use of these devices, any missed orders will default to the next round, which allows for better tracking of the specimen and is a better indicator of turnaround time from collection to results.

STAT and other special collection requests are a big part of everyday work. It is impossible to predict how many requests there will be or when these requests will be received. Each shift should have a "team leader" to track when phlebotomists finish their assigned rounds and assign them to help other phlebotomists or address STAT requests. A satisfactory system for responding to STATs will be unique to each department. It is preferable that the person or persons who should respond to STATs must be decided before, *not* after, the STAT request is received. It is imperative to distribute the STAT assignments as equitably as possible. Special and timed collections can be integrated into the routine collections when possible.

Some hospitals require nurses on the units to draw STAT and timed tests. It is the responsibility of the phlebotomy department team leader or assigned staff to monitor these collections and remind the nurses if not done.

▎MOBILE PHLEBOTOMY

Mobile phlebotomists travel to various locations, such as facilities and patients' homes, to draw blood samples and collect nonblood specimens for laboratory analysis. Mobile phlebotomy services are convenient for nursing facilities, mental health facilities, or other facilities that sometimes have difficulty or are unable to take residents to the hospital or other outpatient draw sites. House calls are made by mobile phlebotomists for those with chronic illnesses, people who are physically challenged, the elderly, and the immunocompromised. The specimens are transported by the phlebotomist to the hospital for processing. Mobile phlebotomy daily schedules may vary so employees must be flexible, adaptable to changes in their environment, professional, and very organized.

STAFFING

The staffing pattern is different for each facility based on the responsibilities of the department. To make this determination, the following factors should be considered:

1. Number and location of patients
2. Types of patients—that is, ambulatory patients or inpatients (for inpatients, the time required to reach their room or to go from room to room must be considered. Even in regular rooms, the problems that the phlebotomist encounters in accessing the patient because of the arrangement of furniture, equipment in use, and the presence of visitors should be considered. Children, older adult patients, and burned or trauma patients may also require more time.)
3. Number of patients requiring enhanced precautions (donning and doffing PPE adds time to each venipuncture when going to isolation rooms and the intensive care unit)
4. Amount of work that can be done at scheduled collection times
5. Number of STAT or special collections that are required
6. Hours of operation (consider whether the department offers 24-hour coverage or has another department cover evening and night hours)
7. Size of the emergency department, trauma unit, and other specific patient units (in some hospitals, one or more of these units may be large enough to warrant dedicated staff)
8. Duties other than collecting specimens (that is, transporting, logging-in, centrifuging specimens, and preparing specimens to be picked up or mailed)

Experience has proven that it is most efficient to have a core of full-time employees to cover the basic needs and a staff of part-time employees for peak hours and other times of staff shortages. The manager should aim to schedule enough phlebotomists to efficiently and properly handle the workload. It is important for the manager to be realistic when allotting time that is required to collect specimens, and therefore, align the number of phlebotomists to the demand for collections at each scheduled round.

OPERATIONAL PLAN

The hospital or clinic will have general goals with which you will be expected to identify, but it is important to develop specific goals and objectives to manage an efficient and successful department. The primary goal of every phlebotomy department is to contribute to optimal patient care by obtaining proper specimens for the test that is requested by the physician. This means that specimens must be collected from the proper patient, at the correct time, using the proper technique. All specimens must be labeled correctly and transported in a timely manner to the testing department. Therefore carefully established procedures and processes need to be in place to coordinate and accomplish the initial requests through the specimen collection.

Occasionally, reorganization of a well-functioning operational plan will be necessary to accommodate changes in the hospital, laboratory, or phlebotomy department. It is recommended that all departments review the proposed changes for possible conflicts. If any conflicts arise, resolve them before instituting the change. Provide all departments with the necessary facts of the change and when it will become effective, and distribute this information in writing.

It is important that all staff members feel that they are part of a team and work as such. This necessitates that each department understand and respect the work requirements of others. Regular meetings with managers or representatives from all departments are recommended. The requirements of the procedures in each department should be discussed. When there are conflicts, reasons why changes can or cannot be made should be presented. Departments must work together to reach solutions that allow each department to organize its work satisfactorily. If phlebotomists are honest about the needs and willing to be flexible, others will usually follow this example, and a mutually satisfactory work organization can be developed.

Lastly, a manager should explain to the employees the reasons for any compromises either by your department or by others. This will develop a good rapport among all departments. This approach helps create an understanding and respect for the employees and needs of all departments, yours included.

EQUIPMENT MANAGEMENT

The equipment, both consumable and nonconsumable, used in the phlebotomy department should be chosen carefully. The decision regarding what collection equipment is purchased and used should be made in cooperation with the phlebotomists and your facility's product review committee in line with budget considerations. All equipment should be monitored and records kept so equipment can be evaluated and changed or updated if indicated.

CONSUMABLE EQUIPMENT

Consumable equipment consists of items that have a one-time or limited use. Consumables should be chosen carefully after the unit manager and the phlebotomists have used them and discussed their advantages and disadvantages. It is recommended to choose only one kind of equipment because the greater the variety of equipment, the more complex and riskier the procedure becomes, disallowing the phlebotomist to gain expertise in its use. For example, each needle manufacturer has a different system for securing the needle after the draw. Using one brand of needle creates a comfortable repetition and ease of use. Using different brands of needles may be awkward because the phlebotomist's movements are less smooth and sure, making a needle stick injury more likely. Uniformity of equipment is also economical, space saving, and important to the operation of the department. It is recommended that you do not buy based on price alone. Stock the various sizes that you need from the same manufacturer whenever possible. See Box 12.1 for a list of expendables.

Storage space is often a problem. All products are dated, and the unit should have approximately a 2- to 3-week supply on hand. Determine from statistics and operating experience what the yearly need will be. Rotate stock to ensure that the oldest stock is used before its expiration date. An employee should be assigned to check expiration dates on a monthly basis.

NONCONSUMABLE EQUIPMENT

Nonconsumable equipment should be evaluated carefully before purchasing and while in use. Consider the following:
1. How well it meets your needs

BOX 12.1   Examples of Consumable Equipment

- Needles
- Syringes
- Lancets

- Tubes
- Tourniquets
- Alcohol, alcohol pads
- Povidone-iodine swabs
- Adhesive tape

- Adhesive bandages
- Glass slides
- Gloves
- Face masks
- Biohazard and sharps containers
- Labeling pens
- Special labels and precautions
- Puncture site warmers
- Gauze, sterile pads

BOX 12.2   Examples of Nonconsumable Equipment

- Collection trays or carts
- Venipuncture chairs
- Beds or other reclining surfaces
- Utility carts and cabinets
- Refrigerators
- File cabinets
- Printers

- Blood pressure cuffs
- Racks for tubes
- Beepers or communication system
- Computer
- Centrifuges
- Stopwatches
- Fax machines

---

2. Accuracy
3. Safety features, if required
4. Reproducibility
5. Ease of operation
6. Ease of maintenance
7. Available service

Nonconsumable equipment consists of items that are repeatedly used and not immediately disposed. Collection trays or wheeled carts are a necessity and, if possible, each phlebotomist should have their own. The volume of specimens to be collected and the space in which they are used and stored must be considered when selecting the size and shape of the trays. The construction and weight of the tray is also an important consideration. It is important to see the equipment demonstrated and, when possible, to obtain opinions from other users. See Box 12.2 for a list of nonconsumable equipment that may be needed for a phlebotomy unit.

MAINTAINING QUALITY

QUALITY IMPROVEMENT

Practical and useful systems for monitoring the safety, quality control, and quality assurance programs of the department should be established. Such monitoring can point out weak areas in planning and organizing, as well as the progress and successes of the department. When developing a quality plan for your department, it is imperative to ask staff for their input, explain why the indicators are being monitored, and share the data with the department.

Items that can be monitored for quality assurance are specimen rejection rates, response time for STAT collections, proper patient identification, and patient satisfaction. Benchmarks need to be established, and corrective actions need to be taken if a benchmark is not met.

Be sure to commend staff members when results are good, and thoroughly discuss any indicated improvement when results are less than acceptable. There is a more extensive discussion of quality in Chapter 13.

CONTINUING EDUCATION

As discussed in Chapter 11, a system of continuing education should also be developed and implemented. Information should be made available to employees about advances in the areas of health care in which they are involved. Encourage them also to become familiar with developments in other areas of health care. Encourage attendance at seminars and workshops by providing financial aid and an equitable distribution of opportunity. It is expected that a manager will attend seminars and workshops and keep informed of advances in the field.

COMMUNICATION

When you meet with other department managers to discuss new techniques or problems, take a representative from your department with you. Your staff members are often more aware of conflicts with their work than you are. Including them also strengthens team effort.

Have formal, documented in-service programs for all changes in techniques, supplies, or work routines. Encourage questions and discussion to prevent misunderstandings. Regular department meetings should be conducted to share any information about the department or issues that might affect the department operations. Encourage employees to share any information, problems, or concerns they might have about the department. In this way, you can proactively address potential problems and issues leading, ideally, to a well-functioning department.

EMPLOYEE PERFORMANCE AND REVIEW

Develop job descriptions and, when possible, create position levels. The levels may be based on responsibilities, education, kind of work, and so on. This provides management with a basis for recognizing exceptional employee performance and provides employees with clear expectations and goal setting. Any issue with employee performance should be periodically addressed and discussed and not held until the performance review.

Keep complete and accurate records of the performance of each employee, and discuss all entries with them. Performances that meet or exceed expectations should be commended and encouragement given. The reason for a less-than-satisfactory performance should be clarified and help offered to correct the problem. These records should be maintained for the duration of employment and retained for the periods dictated by law. Usually, the personnel department will have guidelines for records retention.

BUDGETING

Budgeting, which is a part of every manager's responsibility, is a way of putting a dollar value on your plans. Anticipated revenues, the amount of money collected or brought into a department as a result of sales or services provided, and expenditures, the cost of doing business, are closely monitored by laboratory managers. Hopefully, the revenues are larger than the expenditures; if not, there may be a need to cut costs or raise revenue. Revenues and expenditures are determined by considering the following:

1. Volume of work (revenue generator)
2. Wages and benefits (expenditure)
3. Materials (expenditure)
4. Equipment (expenditure)
5. Historical records (used to predict future revenue and expenditure)

6. Future plans (used in conjunction with historical records to predict future revenue and expenditure)
7. Outside services (may be an expenditure or revenue generator)

SUMMARY

Obviously, there are multiple volumes of books and educational programs on management and budgeting. The preceding brief overview discussion pertains to phlebotomy units that are part of a hospital or clinic; the details vary depending on the size and type of institution. A phlebotomy unit that is not within a hospital or clinic will require the same basic management, although there will be fewer departments with which to coordinate your work. Usually there will be less variety of specimens collected and fewer STAT requests. It will be necessary to have a plan to care for patients who become ill or have adverse reactions. Staffing and scheduling will be based on the needs of the off-site unit. Supplies should be readily available. Otherwise, the rules and requirements remain the same as those within a facility. Employees will still need orientation, training, and evaluations. There will be goals and expectations that must be managed no matter the location of the phlebotomy unit.

CASE 12.1 Critical Thinking

You have been instructed to create a Quality Improvement Program for your department. What steps should be taken to develop the program? List three indicators that can be used.

CASE 12.2 Critical Thinking

You are planning an outpatient collection station in your facility. Where should this be located and how would you design the area?

REVIEW QUESTIONS

1. True or false: The public's opinion of the clinical laboratory is often based on their treatment by the phlebotomy department: _____
2. How may a computer system be used in phlebotomy units? _____

3. What is a consideration when planning a phlebotomy department? _____
4. List several expenditures that may calculate into a budget: _____

BIBLIOGRAPHY

Barker K. *At the Helm: Leading Your Laboratory.* 2nd ed. Seattle: Cold Spring Harbor Laboratory Press; 2010.

Varnadoe L. *Medical Laboratory Management and Supervision.* 2nd ed. Upper Saddle River, NJ: Priority Ed; 2008.
1. Harmening DM. In: *Laboratory Management: Principles and Processes.* 4th ed. DH Publishing; 2020.

Total Quality in Phlebotomy Service

*Linda R. Rehfuss**

"Quality is never an accident; it is always the result of intelligent effort."
—*John Ruskin (1819–1900)*

OBJECTIVES

At the conclusion of this chapter, the student should be able to:
- Define:
  - Quality
  - Quality control
  - Quality assurance
  - Quality improvemen

- Explain the importance of a well-defined quality program.
- List preanalytical errors associated with phlebotomy.
- Discuss the importance of a procedure manual.
- Explain the role of the phlebotomist in the quality of phlebotomy service.

OUTLINE

* The author gratefully acknowledges the previous contributions of Mary P. Nix on which portions of this chapter are based.

KEY TERMS

corrective action

indicators

postanalytical

preanalytical

quality

quality assurance (QA)

quality control (QC)

quality improvement (QI)

thresholds

INTRODUCTION

Quality is a core business strategy, regardless of the industry. The health care industry adopted formal **quality assurance (QA)** policies and monitoring practices in the latter part of the 20th century when it became clear that the science and statistics of quality used in other industries could be applied. When managed care and capitation (a set fee per procedure or patient) emerged, health care shifted its focus from ensuring quality to continuously improving it, applying further what other industries had learned from their efforts to achieve perfection and reduce costs.

Currently, from a scientific perspective, health care in the United States is cutting edge and top notch. However, delivery of and access to patient care are not of the same caliber. A 1998 RAND report and a 1999 report from the Institute of Medicine (IOM) supplied convincing evidence that health outcomes in the United States could be improved. RAND discovered a large gap between the care that patients should receive and the care that they do receive, noting that the gap was applicable to overuse and underuse of services. The IOM report placed medical error and patient safety in the spotlight, estimating a negative effect of medical errors on health care quality and patient outcomes.

A second IOM report, in 2001, presented strategies for improving the quality of care delivered to patients and their access to it. As a result of that report, the U.S. Agency for Healthcare Quality and Research was charged with leading the health care industry in improving the quality of care provided, including patient safety, and identifying ways to improve access to health services.

Currently, the health care industry in the United States is involved in major initiatives to raise the caliber of service provided and to make needed care available to every citizen.

The purpose of this chapter is to provide an orientation to quality; to present the principles of **quality control (QC)**, QA, and **quality improvement (QI)**; and to apply them to phlebotomy.

QUALITY: DEFINITION AND PRINCIPLES

What is quality? To strive for quality, it is important to know what it is. **Quality** is best defined as a degree of excellence. This definition tends to be most applicable not only to businesses but also to societal issues.

The principles of quality in business lie in fact and perception. Doing the right thing, doing it the right way, doing it right the first time, and doing it on time are the facts of quality. These facts of quality, when applied to the health care setting, are often driven by outside agencies, both governmental (such as the Food and Drug Administration [FDA]) and voluntary accrediting agencies (such as the Joint Commission).

Quality begins with the recipient. The laboratory's customers can include coworkers, physicians, and patients. The customer is why we are here. Quality occurs when we meet or exceed the customer's expectations. The perceptions of quality include delivering the right product; satisfying the customer's needs; meeting the customer's expectations; and treating every customer with integrity, courtesy, and respect. Ultimately in health care, it is the patient who evaluates and drives quality. Even if the facts of quality are met, will they alone be enough to attract and retain customers?

Achieving balance between the facts and perceptions of quality requires constant adjusting. Xerox, FedEx, Southwest Airlines, and Motorola are examples of quality, award-winning companies. These and others serve as role models for health care–oriented businesses.

Refer to Box 13.1 for a snapshot of the facts and perceptions of quality.

QUALITY APPLIED TO HEALTH CARE

Technology today provides consumer access to a wealth of information about health care services, organizations and practitioners providing those services, and standards governing practices of the overall industry. Health care organizations have responded to this increased consumer awareness by implementing ways to ensure quality patient care by identifying and reducing patient and employee risks in their policies and practices. These ongoing practices, known as *QI*, are further reinforced by national standard and regulatory agencies, such as The Joint Commission (formerly the Joint Commission on Accreditation of Health Care Organizations [JCAHO]), College of American Pathologists (CAP), Clinical Laboratory Improvement Amendments of 1988 (CLIA '88), and the Clinical Laboratory Standards Institute (CLSI) (formerly the National Committee for Clinical Laboratory Standards [NCCLS]).

Phlebotomists, like other health care professionals, must focus on processes that allow continuous improvements in the quality of services that they provide to patients. The processes concentrate on evaluation of the frequency of hematomas, specimen hemolysis, and redraw and recollection rates resulting from specimen contamination. Minimizing these negative phlebotomy outcomes can reduce health care costs and be extremely beneficial to quality patient care.

A widely accepted definition of *quality of health care*, formulated by IOM, is "the degree to which health services for individuals and populations increase the likelihood of desired health outcomes and are consistent with current professional knowledge." A health outcome is the health state of a patient resulting from health care. Examples of outcomes include adverse outcomes (e.g., an injury caused by a medical treatment such as perforation of a viscus during surgery); clinical outcomes (e.g., serum cholesterol level [a marker for coronary artery disease], change in symptoms, or mortality); and functional status (a measure of an individual's ability to perform normal activities of life). Quality measures and equations (i.e., ways to quantify health outcomes) have been and are being developed. These measures assess the degree of accomplishment of desired health objectives by a clinician or health care organization.

Most health care organizations use a combination of quality measurements to ensure quality care for patients. A Quality Management System (QMS) is developed to organize and direct quality. The first step in organizing a QMS is to determine the evaluation system that will be used. The CLSI has 12 quality system essentials that can be used to establish an evaluation system for laboratory QMS. Refer to Box 13.2 for a list of the 12 laboratory quality system essentials.

QUALITY CONTROL

Clinical laboratory scientists performed quality work and provided quality results long before the term *QA* became popular. How? By performing QC. **QC** is the process that validates final results and quantifies variations. When a test (such as serum glucose) is performed on a patient specimen, control samples representing high, low, and normal results are also tested. Decisions about the reportability of the patient's results are made based on a comparison with the results of the control testing. QC enables laboratory scientists to confidently report accurate and reproducible test results. In phlebotomy, QC relates to ensuring that correct criteria for specimen integrity are met. These include heating or icing specimens, determining that patient preparation is appropriate (such as fasting for glucose tolerance test), and accuracy of timed draws.

Because most clinical laboratory practitioners have a close association with quality, why the increased attention to ensuring it? In addition to economic survival, the pressures of external forces such as accrediting agencies, government regulations, and the public have increased. Since the mid- to late 1980s, every health care organization has been striving to provide high-quality,

BOX 13.2   **The 12 Laboratory Quality System Essentials**

I. The Laboratory
  A. Organization (Quality System Essential [QSE] 1)
    a. Personnel roles and responsibilities
    b. Quality planning and risk management
    c. Review and assessment of goals
  B. Facilities and Safety (QSE 2)
    a. Design/layout of laboratory
    b. Adequate storage space and work space
    c. Required safety equipment availability
    d. Safety training
  C. Personnel (QSE 3)
    a. Qualifications
    b. Job descriptions
    c. Orientation
    d. Competency assessment
    e. Continuing education
  D. Equipment (QSE 4)
    a. Selection criteria
    b. Ongoing maintenance
    c. Service and repair records
  E. Purchasing and Inventory (QSE 5)
    a. Laboratory supplies available
    b. Service contracts
    c. Inventory
II. The Work System
  A. Process Control (QSE 6)
    a. Identification of all processes
    b. Procedure manuals
    c. Test method verification
    d. Quality control and statistics
  B. Documents and Records (QSE 7)
    a. Availability of all documents
    b. Periodic review of all documents
    c. Access to quality control records
    d. Record of storage and retention monitoring
  C. Information Management (QSE 8)
    a. Patient record availability
    b. Patient record security
    c. Patient information methods
    d. Prevention of Medicare and Medicaid fraud
III. Measurement QSEs
  A. Occurrence Management (QSE 9)
    a. Event management
    b. Identification of all events
    c. Reporting of all events
    d. Actions taken in response to events
    e. System in place to reduce future events
    f. Introduction of changes
  B. Assessment: Internal and External (QSE 10)
    a. Licensing and accreditation
    b. External proficiency testing
    c. On-going auditing by accrediting agencies
    d. Development of quality measurements for all phases of testing
  C. Customer Service (QSE 11)
    a. Feedback from customers
    b. Feedback from employees
    c. Feedback from offsite customers
  D. Process Improvement (QSE 12)
    a. Monitoring all QSEs
    b. Root cause analysis

cost-effective patient care. What has changed over the years is the increased emphasis on customer satisfaction and, more recently, the issues of health outcome and patient safety.

QUALITY ASSURANCE

QA, to the health care practitioner, is the process of ensuring that standards of care have been maintained. The use of laboratory tests to diagnose disease and monitor treatments has significantly increased over time, resulting in a proportionate increase in the importance of ensuring overall laboratory quality. QA takes on a broad view, unlike QC, which is specific (e.g., test or product related). Ensuring quality in the laboratory means assessing the entire department's

operation to identify areas of weakness and those of strength. QA involves all aspects of the process, including nonanalytical factors (phlebotomy) and analytical (testing). To accomplish quality, **indicators** (that is, specific, measurable variables) and **thresholds** (that is, points or values prompting study of an aspect of care) are established, data are collected and analyzed, **corrective action** is taken, the effectiveness of the corrective action is monitored, and information is reported to the appropriate personnel. All laboratories, no matter how small, must have a QA program as required by CLIA.

QC then becomes a part of a QA program. It is possible to have QC without having a QA program; this is how laboratories operated for many years. However, it is not possible to have a QA program without QC.

QUALITY IMPROVEMENT

QI is the constant search for ways to improve product, service, and performance. QI is sometimes referred to as *continuous quality improvement.* When QA and QC imply a problem, QI procedures can be used to determine the cause and develop a plan of improvement. This can be seen in examples such as making health care services easier to access or friendlier, as in one-stop shopping. The transition to safer products, such as latex-free tourniquets and gloves, and safer medical devices, such as needles designed to prevent needlestick injuries, are additional examples of searching for excellence (quality). Consider also the use of barcode labels in the laboratory to increase efficiency and reliability.

A major component of QI is performance, such as the phlebotomist's responsiveness to patients' concerns, satisfaction, and the quality of care given. There is a continuous effort to heighten phlebotomists' awareness and sensitivity through various mechanisms, such as feedback from patient surveys and continuing education programs, as discussed in Chapter 11. All employees should also undergo periodic performance review. This gives the supervisor the opportunity to review the overall performance of the phlebotomist and set goals and objectives for the next review period (generally a year). Of course, if there is an immediate concern, it should be addressed with the employee as soon as possible and not withheld for the periodic review.

A well-directed quality program will enable one to see the components of an operation that need to be corrected to meet and adhere to the standards of care. Just as important, a well-directed program enables one to see the components of an operation that are already high in quality, efficient, and cost-effective (that is, not requiring corrective action). Many times, the need to improve an aspect of care for one section of a health care facility requires interdepartmental involvement and teamwork. Anticipated benefits from this type of activity are significant improvement in the quality of care delivered by that facility and increased satisfaction.

The following quality tools can be found in a facility that has an effective quality management program as its focus:

1. Information important to decision making is communicated (usually by memorandum, newsletter, staff meetings, or logbook).

2. Orientation and training are well structured and consistently and efficiently implemented and evaluated (not too long, not too short, and with checklists pertaining to important aspects of the job).
3. Continuing education is strongly encouraged and, ideally, provided.
4. Respect and care for all are promoted through cultural and diversity awareness.
5. Performance is monitored by supervisory personnel and compared with standards (not with the performance of coworkers), and appraisals are conducted.
6. Standard operating procedure (SOP) manuals are up to date, written by supervisory personnel citing accrediting and governing agencies' regulations when necessary, reviewed by the director annually, and used as a reference for all employees.
7. Each employee has a personnel file on record containing items of no surprise to the employee (e.g., job description, performance evaluations, counseling documentation, letters of commendation).
8. Proficiency and competency tests are distributed to the staff on a rotational basis or given to all staff when sufficient quantity exists to do so.
9. Individual participation in scheduled quality activities is included in the job description.
10. Equipment and instruments are calibrated, maintained, and serviced as scheduled.
11. Computer systems are validated before use and monitored thereafter.
12. The workplace and environment are safe.
13. Department leaders actively seek suggestions and communicate objectives.
14. Documentation of all these items is expected (Box 13.3).

Additional information about these items can be found in Chapters 11 and 12. As you may be able to see, QI expands on the foundations of QC and QA, needs to be organization-wide, seems daunting at times, and is inevitably never ending.

FACTS OF QUALITY IN PHLEBOTOMY SERVICE

Performing the right type of phlebotomy (venipuncture vs. skin puncture), doing it the right way (that is, per procedure), doing it correctly the first time, and doing it

BOX 13.3   **Tools for Quality Improvement**

1. Active two-way communication
2. Well-structured orientation and training
3. Periodic continuing education
4. Promotion of respect and caring
5. Monitored and appraised performance
6. Standard operating procedure manuals
7. Accurate personnel file
8. Periodic proficiency or competency testing
9. Participation in quality control and quality assurance activities
10. Properly functioning and maintained equipment and supplies
11. Validated and monitored computer systems
12. Safe work environment
13. Leaders who seek suggestions
14. Documentation

on time are the facts of quality in phlebotomy. Many of these facts have already been detailed elsewhere in this textbook. Adhering to these procedures is one step toward quality patient care.

These facts of quality phlebotomy are paramount to providing a valid test result. Phlebotomy is one component of the **preanalytical**, and first phase, of clinical laboratory work. The preanalytical phase also includes transportation, handling, and accessioning of the specimen. (The analytical [testing the specimen] and **postanalytical** [reporting the result] phases are the second and third phases of laboratory work, respectively.) Having quality technicians or technologists, quality procedures, and quality instrumentation means little if the specimen received in the laboratory is of poor quality. Specimens of low quality can produce inaccurate and potentially dangerous results. Indeed, many errors in laboratory medicine occur in the preanalytical phase.

Examples of preanalytical errors related to phlebotomy include the following:

- Hemolyzed sample
- Insufficient sample
- Incorrect sample
- Clotted sample
- Incorrect preparation of the patient (such as fasting)
- Incorrect identification
- Lack of signature on tube, when appropriate
- Empty tube
- Sample not on ice
- Sample not protected from light

Preanalytical errors can have a negative and possibly expensive outcome on patient care. The wrong treatment may be administered, the wrong patient may be treated, the wrong dosage may be given, the wrong blood type may be transfused, and patient death may even occur as a consequence of an improperly collected specimen. It is crucial that phlebotomists know and understand their critical role in laboratory testing as a major part of providing quality patient care.

Obviously, both the patient and the health care facility want to avoid these situations. Phlebotomists directly affect these preanalytic variables and should strive for quality in their work so that these negative outcomes can be avoided.

Interestingly, four phlebotomy errors have been identified as indefensible in a court of law: patient misidentification, improper angle of insertion, improper vein selection, and ineffective training and evaluation of those performing venipunctures. These errors relate to "doing it the right way, every time." As increased consumer awareness has led to an increase in lawsuits within the health care industry, phlebotomists, as with other health care providers, can be held legally responsible for their actions. (Chapter 14 covers medical-legal issues in phlebotomy.)

Because blood and other body fluids begin to change immediately after collection from the body, the specimen collector should be trained to take steps that will minimize these changes. These steps include the following:

1. Using and referring to clearly written procedures
2. Ensuring the completeness and accuracy of information on requisition forms
3. Using the correct collection technique and tube types
4. Meeting all specimen and labeling requirements
5. Transporting the specimen to the laboratory according to procedure

THE PROCEDURE MANUAL FOR SPECIMEN COLLECTION

The laboratory that performs the tests is responsible for preparing the procedure manuals and other important information regarding procurement of blood or body fluid specimens. The CLSI provides a template for

BOX 13.4   Specimen Collection Manual: Contents Useful in Ensuring Quality Specimens

1. The following should be included for each test:
   a. Test name and alternative names
   b. Patient preparation
   c. Type of specimen
   d. Timing requirements
   e. Type of tube or container
   f. Transportation requirements
   g. Labeling requirements
   h. Test requisition form or code
   i. Name and telephone number of laboratory
2. Criteria for unacceptable specimens
3. Steps for handling inability to collect specimen
4. Requirements for acceptable newborn or pediatric samples

organizing the content necessary for procedure manuals, and accrediting agencies such as the CAP and The Joint Commission require annual updating of procedure manuals. Information in the procedure manuals should be provided to every health care professional involved in the phlebotomy process. Adherence to these steps ensures that the specimen, and ultimately the test result, will be an accurate reflection of the patient's condition and lead to a positive patient outcome.

The most important step in ensuring quality phlebotomy is using and referring to the procedures that describe, outline, and detail specimen collection. Box 13.4 summarizes the contents of specimen collection manuals useful in ensuring quality blood specimens.

Professionals are not expected to remember all the details in the procedure manual. However, they should know its general content, know where to readily locate it, and remember that the manual exists for their reference. It contains answers for most specimen-related questions and should be used when the patient's life is not in jeopardy.

Most phlebotomy errors occur because SOPs are not followed. After the training period, when a question comes to mind, the specimen collection manual should be consulted for the answer. In the hospital setting, all nursing units should have a specimen collection manual because nurses, medical students, and physicians sometimes procure specimens. Therefore the manual should be accessible to them, as well as to the phlebotomist, at all times. The laboratory supervisor should be contacted when the procedure is unclear, thought to be outdated, or difficult to find. Computer systems might allow the manual to be provided online and to be searchable so that questions can be quickly answered.

Each test performed in the laboratory is addressed in the specimen collection manual. The test name, including alternative names, notes on how to prepare the patient for the test (e.g., fasting), the type of preferred specimen (e.g., venous), notes on timing requirements (e.g., for glucose tolerance tests), and the type of container in which to collect the specimen (e.g., an ethylenediaminetetraacetate Vacutainer tube) should be included. Specimen transportation requirements emphasizing the effects of time, temperature, exposure to light, and excessive vibration or rough handling can be found in this manual. Adherence to these requirements is critical to certain tests (such as bilirubin). Adherence to specimen labeling requirements is also critical for some tests, especially those performed by the blood bank; therefore labeling procedures are included in the specimen collection manual. Fig. 13.1, a sample page from an existing manual, illustrates many of these items.

The appropriate test requisition form and the name of the laboratory performing the test can be found in the manual, along with the laboratory's telephone number. Interestingly, the test requisition form may be another, more practical source of specimen collection information. As shown in Fig. 13.2, many of the items found in the collection manual are also found on the test requisition form. In a computerized facility, where computer-generated labels are used in lieu of paper requisitions, this information can be found on the computer label.

Unacceptable Specimens

Some specimen collection manuals include, for each test, the criteria for an unacceptable specimen. Improper collection procedures can significantly increase error in laboratory testing. Collection-related error is the most common cause of invalid laboratory results. Specimen rejection may occur, for example, when (1) labeling is inadequate or improper; (2) collection is not timely (such as within a certain

TEST	SPECIMEN INSTRUCTIONS	HP*	REFERENCE RANGE	CODE	FEE
BETA-SUBUNIT PREGNANCY TESTS-See HCG listings.					
BETA-2 MICROGLOBULIN, SERUM	3 mL blood, red top tube.		20-39 yr: 0-2.0 mg/L 40-59 yr: 0-2.6 60-79 yr: 0-3.1	B2M	64.00
BETA-2 MICROGLOBULIN, URINE (Referral Lab)	10 mL urine, random specimen.		5-154 mcg/L	B2UR	32.00
BILIRUBIN, TOTAL AND DIRECT	2 mL blood, red top tube.		Total: 0.2-1.2 mg/dL Direct: 0.0-0.4	BIL	37.00
BILIRUBIN, TOTAL MICRO (NEONATAL BILIRUBIN)	Blood; 1 red or green Microtainer. Protect from light.			MBL	84.00
BIOPSY-See Surgical Pathology.					
BLASTOMYOCOSIS ANTIBODY	5 mL blood, red top tube. Consultation with lab suggested (955-6363). Fill out Microbiology request and case history form.			BLY	134.00
NOTE: Antibody to blastomyces may be significant when interpreted in light of a suggestive clinical picture. CF titers of 1:8 are also suggestive. Higher titers or rising titers are more significant.					
(Referral Lab)					
BLASTOMYOCOSIS CULTURE	7-10 mL blood, isolator tube.				
BLEEDING TIME (TEMPLATE)	Performed Monday-Friday on day shift. Schedule with lab 1 day in advance (955-7687).		2-8 minutes	BT	84.00
***HP:** Highest lab priority available (S=Stat, A=ASAP)					

Fig. 13.1 Sample page from a laboratory specimen collection manual. (Courtesy the Hospital of the University of Pennsylvania, Philadelphia.)

number of hours after treatment); (3) the sample volume is insufficient for the test being ordered, especially when the specimen container includes an additive; (4) the wrong collection tube or container is used; (5) a collection tube is used after its expiration date; (6) the sample is transported incorrectly (e.g., not sent on ice); and (7) the specimen is found to be hemolyzed (which can adversely affect tests such as potassium). When a specimen is deemed to be unacceptable, it usually must be recollected. Unacceptable specimens, recollected specimens, and duplicate specimen collections are central to the phlebotomy quality process.

Unsuccessful Collection Attempts

In addition to unacceptable specimen criteria, the specimen collection manual should include a procedure that lists the steps the phlebotomist can take when unable to collect a blood specimen. This procedure should address unsuccessful venipunctures, patient unavailability, and patient refusal to be tested. In each scenario, documentation (Fig. 13.3) is important for quality review because the problem must be identified and corrected. Therefore the number of collection attempts is included as an indicator in the inpatient phlebotomy quality program. An outpatient phlebotomy program may include the following as quality indicators: patients not fasting as directed, phlebotomy orders missing, patients difficult to draw, and patients who left collection area before specimen collection.

Newborn and Pediatric Patients

Finally, the unique handling of newborn and pediatric patients should be covered in the specimen collection procedure manual. Specifically, the minimum amount of blood needed to perform a laboratory test on one of these patients should be highlighted in the manual. An

THOMAS JEFFERSON UNIVERSITY HOSPITAL
CLINICAL LABORATORIES

❏ EMERGENCY   ❏ PHONE   ❏ FAX _____ (SPECIFY WHICH)

NOTE: STAT SPECIMENS MUST BE BROUGHT DIRECTLY TO LAB (3RD FLOOR, PAVILION)

SPECIMEN COLLECTED (REQUIRED BY STATE LAW)	DATE	TIME	❏ AM ❏ PM

NAME OF COLLECTOR

MEDICATION
❏ COUMADIN   ❏ HEPARIN   ❏ ASPIRIN   ❏ OTHER _____

ICD-9 CODE: | | | | | | | | | | | | |

(TO SPECIFY COMMON ICD-9 CODES, SEE REVERSE)
ORDER CANNOT BE PROCESSED WITHOUT DIAGNOSIS

To the Physician: Clinical consultants from the laboratory are available to help in the selection of appropriate tests.
Call (215) 955-6545 or - 6381

OUTPATIENT ONLY - PLEASE PRINT

PATIENTS NAME - LAST	FIRST	SEX	DATE OF BIRTH

STREET ADDRESS

CITY	STATE	ZIP CODE

PHYSICIAN ORDERING TEST - LAST NAME	FIRST

STREET ADDRESS

CITY	STATE	ZIP CODE

USE ADDRESSOPLATE OR PRINT THE ABOVE

SPECIMEN MUST BE LABELED WITH PATIENT'S NAME

SPECIMEN NOTES (SEE REVERSE) →

CHEMISTRY TEST GROUPS

❏SM7	BASIC METABOLIC PANEL(80049) R5	
❏CO2	CARBON DIOXIDE (82374) R2	
❏CL	CHLORIDE (82435) R2	
❏CRT	CREATININE (82565) R2	
❏GLF	GLUCOSE (82947) R2	1
❏K	POTASSIUM (84132) R2	
❏NA	SODIUM (84295) R2	
❏BUN	UREA-N (84520) R2	
❏MCM	COMPREHENSIVE METABOLIC PANEL (80054) R5	
❏ALB	ALBUMIN (82040) R1	
❏TBIL	BILIRUBIN, TOTAL (82250) R2	
❏CA	CALCIUM (82310) R2	
❏CL	CHLORIDE (82435) R2	
❏CRT	CREATININE (82565) R2	
❏GLF	GLUCOSE (82947) R2	1
❏ALP	ALKALINE PHOSPHATASE (84075) R2	
❏K	POTASSIUM (84132) R2	
❏PRO	PROTEIN, TOTAL (84155) R2	
❏NA	SODIUM (84295) R2	
❏AST	AST (SGOT) (84450) R2	
❏BUN	UREA-N (84520) R2	
❏ELC	ELECTROLYTES (80051) R5	
❏CO2	CARBON DIOXIDE (82374) R2	
❏CL	CHLORIDE (82435) R2	
❏K	POTASSIUM (84132) R2	
❏NA	SODIUM (84295) R2	
❏HPM	HEPATIC FUNCTION PANEL (80058) R5	
❏ALB	ALBUMIN (82040) R2	
❏BIL	BILIRUBIN (82251) R2 TOTAL AND DIRECT	
❏ALP	ALKALINE PHOSPHATASE (84075) R2	
❏AST	AST (SGOT) (84450) R2	
❏ALT	ALT (SGPT) (84480) R2	
❏CRK	LIPID PANEL (80061) R5	1,9
❏COL	CHOLESTEROL (82465) R2	1,9
❏HDL	HDL-CHOLESTEROL (83718) R5	1,9
❏GLC	TRIGLYCERIDES (84478) R2	1,9

NON-FDA APPROVED TESTS: Medicare will not provide reimbursement for tests which are not approved by the FDA for patient care. These include, among others: CA 19-9, P24 Antigen, Cyclosporine (Non-Specific), Erythropoietin, etc. In addition, Medicare will not provide reimbursement for tests ordered for screening purposes only.
(1) This test includes interpretation; if interpretation is **not** required, please circle test name.
(2) If the initial result for this test is positive, the laboratory will automatically perform normal and usual follow-on test(s). If you do not want the laboratory to perform these test(s), or require that your advance approval be obtained please circle the test name, and write in your instructions.

SPECIMEN NOTES (SEE REVERSE) →

BLOOD

❏ACN	ACETONE (82010) R1	
❏ACPR	ACID PHOSPHATASE (84060) R3	11
❏ACT	ACTH (82024) L3	11
❏AP2	AFP+2 (TRIPLE SCREEN) (82105, 84233, 84702)	R10
❏MA	MICROALBUMIN (82043) UR XLT	
❏ALO	ALCOHOL ETHYL (82055) R5	
❏ATN	ALDOSTERONE (82088) R2	
❏APN	ALPHA FETOPROTEIN (1) (82105) R5 MATERNAL SCREENING	
❏APM	ALPHA FETOPROTEIN (82105) R5 TUMOR MARKER	
❏AML	AMYLASE (82150) R2	
❏AND	ANDROSTENEDIONE (82157) R2	
❏ACE	ANGIOTENSIN (82164) R2 CONVERTING ENZYME	
❏DNA	ANTI dsDNA AB (86225) R5	
❏ANA	ANTINUCLEAR AB (86038) R5	
❏ATA	ANTI-THYROID ABS (86800) R5	
❏CGF	HCG, BLOOD (84702) R2 FULL TITER	
❏MBL	BILIRUBIN, NEONATAL (82250) GM OR PM	12
❏CAO	CA 125 (86316) R2	
❏CAI	CALCIUM, IONIZED (82330) G5	11
❏CEA	CEA (82378) R2	
❏CPK	CK (82550) R2	
❏C34	COMPLEMENT (C3, C4) (86160) R5	
❏CBC	CBC WITH PLATELETS (85029) L3 (NO DIFF)	2
❏CBA	CBC W/DIFF & PLT (85025,85023) L3	
❏PTR	PATHOLOGIST REVIEW OF BLOOD SMEAR	10
❏COR	CORTISOL (82533) R2	
❏CLS	CYCLOSPORINE (80158) L3	3
❏DHE	DHEA-S (82627) R2	
❏DIG	DIGOXIN (80162) R2	
❏DIL	DILANTIN (80185) R2	
❏EST	ESTRADIOL-17B (82670) R5	
❏FER	FERRITIN (82728) R2	
❏FOA	FOLATE (82746) R2	
❏FSH	FSH (83001) R2	
❏GGT	GGT (82977) R2	
❏	GLUC TOL_____ HR R2	
❏GLH	GLYCOHEMOGLOBIN (83036) L5	
❏HGE	HEMOGLOBIN (1) (83020) L2 ELECTROPHORESIS	
❏HPA	HEP A AB PROFILE (1) (86296) R3	4
❏HBC	HEP B CORE AB (1) (86289) R2	
❏HBS	HEP B SURF AB (1) (86291) R2	
❏HAA	HEP B SURF AG (1) (86287) R2	
❏HPC	HEPATITIS C AB (86302) R3	
❏IGE	IMMUNOGLOBULIN-E (82785) R2	
❏IME	IMMUNOFIXATION (84165, 86320) R4 ELECTROPHORESIS (1)	

SPECIMEN NOTES (SEE REVERSE) →

❏IMG	IMMUNOGLOBULINS (86329) R2 QUANTITATIVE	
❏IIB	IRON + IRON (83540, 83550) R5 BINDING	
❏LDH	LD (83615) R2	
❏LH	LH (83002) R2	
❏LSE	LIPASE (83690) R2	
❏LTH	LITHIUM (80178) R2	
❏DRVT	LUPUS INHIB (85613) B3	
❏LYA	LYME ANTIBODY (86618) R5	
❏MG	MAGNESIUM (83735) R2	
❏FTA	FTA TREPONEMA (86781) R10	
❏MNO	MONONUCLEOSIS (86308) R5 SCREEN	
❏OSM	OSMOLALITY (83930) R1	
❏PHE	PHENOBARBITAL (80184) R2	
❏PHO	PHOSPHATE (84100) R2	
❏PRG	PROGESTERONE (84144) R2	
❏PCN	PROLACTIN (84146) R2	
❏PSA5	PROSTATE SPECIFIC (84153) R3 ANTIGEN	
❏PRE	PROTEIN (1) (84165) R3 ELECTROPHORESIS	5
❏PT	PROTHROMBIN TIME (85610) B3	6
❏PTT	PTT [PARTIAL, (85730) B3 THROMBOPLASTIN TIME (ACTIVITY)]	6
❏PTH	PTH, INTACT, (83970) R5 (INCL CALCIUM)	
❏RPR	RAPID PLASMA REAGIN (86592) R5	
❏REN	RENIN ACTIVITY (84244) L5	
❏RTC	RETICULOCYTES (85045) L2	
❏RHF	RHEUMATOID FACTOR (86430) R5	
❏RUB	RUBELLA SCREEN (86762) R5	
❏SED	SED RATE (85651) K5	
❏SIK	SICKLE CELL (85660) L2	
❏T3R	T3 TOTAL (84481) R2	
❏T3U	T3 UPTAKE (84479) R2	7
❏FT4	FREE T4 (84439) R2	
❏T4R	T4 (84436) R2	7
❏T7	T7 (84479, 84436) R2	
❏TEG	TEGRETOL (80156) R2	
❏FTS	TESTOSTERONE, (84402) R3 FREE AND TOTAL	
❏TES	TESTOSTERONE, TOTAL (84403) R2	
❏THE	THEOPHYLLINE (80198) R2	
❏TFR	TRANSFERRIN (84466) R1	
❏TSH	TSH (THYROID SCREEN) (84443) R2	8
❏URC	URATE (84550) R2	
❏VAL	VALPROIC ACID (80164) R2	
❏B12	VITAMINE B12 (82607) R2	

URINE

❏CGI	HCG (QUAL) (84703) UR	
❏UCA	CALCIUM (82340) UT	
❏UCR	CREATININE (82570) UT	

SPECIMEN NOTES (SEE REVERSE) →

❏UCC	CREATININE CLEARANCE (82575) US *	
❏UOS	OSMOLALITY (83935) UR	
❏UPR	PROTEIN (84155) UT	
❏UEL	PROTEIN (1) (84155) UT ELECTROPHORESIS	
❏UMAC	URINALYSIS (2) (81003) UR MACROSCOPE ONLY	
❏UA	URINALYSIS, (81001) UR INCL MICROSCOPIC	
❏VMA	VMA (84585)U24	14

OTHER FLUIDS

❏SFG	GLUCOSE, CSF (82947) C1
❏SFP	PROTEIN, CSF (84155) C1

OTHER TESTS - WRITE IN
_____
_____
_____
_____
_____
_____
_____
_____
_____
_____
_____
_____
_____

URINE TIMES

	MON	DAY	TIME
BEGUN			❏ AM ❏ PM
ENDED	MON	DAY	TIME ❏ AM ❏ PM

LAB USE ONLY
TOTAL TIME _____ HR
VOLUME _____ ML

BLUE BACKGROUND - AVAILABLE AS STAT PROCEDURE

BILLING INFORMATION - REVERSE P.2

LAB USE ONLY
ACCO. NO. _____

_____
_____
_____

LAB I.D.

★★SPECIMEN INFORMATION - SEE REVERSE★★

PATIENT MUST READ AND SIGN STATEMENT ON REVERSE OF FORM

Fig. 13.2 Sample test requisition form. (Courtesy the Hospital of the University of Pennsylvania, Philadelphia.)

SPECIMEN NOTES

1. Fasting specimen.
2. Consists of WBC, RBC, HGB, HCT MCV, MCH, MCHC, RDW, and Platelets (Quant)
3. Submit whole blood only.
4. Profile includes IgG and IgM
5. Includes Protein Electrophoresis and Total Protein.
6. Tube must contain 2.7 mL (in 3 mL Hemogard Blue Top Tube).
7. If T3 Uptake and T4 are both ordered, T7 will be calculated by the lab.
8. TSH is the recommended Thyroid screening test.
9. If all 3 Components of the Lipid Panel are ordered, LDL-Cholesterol is calculated.
10. CBA order is required.
11. Collect on ice.
12. Protect from light.
13. Heparinized whole blood; rush to lab on ice.
14. Collect with 4 Boric Acid tablets.

SPECIMEN TYPE AND AMOUNT

A - ARTERIAL
AF - AMNIOTIC FLUID
B - BLUE TOP TUBE (ALWAYS FILL TUBE)
C - CEREBROSPINAL FLUID
G - GREEN TOP TUBE
K - BLACK TOP TUBE (ALWAYS FILL TUBE)
L - LAVENDER TOP TUBE
M - MICROTAINER

R - RED TOP TUBE
GAST - GASTRIC CONTENT
UR - URINE, RANDOM SAMPLE
UT - URINE, TIMED COLLECTION
U24 - URINE, 24 HOUR COLLECTION

(FOR UT AND U24 - INDICATE "BEGIN" AND "ENDED" TIMES IN "URINE TIMES" BOX ON FRONT OF FORM)

NUMBER FOLLOWING THE SPECIMEN OR TUBE CODE ON THE FRONT OF THIS FORM INDICATES THE MINIMUM AMOUNT OF SPECIMEN TO BE DRAWN, IN ML. FOR EXAMPLE, R5 REPRESENTS 5ML BLOOD IN A RED TUBE

LABORATORY INFORMATION 955-6545
MICROBIOLOGY USE LAB FORM 0473-01
CYTOLOGY USE LAB FORM 0476-00
FLOW CYTOMETRY USE LAB FORM 0489-00
HIV TESTING USE LAB FORM 0473-02

COMMON ICD9 (DIAGNOSIS) CODES - CHECK ALL THAT APPLY: The codes listed are some of the frequently used diagnosis codes and are provided for convenience **only**. It is the physician's responsibility to assign the most appropriate and specific diagnosis code for the tests ordered, and it may be necessary to consult the current ICD-9-CM manual for additional, more specific, or more appropriate codes.

Code	Description	Code	Description	Code	Description	Code	Description
78900	Abdomen Pain Unspec Site __	3058	Cocaine abuse __	075	Infectious mononucleosis __	29534	Paran Schizo-Chr/Exacarb __
7890	Abdominal Pain __	30580	Cocaine Abuse Unspec __	5899	Intestinal disorder NOS __	29532	Paranoid schizo-chronic __
64880	Abn Glucose in Preg, Unsp __	30460	Comb Drug Dep NEC Unspec __	129	Intestinal Parasitism Unspec __	436	Pneumonia organism NOS __
7945	ABN Thyroid func. Study __	2860	Coag Factor VIII Disord __	984	Lead, Toxic Effect __	9583	Posttraum Wnd Infec NEC __
7919	Abn Urine Findings Nec __	4280	Congestive Heart Failure __	2729	Lipoid metabol. Dis. NOS __	V222	Pregnancy State, incidental __
7832	Abnormal loss of weight __	920	Contusion Face/Scalp/Nck __	5738	Liver Disorder NOS __	6029	Prostate Disorder NOS __
8260	Absence of menstruation __	7803	Convulsions __	V427	Liver transplant status __	2989	Psychosis NOS __
30300	Ac alcohol intox Unspec __	4140	Coronary Atherosclerosis __	1628	Mal. Neo Bronch/Lung NEC __	2720	Pure Hypercholesterolem __
3030	Ac Alcohol intoxication __	7820	Cough __	1729	Malig. melanoma skin NOS__	59080	Pyelonephritis NOS __
7061	Acne NEC __	464.4	Croup __	1918	Malig. Neo Brain NEC __	7806	Pyrexia Unknown origin __
482	Acute Pharyngitis __	5959	Cystitis NOS __	1919	Malig. Neo Brain NEC __	5939	Renal and Ureteral Dis NOS __
481.9	Acute Sinusitis, Unspecified __	2963	Depr Psych, Recur Episod __	1869	Malig. Neo Testis NEC __	5199	Resp System Disease NOS __
4559	Acute URI NOS __	29620	Depress Psychosis Unspec __	1748	Malign. Neopl Breast NEC __	78809	Respiratory abnorm NEC __
30928	ADJ React mixed emotion __	311	Depressive Disorder NEC __	185	Malign. Neopl Prostate __	714.0	Rheumatoid Arthritis __
3099	Adjustment reaction NOS __	2500	Diabetes Mellitus Uncomp __	1539	Malignant Neo Colon NOS __	V700	Routine Medical Exam __
30500	Alcohol Abuse, Unspec __	2469	Disorder of thyroid gland __	1538	Malignant Neo Colon NEC __	29572	Schizoaffective Chronic __
2858	Anemia NOS __	7804	Dizziness and Giddiness __	1749	Malignant Neopl Breast NOS __	29570	Schizoaffective, Unspec __
V289	Antenatal Screening NOS __	30590	Drug Abuse NEC Unspec __	1541	Malignant neopl Rectum __	29590	Schizophrenia NOS Unspec __
30000	Anxiety State NOS __	3059	Drug Abuse NEC/NOS __	V703	Med Exam NEC Admin Purp __	V789	Scree Blood Dis NOC __
71690	Anthropathy NOS Unspec __	304.9	Drug dependence, Unspec __	6268	Menstrual disorder NEC __	282.6	Sickle Cell Anemia __
49390	Asthma w/o status esthm __	2929	Drug mental disorder NOS __	632	Missed abortion __	8470	Sprain of neck __
42731	Atrial fibrillation __	995.2	Drug Substance Adverse Effect __	075	Monoucleosis, infectious __	V252	Sterilization __
040	Bacterial Diseases, other __	5339	Ectopic Pregnancy NOS __	340	Multiple sclerosis __	5369	Stomach function dis NOS __
4011	Benign Hypertension __	79093	Elevated PSA (Prostate) __	3009	Neurotic Disorder NOS __	0340	Strep sore Throat __
2957	Bipolar affective NOS __	2599	Endocrine Disorder NOS __	25000	NIDDM w/o complication __	V221	Supervis Oth normal preg __
2984	Bipolar Affective, Manic __	34690	Epilep NOS w/o intrac EP __	788.43	Nocturia __	7802	Syncope and collapse __
2899	Blood disease NOS __	6149	Fem Pelv Inflam Dis NOS __	5586	Nonint Gastroentarit NEC __	7100	Syst Lupus Erythematosus __
30183	Borderline personality __	V708	General Exam NEC __	6238	Noninflam dis vagina NEC __	64003	Threat Abort Antepar COM __
85400	Brain injury NEC __	7809	General symptoms NEC __	7821	Nonspecif skin erupt NEC __	24290	Thyrotox NOS No Crisis __
3090	Brief Depressive React __	2409	Goiter NOS __	2410	Nontox Uninodular goiter __	130	Toxoplasmosis __
490	Bronchitis NOS __	V723	Gynecologic examination __	V22	Normal pregnancy __	13101	Trichomonal vaginitis __
2349	CA in Situ NOS __	7840	Headache __	278	Obesity __	59780	Urethritis NOS __
5920	Calculus of kidney __	4299	Heart Disease NOS __	V715	Observ following rape __	5990	Urine Tract infection NOS __
1121	Candidal vulvovaginitis __	5997	Hematuria __	V718	Observ Suspect Cond NEC __	7889	Urinary Sys Symptom NEC __
6160	Cervicitis __	054	Herpes Simplex __	30401	Opiod dependance Contin __	8151	Vaginitis __
75249	Cervix / Fern Gen Anom NEC __	042	HIV __	73300	Osteoporosis NOS __	81510	Vaginitis NOS __
78859	Chest pain NEC __	5733	Hepatitis, Unspecified __	118	Opportunistic Mycoses __	0999	Venereal Disease NOS __
78660	Chest pain NOS __	2724	Hyperlipidemia NEC/NOS __	65370	Oth Abn Fet Disprop Unsp __	0068	Viral enteritis NOS __
496	Chr Airway Obstruct NEC __	600	Hyperplasia of prostate __	V5849	Other Spec Surg Aftercare __	0799	Viral/Chlamydi Infec NOS __
585	Chronic Renal Failure __	4019	Hypertension NOS __	6202	Ovarian Cyst NEC/NOS __	070	Viral Hepatitis __
4739	Chronic sinusitis NOS __	2449	Hypothyroidism NOS __	7295	Pain in Limb __		
2889	Coagulat Defect NEC/NOS __	009	Ill defined intestinal infection __	7851	Palpitations __		

NEC: Not Elsewhere Classifiable
NOS: Not otherwise specified

Fig. 13.2 cont'd

Uncollected specimen notice Thomas Jefferson University Hospital Clinical Laboratories	Room no.
Patient's name	
Test(s)	
Specimens requested were not collected because: ☐ Patient not in room - Call lab to re-schedule ☐ Patient uncooperative _____ ☐ Unable to draw _____ ☐ Other: _____	

Collector	Time ☐ a.m. ☐ p.m.	Date

Fig. 13.3 Sample uncollected specimen notice. (From Laboratory Information Handbook. Philadelphia, Thomas Jefferson University Hospital Clinical Laboratories, October 1998, pp. 9, 100.)

example of pediatric specimen requirements is shown in Fig. 13.4. Many premature infants undergo transfusion merely to replace blood removed for laboratory testing (known as *iatrogenic blood loss*). By collecting the smallest amount of blood required for testing, significant blood loss can be avoided. Because of the small blood volumes in newborns and children, the number of times blood is collected, and the amounts removed from these patients should be monitored and included in the phlebotomy quality program.

QUALITY CONTROL OF SUPPLIES AND INSTRUMENTS

The best QA and QI practices in phlebotomy depend on the phlebotomists who are trained to perform blood collection procedures. Reports from phlebotomists that evacuated tubes are not working properly (e.g., not drawing the appropriate amount) may result in the performance of a blood collection QC procedure. The implementation of a new brand of tube or of a modified evacuated tube may also be reason to perform a QC procedure.

Blood collection QC procedures may be included in a phlebotomy QA program, depending on the particular facility's interests and experiences. If difficulties are encountered by the workers who use the vacuum tubes, or if new technologies are implemented, the supplier or

manufacturer may be contacted and asked to assist with corrective action or provide consultation.

Whether performed by the laboratory or by the manufacturer, phlebotomy QC may include one or more of the following four procedures.

Evaluating Evacuated Test Tubes

The purpose of evaluating evacuated test tubes is to measure the amount of vacuum draw and compare it with expected results under standard test conditions.

Evaluating the Stopper Assembly

The purpose of evaluating the stopper assembly is to ensure that it will function as expected during collection and sample mixing. Stoppers that pull out, fall out, are loose, or leak during the steps of this test procedure are defective and can lead to contamination and compromising the specimen quality. They may also pose a safety hazard.

Centrifuge Test

In the centrifuge test, the ability of an evacuated tube to withstand the centrifugation needed to separate whole blood into its components is evaluated. After the vacuum tubes are completely filled with water, they are placed in centrifuge carriers, following the centrifuge manufacturer's directions. The tubes are spun for 10 minutes with a 2200 relative centrifugal force. Tube breakage of any degree indicates a defect.

CAPILLARY SPECIMEN REQUIREMENTS

Pediatric specimens are accepted for a number of tests. This section lists all the common ones for which pediatric specimens can be used, and indicates the number of Microtainer blood tubes which are needed. This list is classified by general test type, i.e., chemistry, hematology, and so forth. Most specimens are serum (red top Microtainer), however please note that some require EDTA (lavender top tube).

Specimen amounts indicated apply where the hematocrit of the patient is normal. If the hematocrit is high, it is suggested that the amounts shown be doubled.

	NUMBER OF MICROTAINER(S)	COLOR
CHEMISTRY		
Acid Phosphatase	2	Red/Green
Albumin	1/3	Red/Green
Alkaline Phosphatase	2/3	Red/Green
ALT	2/3	Red/Green
Amylase	1/3	Red/Green
AST	2/3	Red/Green
Bilirubin (Fractionated)	1/2	Red/Green
Calcium	1/3	Red/Green
Chem-7 Panel (SMA7)	1	Red/Green
Chloride	1/3	Red/Green
Cholesterol	1/3	Red/Green
CO_2	1/3	Red/Green
Complement C3, C4	1	Red
CK	2/3	Red/Green
CK Isoenzymes	1	Red
Creatinine	1/3	Red/Green
Enzymes	1	Red
GGT	2/3	Red/Green
Glucose	1/3	Red/Green
Health Screen-12 (SMA 12)	1	Red/Green
Hemoglobin, Plasma Free	1	Lavender
Immunoelectrophoresis	1	Red
Immunoglobulins	1	Red
LD	2/3	Red/Green
LD Isoenzymes	1	Red
Lipase	1	Red/Green
Magnesium	1/3	Red/Green
Microbilirubin	1/2	Red/Green
Osmolality	2/3	Red/Green
Phosphate	1/3	Red/Green
Potassium	1/3	Red/Green
Protein Electrophoresis	1	Red
Protein, Total	1/3	Red/Green
Sodium	1/3	Red/Green
Total Protein	1/3	Red/Green

Fig. 13.4 Sample pediatric specimen requirements. (From Laboratory Information Handbook. Philadelphia, Thomas Jefferson University Hospital Clinical Laboratories, October 1998, pp. 9, 100.)

Additive Test

The additive assay determines the quantity and identity of the chemical (such as anticoagulant) added to the evacuated tube. Assays follow U.S. Pharmacopeia or other appropriate chemical methods.

More detailed instructions for any of these QC procedures can be obtained from the CLSI guidelines at *www.clsi.org.*

PERCEPTIONS OF QUALITY IN PHLEBOTOMY SERVICE

Delivering the right product or service (e.g., collection of blood specimens); satisfying the customer's needs and concerns; meeting the customer's expectations; and treating every customer with integrity, courtesy, respect, and care directly affect the perceptions of quality in phlebotomy. Who are the customers of a phlebotomist? Patients are not the only customers; the patient's family, doctors, nurses, and other departments' employees are also customers.

What are the needs of these customers? Regardless of the customer, the need is professional service and assistance in detecting or treating an illness. All customers expect a relatively painless venipuncture, proper timing, clear instructions, use of proper technique, adherence to SOP (consistency), efficiency, effective interpersonal communication skills, and teamwork. Customers do not want or expect additional stresses. They want to be treated with integrity, courtesy, and respect. Using the best venipuncture technique means nothing to the customer who has been mistreated (yelled at, forced, or coerced to permit testing, lied to, given false hopes, made the recipient of prejudice, and so on). Professional behavior is a key to quality patient care.

It is important to remember that phlebotomists are usually the only representative of the clinical laboratory who have direct patient contact. Patients, doctors, nurses, and others who have had an unpleasant experience with a phlebotomist are likely to have a negative image of the laboratory and its ability to provide quality services. However, the converse is also true. Positive experiences tend to yield positive patient outcomes. Members of a phlebotomy team can be considered the laboratory's public relations officers. Therefore a laboratory quality-monitoring program may include customer satisfaction surveys and incident report monitoring.

At times, extraneous situations arise that can interfere with quality work. Examples include, but are not

limited to, patients who are being resuscitated, patients with traumatic injuries, combative patients, uncooperative family members, belligerent doctors or nurses, and frequent experiences of heavy workload and low staffing. Each of these, or any combination, tend to be stressful for the phlebotomist.

When these extraneous situations occur, effective coping tactics are needed. Maintaining focus, adhering to SOPs and referring to the manual when questioned, practicing assertive behaviors (neither aggressive nor passive), being empathetic, and displaying a caring professional image will enable phlebotomists to handle these stressful occasions with pride and a positive outcome.

SUMMARY

A phlebotomy total quality program is designed by combining the technical aspects of blood collection and the customers' perceptions of quality of service with regulatory requirements for monitoring, evaluating, and continuously improving service. Quality performance processes and outcomes should be tracked through quality indicators and threshold values to continuously identify and evaluate performance practices that can reduce and eliminate errors, as well as patient and employee risk. Positive patient outcomes are the goal of any health care delivery service. Using and referring to the procedures in the specimen collection manual and reporting problems to supervisory personnel are important to ensuring quality. The number and types of specimens rejected, the number of specimens recollected, the number of duplicate draws, the number of collection attempts, the number of specimens drawn from newborn and pediatric patients, incidents of untimeliness, and cases of customer complaints are usually the indicators

---

BOX 13.5   Indicators of Quality Phlebotomy

- The number and types of specimens rejected
- The number of specimens recollected
- The number of duplicate draws
- The number of collection attempts
- The number of specimens drawn from newborn and pediatric patients
- Incidents of untimeliness
- Cases of customer complaints

included in the phlebotomy quality plan (Box 13.5). Factors contributing to poor-quality services are identified and analyzed; corrective action is taken, when indicated; and the effectiveness of this action is studied. The search for ways to maintain quality standards and keep costs down, retain existing customers, and attract new customers is crucial to survival in today's business world.

Each employee's involvement in the entire process is fundamental to successful QC, QA, and QI plans. Monitoring and evaluating quality is a time-consuming process. However, the benefits (positive outcomes, satisfied customers, improved teamwork, improved profitability and market share, and so on) are worth the investment. Commitment, enthusiasm, and focus on quality patient care are integral to the success of the health care profession and organizations.

CASE 13.1   Critical Thinking

You have been asked to review your laboratory's procedure manual. Under the section for specimen rejection, it states only, "Specimens may be rejected if they are not labeled properly." What feedback are you going to give to the supervisors?

REVIEW QUESTIONS

1. Doing the right thing, doing it the right way, doing it right the first time, and doing it on time are the _____ of quality.
2. Reducing medical _____ and improving patient safety are the current focus of overall health care quality improvement.
3. The document with which every phlebotomist must be familiar is the _____.
4. Quality _____ is the process of making sure that standards of care have been maintained.
5. Customer _____ surveys are part of quality monitoring programs.
6. The number of collection _____ is an indicator of an inpatient phlebotomy quality program.
7. Why is the phlebotomist important to the perception of quality for the entire laboratory?
8. Discuss the following statement: Quality in regard to phlebotomy is the responsibility of the phlebotomy supervisors.

Howanitz PJ, Renner SW, Walsh MK. Continuous wristband monitoring over 2 years decreases identification errors. A College of American Pathologists Q-Tracks study. *Arch Pathol Lab Med.* 2002;126:809–815.

BIBLIOGRAPHY

Bishop ML, Fody EP, Schoeff LE. Phlebotomy and specimen considerations. In: *Clinical Chemistry: Techniques, Principles, Correlations.* 2nd ed. Philadelphia: Lippincott Williams & Wilkins; 2010:33–72.

Bonini P, Plebani M, Ceriotti F, Rubboli F. Errors in laboratory medicine. *Clinical Chemistry.* 2002;48(5): 691–698.

Clinical and Laboratory Standards Institute (CLSI). *Development and Use of Quality Indicators for Process Improvement and Monitoring of Laboratory Quality. Approved Guideline. CLSI Document GP35-A.* Wayne, PA: Clinical and Laboratory Standards Institute; 2010.

Dale JC, Novis DA. Outpatient phlebotomy success and reasons for specimen rejection. A Q-Probes study. *Arch Pathol Lab Med.* 2002;126:416–419.

Ernst DJ. Four indefensible phlebotomy errors and how to prevent them. *J Healthc Risk Manage.* 1998;18(2):41–46.

Institute of Medicine. *The Committee on the Quality of Health Care in America: Crossing the Quality Chasm: A New Health System for the 21st Century.* Washington, DC: The National Academies Press; 2001.

National Committee for Clinical Laboratory Standards. *A Quality Management System Model for Healthcare.* 5th. Wayne, PA: NCCLS/CLSI; 2019.

Schuster MA, McGlynn EA, Brook RH. How good is the quality of healthcare in the United States? *Milbank Quarterly.* 1998;76(4):517–563.

Sirota RL. The Institute of Medicine's report on medical error. Implications for pathology. *Arch Pathol Lab Med.* 2000; 124:1674–1678.

Turgeon ML. *Concepts, Procedures and Clinical Applications. Linne & Ringsrud's Clinical Laboratory Science.* 8th ed. St. Louis: Mosby; 2019.

Medical-Legal Issues and Health Law Procedures

Edited by John C. Flynn, Jr. *

> *"Ignorance of the law excuses no man."*
> —*John Selden (1584–1654)*

OBJECTIVES

At the conclusion of this chapter, the student should be able to:

- List the different types of laws.
- Define standard of care as it relates to phlebotomy.
- Explain the difference between plaintiff and defendant.
- Define:
  - Assault
  - Battery
  - Negligence
- Explain the difference between circumstantial evidence and direct evidence.
- Explain the Health Insurance Portability and Accountability Act of 1996 (HIPAA).
- Explain the importance of the Patient Care Partnership.
- Describe Chain of Custody and explain why it is important in specimen collection.

OUTLINE

---

* This chapter has been edited from a contribution to the fourth edition by Shirley E. Greening.

KEY TERMS

burden of proof
circumstantial evidence
consent
informed consent
defamation
defendant
direct evidence
discovery
evidence
fiduciary

HIPAA
immunity
litigation
negligence
negligence per se
plaintiff
rulemaking
standard of care
testimony

INTRODUCTION

The term *medical-legal* describes the interrelationship of the professions and practices of law and medicine. The medical-legal field is sometimes called "medical law" or "legal medicine." Early medical law most often concentrated on forensic medicine, which is the presentation of medical data or evidence in courts of law. Medical law has now expanded to encompass such fields as pathology, psychiatry, toxicology, public health regulation, health care legislation, court rulings, and administrative regulation of medical professional practice and medical service programs. Health law is a specialty area of law that relates to practitioners in medicine, dentistry, nursing, hospital administration, environmental health and safety, and allied health. The allied health professions include those individuals who work in laboratories located in hospitals, public health facilities, private or commercial enterprises, and research settings; thus they include phlebotomists.[1]

Phlebotomists, as members of the laboratory health care team, are in a unique position in relation to most other laboratory personnel. In many health care settings phlebotomists may be the only laboratorians who have direct contact with patients or blood donors.

Phlebotomists are also often the only laboratorians who perform specimen collection procedures on patients or donors, and one of only a few laboratorians who deal with the patients' perceptions of fear of infection, illness, and death and dying. Phlebotomists must have a strong educational background and good training; be technically proficient; follow laboratory procedures; be in compliance with government rules and regulations; and at the same time be good listeners, good communicators, good empathizers, and good public relations representatives. If phlebotomists become inattentive to, careless about, or unaware of their professional roles and duties, they may increase the risk of errors in the practice of their profession and thus increase the risk of being held legally liable for those errors. Examples of the most common errors are injury to a blood donor or patient, misidentification of a patient, misinterpretation of a physician's orders, mislabeling of a specimen, and transmission of disease.

Phlebotomists now practice their profession at a time when patients and clients have high expectations for the success of their health care. Patients and clients are increasingly likely to question the quality of care or to object to treatments or procedures that they perceive as harmful, injurious, or damaging to them. One result of this questioning may be that the patient or client takes legal action by filing a malpractice claim against the health care institution, the laboratory, and any individuals involved in their care, including phlebotomists.[2,3]

Another result may be that government regulatory agencies or laboratory accreditation organizations may call into question the way that a laboratory supervises its personnel or the ways in which a laboratory ensures that it is providing quality services and care to patients and clients.

It is important that phlebotomists be familiar with the various legal principles and regulatory framework that affect their activities as members of the health care team. Phlebotomists should not have to conduct their professional activities in constant fear of legal liability (what some have termed *defensive medicine*). Rather, an understanding of why and how medical-legal issues arise in the day-to-day performance of phlebotomists' duties is part of phlebotomy education and practice.

SOURCES OF LAWS

Common law consists of those principles and rules of action that derive their authority solely from usages and customs that have evolved from ancient, unwritten laws of England. The common law is all the statutory and case law background of England and the American colonies before the American Revolution and is distinguished from statutory or legislative law, which developed after the American Revolution. Many common law principles have been incorporated into more formalized bodies of law governing cities, states, and nations.

Statutory law (also called *legislative law*) is the body of law that is voted on and passed by the U.S. Congress or by a state legislature as an outcome of the political process or societal influences. Legislatively enacted laws are called *statutes*. A municipality may also enact laws, which are usually called *codes* or *ordinances*.

Administrative law (also called *regulatory law*) is not technically a set of laws but instead consists of the rules and regulations that are written by government agencies to implement statutes or public laws. The U.S. Congress delegates authority to various government agencies that then write the specific provisions of the statutes in a process known as **rulemaking.** Most agencies also have the power to monitor compliance with these rules and enforce penalties for

noncompliance. In contrast to courts or legislatures, government agencies employ and consult with experts who have special knowledge about the areas covered by statutes. Agencies also have much greater flexibility than courts or legislatures to revise regulations in response to social and economic changes or new scientific information. Courts or legislatures may defer to a government agency for an interpretation of a court rule or legislative statute.[4]

Decisional law (also called *case law*) develops as a result of federal, state, or local courts deciding cases brought by two or more individual parties. Cases are decided based on precedents (a decision in a previous case), which can then be narrowed, expanded, distinguished, or overruled. Case law that is decided "once and for all" is termed *stare decisis*; if an issue had been litigated before by the same parties and cannot be litigated again, it is termed *res judicata*.[5] Case law can become statutory law if local, state, or federal government legislatures vote to incorporate a judicial line of decisions into the form of a statute. By passing legislation, governments recognize that decisions in individual cases have importance and application to all citizens.

Each source of law or method of lawmaking (statutory, case, and administrative) may deal with civil laws, criminal laws, or laws of equity. *Civil laws* are those that relate to private rights and remedies sought by citizens through proceedings termed *civil actions*. Civil actions are brought to enforce, redress, or protect an individual's private rights. *Criminal laws* (also termed *penal laws*) refer to those state and federal statutes that define criminal offenses and specify corresponding penalties, fines, and punishments for offenses against the safety and welfare of the public or wrongs committed against the federal government or a state government. Criminal laws generally apply to misconduct that is willful, intentional, wanton, or reckless. The doctrine of *equity* was developed to administer justice on principles of fairness, especially when a court or an administrative agency does not have the power or the legal precedents to make, carry out, or enforce a decision.

Standards of proof in cases brought before regulatory, civil, or criminal forums are variable and can overlap depending on the severity and extent of a violation. For example, most questions regarding regulatory law are decided based on whether there was substantial compliance with an agency's rule or regulation. In a civil action, a plaintiff must show that it was more probable than not that a defendant caused an injury or other type of harm. Most criminal cases require that evidence of guilt be beyond a reasonable doubt.

AREAS OF LAW APPLICABLE TO PHLEBOTOMY PRACTICE

The phlebotomist's interactions with patients, clients, and other health care professionals can be viewed from different legal perspectives. Health care workers (most commonly physicians) and patients could be viewed as having an implied contractual relationship. A contract is formed when the physician offers or makes available health services, and the patient agrees to the medical care. The contract is formalized when the physician is paid. There is no requirement for an express written agreement between these two parties to the contract—the actions undertaken by the physician and patient essentially imply that a contract has been made. However, the physician-patient relationship thus formed is more than a mere business deal; it is a voluntary arrangement most aptly seen as creating a status or relationship rather than a contract. Thus the physician-patient relationship gives rise to certain professional duties and fiduciary obligations even when there is no payment for services.[6]

A physician or a patient could be in breach of contract if either does not meet their part of the agreement. However, it is rare indeed for a physician to take legal action against a patient for not following medical instructions. In health law, it is overwhelmingly the patient who sues a physician, hospital, or health care worker. Why do patients sue? They believe the health professional has failed to do something that they should have done. This failure to meet a standard of care, when the health professional has a duty of due care to a patient, most commonly falls under the area of law known as *torts*. For various reasons, claims against health care personnel are usually framed in terms of tortious conduct rather than breach of contract. Patients do not claim that a physician or other health care worker violated a contract; they claim that they committed a tort.[7]

A tort (from the Latin word *torquere*, meaning "twisted") is a civil wrong or injury that may be remedied by a court in the form of an action for damages. All torts involve a violation of some duty that is owed by one individual to another individual. When phlebotomists, a phlebotomy service, or a laboratory employing phlebotomists is held liable for an injury or other damage to a patient or client, each may be blamed for intentionally or unintentionally acting, or failing to act, in a manner that caused an injury. The patient or client who claims to be injured is called the plaintiff. The person being blamed is the defendant.

INTENTIONAL TORTS

In the context of health care, claims falling under the category of intentional torts usually arise in conjunction with questions about whether a patient gave permission for or consented to a medical procedure, treatment, or diagnostic test. When these circumstances occur, they are generally framed as a charge of *assault* or *battery*. In most jurisdictions, assault and battery are criminal offenses.

Assault is any active, willful attempt or threat to inflict injury on another person that is coupled with an apparent ability to inflict such harm. Assault can be committed without actually touching or striking; it is the plaintiff's sense of awareness and apprehension of imminent harm that determines whether there is an assault. *Assault* is often defined as an unlawful attempt to commit a battery.

Battery can be viewed as an active intent to cause harm or injury to a person without that person's consent that actually does harm the person. The offer or threat to use harm is an assault; the use of it is battery. Because battery always includes an assault, the two are commonly combined in the phrase "assault and battery." The term *technical battery* is sometimes used to describe those situations in which a physician or other health care worker, in the course of treatment, exceeds the consent given by the patient, although no harmful purpose was intended.

When a patient enters a hospital or a client comes into a blood-drawing center, the presumption is that they have consented to be treated or have consented to be a donor. However, few individuals would give blanket consent to any and all possible medical procedures without being given more information with which to make an informed choice. (See "Consent and Informed Consent" later in this chapter.) If a phlebotomist proceeds to collect blood after a patient has refused to have blood drawn, the patient could claim that the act of the phlebotomist approaching them with a needle was an assault. If the act of drawing blood was perceived by the patient as painful or injurious, they could claim that battery was committed.

It is not uncommon for patients to feel stress when confronted with medical decisions and procedures. However, occasionally the behavior of health care personnel can intentionally or unintentionally produce severe emotional reactions in patients. Intentional behavior (conduct or words) that is particularly outrageous and extreme can lead to a charge of intentional infliction of emotional distress. Even if conduct is not intended to threaten, if the patient perceives a threat, they may claim negligent infliction of emotional distress. Obviously, the phlebotomist must avoid threatening language ("if you don't let me draw blood, you're going to die") or gestures (acting out a painful procedure) that could create such distress.

UNINTENTIONAL TORTS

When a health care worker violates a duty owed to a patient or client, it is called *malpractice. Malpractice* can be defined as professional misconduct, an unreasonable lack of skill in or faithfulness to professional duties, illegal or immoral conduct, ignorance, or neglectful or careless mistreatment that leads to injury, unnecessary suffering, or the death of a patient or client. Most legal actions involving malpractice by health care personnel are grounded in the theory of negligence, which is the failure of a "duty of due care."

Negligence: What Must Be Proved?

In every legal action for negligence, the plaintiff must go through a four-step process to prove that a health care worker is at fault for failing to perform some legal duty. These four steps, called *elements*, are duty, breach of duty, causation, and damages.

Plaintiffs have the burden of proving each of these four elements. In most malpractice cases, if even one element cannot be proved, then the defendant is not held liable for malpractice. However, in some instances, an average reasonable person who has no special professional knowledge could conclude that an injury would not have occurred in the absence of a negligent act. When a breach of duty is obvious to a layperson,

the doctrine of *res ipsa loquitur* ("the thing speaks for itself") can be applied. This has the effect of shifting the burden of proof to the defendant, who must then prove that they were *not* negligent.

Duty

As a citizen, every individual has a duty to behave as a reasonably careful person would, given the same or similar circumstances. This standard of behavior means that individuals must act or refrain from acting so as not to injure or damage another person or that person's property. The duty to meet a standard of behavior or care can arise from a state statute or city ordinance (such as "Do not cross the street when the light is red"). In health care, duty is usually established by standards of care or practice that exist by custom or by professional rules and guidelines. The legal standard of care is "that degree of skill, proficiency, knowledge, and care ordinarily possessed and employed by members in the profession." The standard has to be shown to exist, and the phlebotomist must be performing in the capacity applicable to that standard.

Those persons engaged in professions that require special knowledge and skills are judged according to a standard of care upheld by similar professionals. For phlebotomists, the test to determine what they did or should have done would be, "What would a reasonable, prudent *phlebotomist* have done under the same or similar circumstances?" In the past, physicians and other health professionals were held to standards that existed in their own communities (the so-called *locality rule*). Because health professionals now have access to information outside their own communities, this standard has been expanded to include what would be expected in similar communities. When national standards exist, such as national certification examinations or national accreditation standards for schools, a national standard of care can be imposed. This is true for the profession of phlebotomy—for example, a phlebotomist in California is held to the same standard of care used for a phlebotomist in New York, unless a state regulation requires a standard stricter than the national standard.

Breach of Duty

Conduct that exposes others to an unreasonable risk of harm is a breach of duty. The plaintiff must be able to show what actually happened and that the defendant acted unreasonably. Either direct or circumstantial evidence can demonstrate what happened. If the defendant knew or should have known that there was a reasonable probability that their conduct would cause harm, then the defendant will be found to have breached the duty of due care.

Causation

The cause of harm or injury is both a factual and a legal question. To show *cause-in-fact* (or actual cause), the plaintiff must demonstrate that they would not have been injured but for the conduct of the defendant. There must be a direct line from the conduct to the injury with no intervening circumstances and no other factors or events that contributed to the injury. *Proximate cause* is the term used to distinguish legal causation from factual causation. Legal (proximate) cause is a policy choice that essentially determines who should bear the costs of harm. If an injury was reasonably foreseeable by the defendant, then the defendant will be held legally liable for the injury.

Damages

Once negligence and causation are established, plaintiffs must be able to show that they were actually damaged by the negligent act. The harm to a plaintiff may be physical, emotional, or financial. In these circumstances, courts attempt to place a monetary value on the injury. Compensatory damages attempt to reimburse the plaintiff to the position the plaintiff was in before the injury. Special damages allow recovery of economic losses during the time of injury, which may be for medical bills or lost wages but also can be for future losses. Future losses might include the costs of continuing medical treatment or loss of future wages if the person is unable to return to work. General damages are those costs related to the injury itself. Punitive damages, those assessed to punish a defendant, are usually not awarded in negligence cases, unless the defendant's conduct was reckless or willful.

Liability of Employers for Phlebotomy Personnel

Most phlebotomists are employed by hospitals, independent laboratories, or other health care organizations, and when a phlebotomist is found to be negligent, their employer can also be found negligent. The employer,

employee's supervisor, or a laboratory director may be vicariously liable when the employee's negligent conduct falls within the scope of the employment, regardless of whether the employer was actually present or had the ability to control the employee's conduct. *Respondeat superior* ("let the master answer") is the legal doctrine that places an employer in a position of responsibility for the acts of its employees. An employer has an affirmative duty to control the conduct of employees.

In corporate negligence theory, a hospital, its board of directors, administrators, and reviewing committees, and any other persons who act as agents for the corporation owe a duty of due care to patients. The principles of corporate negligence are similar to those of vicarious liability, but in corporate negligence, liability is imposed on the corporate entity and on nonmedical agents of the corporation rather than on negligent physicians or allied health personnel. Examples of corporate negligence include a commercial laboratory hiring an unqualified laboratorian or a hospital maintaining an unsafe environment for patient treatment.

The types of duties owed by a hospital directly to a patient include a duty to use reasonable care to maintain safe and adequate equipment and facilities, a duty to oversee all who practice medicine within the hospital walls, a duty to select and retain competent physician and nonphysician personnel, and a duty to establish and enforce policies and rules that ensure quality care for patients.[8] Under corporate liability, a hospital cannot avoid liability by delegating these duties to physicians or other individuals who work in the hospital. Clearly, this duty extends to specimen collection stations or satellite laboratories owned, operated, or supervised by the hospital or independent laboratory.

HOW IS THE PHLEBOTOMY STANDARD OF CARE DETERMINED?

Courts and plaintiffs rely on a variety of sources to show that standards of care and practice exist for a particular profession. All states have statutes called *medical practice acts* (MPAs) that define the qualifications and experience necessary to legally practice medicine. MPAs usually delineate which medical procedures or tests can be delegated to other health personnel under a physician's supervision, and they prohibit anyone who is not licensed as a physician or other health professional (such as a nurse or physical therapist) from practicing healing or diagnostic medicine. State licensing boards generally review cases in which a person is engaged in the unauthorized practice of medicine. MPAs are enforced through disciplinary actions imposed by licensing boards and, in extreme cases, by criminal sanctions.[9]

Many states also *license* allied health personnel. Because most state licensing boards require some proof of qualification for licensure, lack of a license may be used to demonstrate a failure to meet a standard of care. Situations may arise in which a person has the appropriate education, training, or experience to practice in an allied health profession but does not have a license to practice. When an individual is not licensed and malpractice is shown, that individual's conduct may be declared to be negligence per se, in which practicing without a license is a violation of a statute.[5]

Hospital and laboratory *certification* or *accreditation standards and guidelines* can be used to demonstrate quality control and quality assurance procedures in phlebotomy practice. Even when standards are voluntary, compliance with or awareness of standards and guidelines can be used to show that a phlebotomy service or a phlebotomist knew or should have known what procedures and conduct were appropriate under the circumstances. Certification and accreditation guidelines are especially effective as evidence of practice standards when they are applicable nationwide and followed by a variety and number of phlebotomy services and phlebotomy practitioners. Examples of organizations that accredit or certify phlebotomy services include The Joint Commission, the College of American Pathologists, and the American Association of Blood Banks.

Mandatory standards in the form of federal, state, and local laws and regulations are commonly used to establish a statutory standard of practice for phlebotomy services. Regulations usually outline minimum standards of performance. Mere compliance with a statutory requirement does not necessarily protect phlebotomy services and personnel from negligent actions, especially if it can be shown that personnel knew or should have known that more comprehensive actions were required, either in general or as related to the specific circumstances surrounding the plaintiff. Examples of federal statutory standards are those contained in the Clinical Laboratory Improvement Amendments of 1988 (CLIA '88)[10] and the Occupational Safety and Health Administration's (OSHA) Rules on Occupational Exposure to Bloodborne Pathogens.[11] States may have health and safety statutes that are similar to or more stringent than federal standards. Cities usually have health and safety codes or ordinances that govern areas such as storage of chemicals and disposal of waste materials. When federal and state laws or regulations apply to laboratory practice, the laboratories are usually required to abide by the more stringent law.

Statements of competencies, such as those contained in the National Accreditation Agency for Clinical Laboratory Sciences' Phlebotomy Programs Approval Guide,[12] or designated skills, such as those listed in the National Phlebotomy Association certification standards,[13] describe tasks and activities required of phlebotomy practitioners. These can be used to show how an individual failed to meet a particular level of performance. For example, if there is a question whether a phlebotomist performed a capillary collection correctly and the competency expects an entry-level phlebotomist to be able to perform the correct procedure for capillary collection, the statement of competency can be used to establish the appropriate standard of care.

Professional practice guidelines, which appear in brochures or bulletins written or endorsed by professional organizations, can be used to show a recommended practice that is viewed by the profession as clinically effective or technically superior. Guidelines may relate to timing of blood collections, collection of patient data, preservation and handling procedures, or follow-up and documentation protocols.

Technical guidelines and standards that describe how to perform a certain test or procedure can be used to show how a phlebotomist was negligent in the collection, handling, or transportation of blood specimens.[14]

Scientific journals and textbooks (learned treatises) can be used to demonstrate that knowledge was available to a practitioner at the time of the negligent act, thereby showing what the practitioner should have known or done.

The testimony of expert witnesses is commonly used to establish the standard of practice in a health profession. In a case involving a phlebotomist, an experienced phlebotomist, a physician, or a phlebotomy supervisor can be asked to state an opinion on what constitutes acceptable quality control or assurance practices.

OTHER LEGAL DOCTRINES AND AREAS OF LAW APPLICABLE TO PHLEBOTOMY PRACTICE

INTERPLAY AMONG THE RIGHTS OF PRIVACY, CONFIDENTIALITY, AND INFORMED CONSENT

Legal disputes involving intentional and unintentional injury to patients and clients by health care workers have their roots in guaranteed individual rights. These rights have their basis in the U.S. Constitution and Bill of Rights, regardless of whether they are specifically enumerated in the Constitution. For example, the U.S. Constitution does not mention a right of privacy; however, the U.S. Supreme Court has recognized that a right of privacy exists and that certain areas of privacy are guaranteed under the Constitution.[7] The right of privacy includes the right to confidentiality, and if this right is waived, consent to the waiver must be informed.

Right of Privacy

An individual's right "to be let alone," recognized in all U.S. jurisdictions, includes the right to be free of "intrusion upon physical and mental solitude or seclusion" and the right to be free of "public disclosure of private facts."[7] Every health care institution and health care worker has a duty to respect a patient's or client's right of privacy, which includes the privacy and confidentiality of information obtained from the patient or client for purposes of diagnosis, medical records, and public health—reporting requirements. If a health care worker conducts tests on or publishes information about a patient or client without that person's consent, the health care worker could be sued for wrongful invasion of privacy, defamation, fraud, false imprisonment, or other actionable torts.

Confidentiality

Health care workers must be vigilant in keeping information about patients and clients confidential. This is especially true in blood banks, transfusion services, and phlebotomy services, where phlebotomists may have access to information about patients who are human immunodeficiency virus (HIV)—positive, who have acquired immune deficiency syndrome (AIDS) or other sexually transmitted diseases, or who may have medical histories that, if disclosed, might cause undue embarrassment to or prejudice or discrimination against that patient. Phlebotomists and their supervisors should understand that they have a legal duty to keep records, documentation, and laboratory test results confidential. This duty may be waived only if a patient has given express permission for the information to be released, if the patient has sued the institution or its health care personnel, or if the health care worker is specifically obligated to release patient information (for example, to the Centers for Disease Control and Prevention [CDC] or other authorized public health department). Even in the last situation, care must be taken to ensure that the confidentiality of patient records and reports cannot be breached while they are being communicated or are in transit.[9] The section on the Health Insurance Portability and Accountability Act of 1996 (HIPAA) provides a deeper understanding of the responsibilities.

Consent and Informed Consent

Physicians and other health care workers are required to obtain a patient's consent before performing any invasive or diagnostic procedure. Consent can take various forms (such as written agreements, spoken words, implicit actions, or making an appointment for a test). In a nineteenth-century case, for example, a plaintiff's failure to object to a vaccine that the defendant was preparing to give to the plaintiff conveyed apparent consent to the injection.[15] In our current health care system, many individuals obtain laboratory test requests from their primary health providers. For instance, consent is implied when a patient then goes to an outpatient test center to have their blood drawn. Implied consent for laboratory specimen collection also applies in critical situations, such as when an individual is brought to an emergency room or trauma center and must have blood drawn as part of the diagnostic workup.

However, to agree to a medical procedure, a patient must first know what they are agreeing to. Thus the doctrine of consent has expanded to include *informed consent*, which emphasizes that health care workers must fully disclose any risks, alternatives, and benefits of a procedure or test so that the patient or client can make an informed decision about whether they want to be treated or tested.[16] "[T]he doctrine of informed consent imposes on a physician, before he subjects his patient to medical treatment, the duty to explain the procedure to the patient and to warn him of any material risks or dangers inherent in or collateral to the therapy, so as to enable the patient to make an intelligent and informed choice about whether or not to undergo such treatment."[17]

The correlate to informed consent is *informed refusal.* Patients may refuse treatment for religious, social, financial, or other reasons, but even in these cases a health care worker may be found negligent for the lack of information given to the patient if the patient didn't have enough information available to make a reasonable decision to forego treatment.[16]

In general, it is the physician who has the duty to disclose adequate information to a patient. Phlebotomists should be wary of volunteering information to a patient in situations in which they do not have the legal or professional authority to do so. These situations may be difficult judgment calls for the phlebotomist because patients often ask phlebotomists questions about their treatment or why they are drawing blood. The phlebotomist should politely refer the patient to their physician or charge nurse for these explanations.

HEALTH INSURANCE PORTABILITY AND ACCOUNTABILITY ACT OF 1996

In passing HIPAA,[18] the U.S. Congress attempted to streamline the health care system and reduce costs. One HIPAA provision was designed to help health care providers more easily transmit health information. However, it became clear that electronic transmission of health information could jeopardize patient privacy.

Subsequently, the U.S. Department of Health and Human Services (DHHS) enacted the HIPAA Privacy Rule, which became effective on April 14, 2003. This ruling protects patients' confidential medical records and personal health information. It limits the use and release of health information that can be identified, gives patients access to their medical records, and restricts disclosure of health information to a minimum needed for the intended purpose. It also establishes safeguards and restrictions about disclosure of records for purposes such as public health, research, and law enforcement.[19] Doctors, nurses, and any other health care providers, including phlebotomists, must comply with the HIPAA Privacy Rule. They must ensure that protected health information (PHI), which is any written, verbal, or electronic "individually identifiable"

information, including laboratory tests, is not intentionally or unintentionally disclosed to unauthorized individuals or companies. Phlebotomists must ensure that customary laboratory fixtures such as patient sign-in sheets, computer screens, accession logs, fax pages, blood collection supplies, and the like are not shared with or viewable by unauthorized persons.[20] Noncompliance is subject to criminal and civil sanctions under HIPAA, and most laboratory employees are required to sign their employer's nondisclosure statement.

PATIENT'S BILL OF RIGHTS AND THE PATIENT CARE PARTNERSHIP

Whereas the HIPAA rule focuses on health care providers, their employees, and business associates, the *Patient's Bill of Rights* is patient centered. The American Hospital Association in the early 1970s developed a policy statement for health care institutions and their patients that incorporated and reflected the individual rights guaranteed under the legal doctrines of privacy, informed consent, and confidentiality. Since that time, many hospitals have adopted the Patient's Bill of Rights into their policy manuals, and some state legislatures have passed Patient's Bill of Rights statutes.[21]

The Patient's Bill of Rights, now termed the *Patient Care Partnership,* is intended to "promote the interests and well-being of the patients and residents of health care facilities."[1] As such, it enumerates the patient's right to respectful care, to adequate information with which to make an informed decision (or refusal) about their care, and to confidentiality in treatment and communication of records about their medical care program. In addition, the document affirms a patient's right to information about medical bills and charges, possible involvement in medical research and experimentation, and hospital rules and regulations (see Box 11.2).

MEDICAL DEVICES AND EQUIPMENT FAILURES

Phlebotomists use many pieces of equipment and/or reagents that are manufactured by medical equipment or pharmaceutical companies and then purchased by the hospital or laboratory from manufacturers, distributors, or retailers. These supplies—whether they be needles, syringes, collection tubes, protective equipment or clothing, chemicals, or blood—may, in unusual situations, be defective or unsafe because of the way they were designed, assembled, or screened, or they may be inherently dangerous even when used under normal conditions. When a patient suffers a needle break during blood draw, has a violent reaction to a drug, or contracts an infectious disease after use of a product, they may sue the manufacturer of that product under various legal theories, including negligence, strict liability in tort, and breach of *implied warranty of merchantability.*

Under negligence theory, plaintiffs must prove that the defendants (the manufacturers) have a duty to conform to certain standards of care in the manufacture of their products and to guard against unreasonable risks. *Strict liability in tort* is imposed when manufacturers are held liable for injuries caused by an unreasonably dangerous or defective product, even if there is no finding of fault. Breach of an implied warranty of merchantability may be found on the basis that manufacturers or sellers of goods should be obligated to provide consumers with products that are fit for the purpose for which they are being sold.

These legal actions fall under the law of *products liability.* Products liability focuses on the liability of suppliers for defective products that cause physical harm. The defect in question may not be the actual product itself; defects may arise because of inadequate packaging, instructions, or warning labels.[22]

The term *product* implies goods that are sold predominantly in commercial settings. Manufacturer liability for defective health care products has received much professional and legal attention because health care treatment and diagnostic testing has traditionally been viewed as a service rather than as a product. Especially in the areas of blood transfusions (which may result in HIV transmission) and genetically engineered pharmaceuticals (such as coagulation components), the distinction between products and services has been challenged by plaintiffs who sue blood banks or pharmaceutical companies to recover damages resulting from transmission of infectious diseases.

Because the availability of blood and blood products is of great importance to public health, many states have passed blood shield statutes that exempt blood transfers, blood derivatives, or blood products from the threat of products liability lawsuits and specifically mandate that blood components are to be considered medical services, not goods or products. Immunity from legal action thus guarantees an adequate blood supply for use in medical emergencies and treatment of chronic blood-related disorders.

CASE LAW

As the range of health care services has expanded and health care personnel have become more specialized, the reach of malpractice litigation is no longer confined to the physician-patient relationship and may include nonmedical personnel as part of the health care team. Although most of the following cases did not specifically involve phlebotomists, the situations can be compared with laboratory and phlebotomy practice. These cases demonstrate how nonphysician health care personnel can become involved in lawsuits and remind phlebotomists of the consequences of poor practice standards and procedures.

- *Shumosky vs. Lutheran Welfare Services and Bayada Nurses*, 2001 Pa Super 285 [Nurse accidentally pricked her finger with a needle used to give a patient with AIDS an injection. The nurse sued for negligent infliction of emotional distress, among other causes of action, stating that her employers failed to inform her that the patient had AIDS.] More recently (2010), a phlebotomist working in an emergency department was stabbed by a mentally unstable and sometimes violent HIV- and hepatitis C-positive patient with the needle he used to draw blood from her. Although treated prophylactically with antiretrovirals, the phlebotomist became emotionally stressed and sued the hospital and supervisor for not communicating to him the dangerous nature of the patient. The jury agreed; the defendant was awarded several hundred thousand dollars.
- *Arbogast vs. Mid-Ohio Valley Medical Corp*, S Ct App WVa, No. 31314, October 31, 2003 [Patient had blood drawn from her outstretched, unsupported arm by a laboratory technician. Later, patient complained of bruising, numbness, and pain. Patient sued, alleging negligence in blood drawing that caused her to develop "complex regional pain syndrome" for which she underwent surgery. National Committee on Clinical Laboratory Standards blood collection standards were used to establish standard

of care. Court concluded that venipuncture as proximate cause of injury was not proved. Judgment for defendant (Mid-Ohio Valley Medical Corp).] With a similar set of facts but with a different result in 2005, a laboratory had made a motion for summary judgment (which would effectively dismiss the case). However, the court found that the laboratory could be held vicariously liable for the plaintiff's injury. *Wilkerson vs. Laboratory Corporation of America*, No. 2:04-CV-03212, U.S. Dist. Ct E Dist Pa. July 13, 2005.

- *Unpublished Opinion*, May 23, 2003, Ky App [Phlebotomist placed tourniquet on plaintiff's arm, then left room for 10 minutes. Plaintiff's arm became swollen and painful, resulting in substantial medical expenses for treatment. Plaintiff successfully sued for negligence—leaving tourniquet in place for extended time did not conform to phlebotomy standard of care.] *http://www.kaiserpapers.org/bloodletter.html* (accessed 11/28/03) [Hospital fined by state for violations of OSHA standards, including Bloodborne Pathogens Standard, for failure to maintain detailed sharps injury log, lack of effective infection control plan, failure to use devices with engineered sharp injury protection, removing needles from tube holders, and phlebotomists reusing tube holders.]
- *Hubbard vs. Fewell et al*, No. COA04-1072, App. Ct, N.C (2005). [Blood drawn by phlebotomist to determine whether patient was a Factor VIII carrier was misdiagnosed as negative. Relying on negative result, plaintiff subsequently delivered son with hemophilia. This case was settled. However, it was further determined that the blood sample may not have been prepared and transported in a timely manner, which may have further contributed to the misdiagnosis. The defendant's grant of summary judgment from the lower court was reversed by this Appellate Court.]
- *Belmon vs. St. Frances Cabrini Hospital*, 427 So2d 541, 544 (LaApp, 1983) [Negligent blood sample collection by a medical technician caused hemorrhage.]
- *Bagent vs. Illini Community Hospital*, et al. S. Ct. Il, docket no. 102430, 2007 [Plaintiff filed complaint against hospital under a theory of *respondeat superior*. The circuit court entered summary judgment

in favor of the hospital. A divided panel of the appellate court reversed that judgment. 363 Ill. App. 3d 916. This court found that the phlebotomist breached duty of health care practitioner—patient confidentiality in violation of that state's Hospital Licensing Act, when phlebotomist disclosed the results of a pregnancy test while off duty after hours in a bar.]

- *Butler vs. Louisiana State Board of Education*, 331 So2d 192, 196 (LaApp, 1976) [A donor fainted and sustained injuries, and a biology professor was held negligent for not giving students previous instructions on blood drawing and donor care.]
- *St. Paul Fire and Marine Insurance Co vs. Prothro*, 590 SW2d 35 (Ark App 1979) [Negligent physical therapy procedures caused a patient to develop a *Staphylococcus* infection.]
- *Simpson vs. Sisters of Charity of Providence*, 588 P2d 4 (Or 1978) [Radiology technician performed a poor-quality radiograph that failed to demonstrate a fracture that subsequently caused paralysis.]
- *Southeastern Kentucky Baptist Hospital, Inc vs. Bruce*, 539 SW2d 286 (Ky 1976) [Misidentification of a patient led to a surgical procedure on the wrong patient.]
- *Wood vs. Miller*, 76 P2d 963 (Or 1983) [Negligent use of diathermy equipment burned a patient.]
- *Favalora vs. Aetna Casualty and Surety Co*, 144 So2d 544 (La App 1962) [A patient fainted and fell, sustaining injuries; a radiology technician and supervising physician were found negligent for not being alert to and prepared for the patient's condition.]
- *McCormick vs. Auret* (Ga 1980) [Failure to use sterile equipment during venipuncture led to nerve damage secondary to infection.]
- *Alessio vs. Crook*, 633 SW2d 770 (Tenn App 1982) [Failure to include an x-ray report in the patient's medical record before patient discharge resulted in more extensive surgery than would have been required had the physician seen the report.]
- *Variety Children's Hospital vs. Osle*, 292 So2d 382 (Fl App D3 1974) [A surgeon failed to label and separate specimens sent to a pathology laboratory. Because the pathologist was unable to determine which of the two specimens was malignant, removal of both of the patient's breasts was necessary.]

- *Jeanes vs. Milner,* 428 F2d 598 (Ark 1970) [A 1-month delay in mailing specimens to a laboratory resulted in delayed diagnosis of cancer; if it had been detected promptly and treated, the pain and suffering of the patient could have been lessened.]
- *Ray vs. Wagner,* 176 NW2d 101 (Minn 1970) [A patient claimed a physician was negligent for failing to notify her of her malignancy in a timely fashion; the patient was found contributorily negligent for giving the physician incomplete and misleading information about how she could be reached.]
- *Thor vs. Boska,* 113 Cal Rptr 296 (1974) [A physician's inability to produce medical records after he had been sued for malpractice created an inference of guilt.]
- *Lauro vs. Travelers Insurance Company,* 262 So2d 787 (La App 1972) [A hospital was not negligent for not using the latest laboratory equipment available, where current standards of care demonstrated that the equipment used was acceptable.]

DEFENSES TO LEGAL CLAIMS

If faced with a lawsuit brought by a patient, the laboratory and the phlebotomist may resort to several defenses to avoid a finding of liability.

STATUTES OF LIMITATION

All states have statutes of limitation that restrict or limit the length of time in which a claimant can file a cause of action after an injury. The purpose of statutes of limitation is twofold. First, they are intended to compel legal actions within a reasonable time so that potential litigants have a fair opportunity to defend themselves while evidence and witnesses are still available.[7] Second, they allow presumably innocent parties to continue their lives and livelihoods without the constant and continuing threat of liability.

In malpractice cases, statutes of limitation can start at several points: at the time of the negligent act, at the time when the injury was discovered, or when the physician-patient relationship ends.

The length of time these statutes run varies from state to state and can be a few months to many years, depending on the cause of action and nature of the injury. Statutes of limitation may also be tolled (suspended or stopped temporarily) if, for example, the

plaintiff is a child, the defendant is absent from the jurisdiction, or the injury in question has been fraudulently concealed.

CONTRIBUTORY NEGLIGENCE

In rare malpractice situations, a patient's own actions may fall below the standard to which a reasonably prudent patient might be expected to conform. For example, if a patient, during the course of a routine blood collection procedure, unreasonably manipulates or otherwise interferes with the venipuncture to the extent that they are injured, and then sues the phlebotomist for the injury, the phlebotomist may raise the affirmative defense of contributory negligence.[23]

In some states, contributory negligence completely bars recovery against the defendant, even if the defendant is found negligent. In other states, a finding of contributory negligence has the effect of reducing the amount of monetary damages against a negligent defendant.

ADEQUATE AND ACCURATE RECORDS AS THE BEST DEFENSE

The importance of detailed, legible, comprehensive record keeping and documentation for laboratory procedures and patient identification cannot be overemphasized. Documentation relating to the laboratory not only is required by federal regulations and accreditation organizations, but it is also essential in the legal arena. Legal action against a laboratory rarely takes place at the moment malpractice occurs; claims may be filed years later. Even after a claim is filed, it may be several more years before all evidence is collected in the discovery process and the claim is litigated in court. During this waiting period, memories fade, contemporaneous records may be misfiled or lost, and laboratory personnel change.

Laboratory notations and records should never be altered without documentation of the reasons for the change. Indeed, poorly maintained, sloppy, or altered records may prejudice a jury against a laboratory or health care professional, no matter how well intentioned the change might have been.

A laboratory's or phlebotomist's best defense is the ability to produce witnesses and records that substantiate adherence to acceptable professional standards of practice for documenting identifiable specimen collection, test procedures, test reporting, records storage and archiving procedures, quality control and quality assurance methods, and remedial or corrective actions when laboratory errors occur.[7]

CHAIN OF CUSTODY IN THE CLINICAL LABORATORY

Chain of custody is a rule of legal evidence that requires an authorized person (e.g., a police officer, attorney, clinical or forensic testing laboratory, or medical examiner) to account for the location, control, and integrity of a specimen, result, or report at all times. Any break in this chain of custody, from specimen collection to the presentation of test results in a court of law, may suggest that the specimen was tampered with or otherwise altered. If continuous and uninterrupted custody cannot be established, the laboratory specimen or the result(s) of testing may not be admissible as evidence in a legal case.[24]

It is not uncommon for phlebotomists to be called on to collect urine or blood specimens from individuals for the purpose of screening for narcotics, alcohol, or infectious agents. Phlebotomists may also be required to transport specimens that may become evidence in a criminal investigation. To establish each link in the chain of custody, each component step of the specimen-testing process (including requisition and report forms) must be documented. Most often this is accomplished by a chain-of-custody form that accompanies the specimen. All individuals who receive, release, or otherwise come into contact with the specimen are required to sign, date, and timestamp the form to show that the specimen was not tampered with. Phlebotomists or other laboratory workers may be asked to testify about their role in maintaining the chain of custody.

Although the primary purpose of establishing a chain of custody is to ensure that evidence is admissible, the documentation required is not unlike the quality and accuracy-based patient test management provisions of CLIA '88 (see later). In legal cases alleging patient misidentification, lost specimens, or missing reports, laboratories may be required to show not only an unbroken chain of custody but also that they have complied with the provisions of CLIA '88.

LEGAL AND PROFESSIONAL PROTECTIONS FOR THE PHLEBOTOMIST

The legal doctrines and statutory provisions covered in this chapter focus on the rights and protections available to patients, clients, and donors when faced with substandard or negligent laboratory and phlebotomy practices. Phlebotomists, too, may be concerned about their own exposure to hazardous or infectious agents or about unsafe working conditions. Phlebotomists do have recourse to address these concerns, in addition to bringing unsafe conditions to the attention of their immediate supervisors.

When phlebotomy services are understaffed, phlebotomists are sometimes called on to perform additional tasks that are either beyond the scope of their expertise or increase workloads to the point at which patient care is compromised. Especially in the area of nursing, *protest of assignment forms* are sometimes used as a means to alert supervisors to potentially dangerous practice situations. These forms usually become part of the employee's file and therefore should not be used casually or merely to complain about a short-term situation. They should be used by the phlebotomist only when an extra work assignment is protracted, excessive, clearly unreasonable, and imminently dangerous to the phlebotomist or to their patients.

The regulations of OSHA and analogous state agencies are specifically designed to protect the health and safety of employees in the workplace. Phlebotomists should report any hazardous or unsafe materials, conditions, or practices to their supervisor and should be active participants in the formulation of workplace policies to avoid or protect against these situations.

It is generally not necessary for phlebotomists to purchase individual professional liability (malpractice) insurance) policies because most health care employers and institutions cover employees under blanket policies. Phlebotomists should check to see whether they are specifically included in or excluded from the employer's insurance policy and whether their employer's policy is an "occurrence" or "claims-made" policy. Occurrence policies protect employees even at a future date, provided that the policy was in effect at the time when the alleged malpractice incident occurred. A claims-made policy is one that must be continually in force at both the time of the incident and the time the claim is made.

Phlebotomists who are self-employed, either as temporary workers placed in positions through an employment agency or as independent contractors, may purchase professional liability insurance through several companies that provide individual or group coverage to allied health practitioners. Liability policies usually cover monetary damages for personal injuries up to preset limits and usually include coverage for attorney fees and court costs. Many companies provide legal counsel as part of the coverage.

REGULATION OF LABORATORIES AND LABORATORY PRACTITIONERS

In the past few years, laboratories, laboratory practitioners, and other health care workers have been subject to heightened scrutiny and oversight by state and federal government agencies, both for the protection of the health and welfare of the public and for their own protection. Although state laboratory regulation is quite diverse, federal regulation is intended to apply to virtually all laboratory and health care settings.

CLINICAL LABORATORY IMPROVEMENT AMENDMENTS OF 1988

In October 1988, the U.S. Congress passed Public Law 100 to 578, CLIA '88, amid a flurry of television and newspaper coverage about poorly run laboratories that were misdiagnosing or mishandling laboratory tests and amid reports of questionable business and payment practices. Congress delegated authority to administer this public law to the Centers for Medicare and Medicaid Services (CMS) (formerly the Health Care Financing Administration). The CDC and CMS's Division of Laboratory Services, within the Survey and Certification Group under the Center for Medicaid and State Operations, now have the responsibility for overseeing the CLIA program.

The federal regulations implementing CLIA '88 went into effect on September 1, 1992. After several revisions, final rules became effective on January 24, 2004. The rules are intended to ensure the quality and accuracy of laboratory testing by creating a uniform set of provisions governing all laboratories that examine human specimens for the diagnosis, prevention, or treatment of any disease or impairment of, or the assessment of the health of, human beings.[10] Virtually every clinical testing laboratory in the United States, whether in a hospital, a physician office laboratory, or an independent facility, must be certified by the federal government. Facilities that only collect or prepare specimens (or both) or only serve as a mailing service and do not perform testing are not considered laboratories.

Laboratories are subject to inspections by federal and state agencies. Government inspectors or their agents can periodically review laboratory operations to ensure compliance with CLIA '88.

Under CLIA '88, the level of regulatory oversight and performance expectations depends on the complexity of a given test procedure, rather than on the location or type of laboratory. All laboratory tests (called *analytes*) are categorized as waived, provider-performed microscopy procedures, moderately complex, or highly complex, with highly complex testing subject to the most stringent regulations. The level of test complexity is determined by assessing the relative simplicity or difficulty of conducting the test and the relative risk of harm to the patient if the test is performed incorrectly. Most specimens collected by phlebotomists are for moderately or highly complex testing in clinical hematology or clinical chemistry laboratories.

The CLIA '88 regulations include provisions for preanalytical, analytical, and postanalytical steps in the testing process. Regulations mandate proficiency testing of laboratories based on the types of tests they perform. In addition, laboratories are required to demonstrate and document their quality control and quality assurance procedures to ensure that patient tests and records are managed appropriately and to demonstrate that testing personnel have adequate education, training, and experience to perform tests. The focus of the CLIA '88 regulations is on *continuous quality improvement* and *outcome measures*. Laboratories must show that the methods used to test specimens lead to accurate, reliable, quality test results.

Laboratories not meeting the conditions required by the CLIA '88 provisions can be subject to various sanctions and penalties. These range from directed plans of correction to withholding of payment from the Medicare and Medicaid programs for laboratory tests. Laboratories that remain out of compliance with the regulations may be shut down or have substantial monetary fines imposed.

Phlebotomists are responsible for performing many of the pre- and postanalytical steps in the blood testing process. The laboratory's overall performance and its ability to maintain consistent and reproducible quality tests rely in large part on the quality and preservation of specimens collected by the phlebotomist. Therefore knowledge of and compliance with these provisions can not only contribute to quality patient care but also provide the phlebotomist and the laboratory with some measure of protection against regulatory sanctions and civil lawsuits.

The current CLIA Regulations can be accessed at *http://wwwn.cdc.gov/clia/regs/toc.aspx*. The following selected provisions of CLIA '88 have special significance to phlebotomists and phlebotomy practice.

Subpart J: Facility Administration for Nonwaived Testing

§493.1101 Standard: Facilities

(a) The laboratory must be constructed, arranged, and maintained to ensure the following:
  (1) The space, ventilation, and utilities necessary for conducting all phases of the testing process.
  (2) Contamination of patient specimens, equipment, instruments, reagents, materials, and supplies is minimized.
(b) The laboratory must have appropriate and sufficient equipment, instruments, reagents, materials, and supplies for the type and volume of testing it performs.
(c) The laboratory must be in compliance with applicable federal, state, and local laboratory requirements.
(d) Safety procedures must be established, accessible, and observed to ensure protection from physical, chemical, biochemical, and electrical hazards, and biohazardous materials.

Subpart K: Quality Systems for Nonwaived Testing
§493.1200 Introduction

(a) Each laboratory that performs nonwaived testing must establish and maintain written policies and procedures that implement and monitor a quality system for all phases of the total testing process

(that is, preanalytic, analytic, and postanalytic) as well as general laboratory systems.
(b) The laboratory's quality systems must include a quality assessment component that ensures continuous improvement of the laboratory's performance and services through ongoing monitoring that identifies, evaluates, and resolves problems.
(c) The various components of the laboratory's quality system…must be appropriate for the…testing the laboratory performs, services it offers, and clients it serves.

§493.1232 Standard: Specimen identification and integrity

The laboratory must establish and follow written policies and procedures that ensure positive identification and optimum integrity of a patient's specimen from the time of collection or receipt of the specimen through completion of testing and reporting of results.

§493.1241 Standard: Test request

(a) The laboratory must have a written or electronic request for patient testing from an authorized person.
(b) The laboratory may accept oral requests for laboratory tests if it solicits a written or electronic authorization within 30 days of the oral request and maintains the authorization or documentation of its efforts to obtain the authorization.
(c) The laboratory must ensure the test requisition solicits the following information:
  (1) The name and address or other suitable identifiers of the authorized person requesting the test…
  (2) The patient's name or unique patient identifier.
  (3) The sex and age or date of birth of the patient.
  (4) The test(s) to be performed.
  (5) The source of the specimen, when appropriate.
  (6) The date and, if appropriate, time of specimen collection.
  (7) Any additional information relevant and necessary for a specific test to ensure accurate and timely testing and reporting of results.

§493.1242 Standard: Specimen submission, handling, and referral

(a) The laboratory must establish and follow written policies and procedures for each of the following, if applicable:
    (1) Patient preparation.
    (2) Specimen collection.
    (3) Specimen labeling, including patient name or unique patient identifier and, when appropriate, specimen source.
    (4) Specimen storage and preservation.
    (5) Conditions for specimen transportation.
    (6) Specimen processing.
    (7) Specimen acceptability and rejection.
(b) The laboratory must document the date and time it receives a specimen.

§493.1283 Standard: Test records

(a) The laboratory must maintain an information or record system that includes the following:
    (1) The positive identification of the specimen.
    (2) The date and time of specimen receipt into the laboratory.
    (3) The condition and disposition of specimens that do not meet the laboratory's criteria for specimen acceptability.
    (4) The records and dates of all specimen testing, including the identity of the personnel who performed the test(s).
(b) Records of patient testing including, if applicable, instrument printouts, must be retained.

§493.1231 Standard: Confidentiality of patient information

The laboratory must ensure confidentiality of patient information throughout all phases of the total testing process that is under the laboratory's control.

§493.1291 Test report

(f) Test results must be released only to authorized persons and, if applicable, the individual responsible for using the test results and the laboratory that initially requested the test.

§493.1250 Condition: Analytic systems

The laboratory must monitor and evaluate the overall quality of the analytic systems and correct identified problems.

§493.1251 Standard: Procedure manual

(a) A written procedure manual for all tests, assays, and examinations performed by the laboratory must be available to, and followed by, laboratory personnel. Textbooks may supplement but not replace the laboratory's written procedures for testing or examining specimens.
(b) The procedure manual must include the following when applicable to the test procedure:
    (1) Requirements for patient preparation; specimen collection, labeling, storage, preservation, transportation, processing, and referral; and criteria for specimen acceptability and rejection…
    (2) Preparation of slides, solutions, calibrators, controls, reagents, stains, and other materials used in testing.

§493.1252 Standard: Test systems, equipment, instruments, reagents, materials, and supplies

(a) Testing must be performed following the manufacturer's instructions and in a manner that provides test results within the laboratory's stated performance…
(b) The laboratory must define criteria for those conditions that are essential for proper storage of reagents and specimens, accurate and reliable test system operation, and test result reporting…and…include the following…:
    (1) Protection of equipment and instruments from fluctuations and interruptions in electrical current that adversely affect patient test results and test reports.
(c) Reagents, solutions…and other supplies…must be labeled to indicate the following:
    (1) Identity…
    (2) Storage requirements.
    (3) Preparation and expiration dates.

(4) Other pertinent information required for proper use.

(d) Reagents, solutions, and other supplies must not be used when they have exceeded their expiration date, have deteriorated, or are of substandard quality.

(e) Components of reagent kits of different lot numbers must not be interchanged unless otherwise specified by the manufacturer.

§493.1254 Standard: Maintenance and function checks

(b) [For] equipment, instruments, or test systems…the laboratory must do the following…:
  (2)
    (i) Define a function check protocol that ensures equipment, instrument, and test system performance that is necessary for accurate and reliable test results and test result reporting.
    (ii) Perform and document the function checks…

§493.1103 Standard: Requirements for transfusion services

(b) Blood and blood products storage and distribution.
  (1) If a facility stores or maintains blood or blood products for transfusion outside of a monitored refrigerator, the facility must ensure the storage conditions, including temperature, are appropriate to prevent deterioration of the blood or blood product.
  (2) The facility must establish and follow policies to ensure positive identification of a blood or blood product recipient.
(c) Investigation of transfusion reactions. The facility must have procedures for preventing transfusion reactions and, when necessary, promptly identify, investigate, and report blood and blood product transfusion reactions to the laboratory and, as appropriate, to federal and state authorities.

Subpart M: Personnel for Nonwaived Testing

§493.1423 Standard: Testing personnel qualifications

Each individual performing moderate complexity testing must:
(a) Possess a current license issued by the state in which the laboratory is located, if such licensing is required; and
  (4)
    (i) Have earned a high school diploma or equivalent; and
    (ii) Have documentation of training that ensures the individual has the skills required for proper specimen collection, including patient preparation, if applicable, labeling, handling, preservation or fixation, and processing or preparation; for performing preventive maintenance and troubleshooting…; a working knowledge of reagent stability and storage; and an awareness of factors that influence test results.[10]

Phlebotomists should note that although their specific duties and functions within their work setting may place them outside the scope of personnel standards for the purposes of federal CLIA '88 regulations, the laws of the state in which their workplace is located may have more specific phlebotomy requirements. Therefore the personnel standards listed here are intended only to provide a general outline.

OTHER REGULATORY AGENCIES GOVERNING LABORATORIES AND PHLEBOTOMISTS

Many state and federal laws and agencies govern laboratory practice in some way. Employment practices, wages and salaries, business practices, facilities construction, intrastate and interstate transportation of specimens, licensing of personnel, and testing methodology are but a sampling of laboratory-related government oversight activities that affect the clinical laboratory. Although a complete listing of these agencies is beyond the scope of this chapter, listed next are the federal agencies, apart from the CMS, that have substantial influence on laboratories in the United States.[25,26]

The Occupational Safety and Health Act of 1970 established *OSHA* within the U.S. Department of Labor. OSHA is the federal agency that sets rules and regulations covering all aspects of employer and employee safety and health. This agency sets workplace standards and regulates such areas as ventilation; noise; fire and electrical safety; labeling and appropriate precautions for flammables; biological, chemical, and radiation hazards; and safe exposure levels.

The *Food and Drug Administration* (FDA) is responsible for the approval of virtually all medical and diagnostic equipment, devices, pharmaceuticals, reagents, and diagnostic tests before they can be marketed for sale and used in health care settings. The FDA, through its process of premarket approval and its content-labeling requirements, has evaluated the safety, clinical efficacy, and medical need of almost all the testing equipment, reagents, and supplies used by the phlebotomist.

The CDC, through its various offices and divisions, serves as a federal resource for developing technical and scientific standards and conducting epidemiological, health and safety, quality assurance, and health evaluation and proficiency studies and programs.

The *Environmental Protection Agency (EPA)* monitors and enforces regulations for the safe disposal of chemical and other hazardous wastes, including biological hazards.

The *U.S. Postal Service* has developed regulations covering the safe packaging and transport of human biological specimens through the mail and requires appropriate warning labels to protect postal workers from potentially hazardous or infectious agents.

Importantly, almost all these agencies or departments (i.e., OSHA, FDA, CDC, DHHS) have some level of oversight over transfusion services and blood banks, in addition to general laboratory oversight.

SUMMARY

The ability to demonstrate sound laboratory management principles and compliance with regulatory provisions, professional accreditation guidelines, and practice standards can provide substantial protection against the threat of litigation. Although it is not expected that entry-level phlebotomists understand in depth all the law and legal language in this chapter, this material is intended to provide a broad overview and demonstrate the importance of always conducting phlebotomy with the utmost care and attention. No laboratory or health care worker can be completely protected from lawsuits, but potential liability can be minimized by conscientious and continuous attention to good laboratory practice. Lastly, all health care workers must understand they will be held accountable in the performance of their jobs.

CASE 14.1   Critical Thinking

Susan Jones, a phlebotomist, was assigned to draw blood from a 46-year-old man. All appropriate patient identification and consent procedures were followed. But during multiple venipuncture attempts, the patient complained of pain. The draw was finally completed on the fourth attempt. Three months later, the man was diagnosed with a median nerve injury that caused partial paralysis. He believed that his injury was related to the multiple, painful venipunctures. He filed a lawsuit against the phlebotomist and her hospital.

On what basis do you think the lawsuit was filed against the phlebotomist and why?
1. Administrative (regulatory) law
2. Negligence
3. Assault and battery
4. Product liability

CASE 14.2   Critical Thinking

During a busy morning of blood draws, Brian, a phlebotomist, collected blood from three patients, left the collection station for another call, and then returned to the station to apply the patient identification labels to the tubes. Because of the distraction, he misidentified the specimens, which were sent to the laboratory where they were typed and crossmatched according to the incorrect patient information on the tubes. As a result of the incorrect identifications, one of the three patients received incompatible blood and subsequently died. The patient's family filed a negligence lawsuit when they found out about the incorrect identification.

Can Brian successfully defend his actions in mis-identifying the patient samples?
- A. *Yes* because he didn't intentionally mislabel the specimens.
- B. *Yes* because there is no standard of practice for phlebotomists that states that all specimens must be properly identified and labeled. If there is no standard, there is no legal basis for negligence.
- C. *No* because he did not meet the phlebotomy standard of practice for ensuring that specimen labeling, patient identification, and matching patient to specimen occur at the point of care.
- D. *Yes* because it is only the phlebotomist's supervisor who is responsible for a phlebotomist's mistakes.

▌REVIEW QUESTIONS

1. The federal agency responsible for approving and regulating medical devices, pharmaceuticals, and diagnostic test kits is the _____.
2. The legal responsibility of an employer for the negligent acts of employees is called _____.
3. The legal doctrine of _____ requires that a patient must be able to make an intelligent and reasoned decision about whether they agree to a medical procedure or diagnostic test.
4. Imposition of liability on manufacturers for defective blood and blood products falls under the law of _____.
5. When a patient who has filed a lawsuit has disregarded a physician's orders or acts unreasonably, thus causing all or part of the injuries sustained, the defendant may use the defense of _____.
6. The rules that prohibit the intentional or unintentional disclosure of any written, verbal, or electronic transmission of patient health information, including laboratory tests, to unauthorized individuals or companies are part of the _____.

REFERENCES

1. Curran WJ, Hall MA, Kaye DH. *Health Care Law, Forensic Science, and Public Policy.* 4th ed. Boston: Little, Brown; 1990.
2. Peterson RG. Malpractice liability of allied health professionals: developments in an area of critical concern. *J Allied Health.* 1985;14:363–372.
3. Oliver R. Legal liability of students and residents in the health care setting. *J Med Edu.* 1986;61:560–561.
4. Gelhorn E, Levin RM. *Administrative Law and Process. A Nutshell.* 4th ed. St. Paul, MN: West Group; 1997.
5. Garner BA, ed. *Black's Law Dictionary.* 9th ed. St. Paul: MN: Thompson/West; 2009.
6. Hall MA, Bobinski MA. *Orentlicher D: Health Care Law and Ethics.* 7th ed. New York, NY: Wolters-Kluwer; 2007.
7. Wadlington W, Waltz JR, Dworkin RB. *Law and Medicine: Cases and Materials.* Mineola, NY: The Foundation Press; 1980.
8. Thompson vs. Nason Hospital, 591 A2d 703 (Pa 1991).
9. Furrow BR, Johnson SH, Jost TS, Schwartz RL. *Health Law: Cases, Materials and Problems.* 2nd ed. St. Paul: MN. West Publishing; 1991.
10. Department of Health and Human Services, Centers for Medicare and Medicaid Services, Centers for Disease Control and Prevention: 42 CFR 493, 68 FR 3639-3714, 2003. See also http://wwwn.cdc.gov/clia/regs/toc.aspx. Accessed February 28, 2011.
11. Department of Labor, Occupational Safety and Health Administration: Occupational Exposure to Bloodborne Pathogens. 29 CFR 1910.1030; 56 FR 64004–64182, 1991.
12. National Accrediting Agency for Clinical Laboratory Sciences. *Phlebotomy Programs Approval Guide: Standards of Approved Educational Programs for the Phlebotomist.* Rosemont, IL: NAACLS; 2009. http://naacls.org/approval/newguide_Approval.asp.
13. National Phlebotomy Association. *Health and Medical Care Services—Medicine: Phlebotomy Technicians.* Washington, DC: NPA; 2003.

14. Clinical Laboratory Standards Institute (formerly National Committee for Clinical Laboratory Standards): Procedures for the Collection of Diagnostic Blood Specimens by Skin Puncture, 4th ed. Approved Standard, Wayne, PA. NCCLS, 1999; Collection, Transport, and Preparation of Blood Specimens for Coagulation Testing and Performance of Coagulation Assays. NCCLS Document H21. Villanova. NCCLS, 1986; Procedures for the Domestic Handling and Transport of Diagnostic Specimens and Etiologic Agents. 2nd ed. Code H5—A2. Villanova. NCCLS, 1985.

15. O'Brien vs. Cunard, 28 NE 266 (Mass. 1891).

16. Swartz M. The patient who refuses medical treatment: a dilemma for hospitals and physicians. *Am J Law Med.* 1985;11:147—194. See also Truman vs. Thomas, 611 P2d 902 (Ca 1980).

17. Sard vs. Hardy, 879 A2d 1014 (Md 1977).

18. HIPAA, PL104-191, August 21, 1996. To amend the Internal Revenue Code of 1986 to improve portability and continuity of health insurance coverage in the group and individual markets; to combat waste, fraud, and abuse in health insurance and health care delivery; to promote the use of medical savings accounts; to improve access to long-term care services and coverage; to simplify the administration of health insurance; and for other purposes. 45CFR160 et seq.

19. American Society of Phlebotomy Technicians. 2004. *ASPT Newsletter,* ©*2003 ASPT*; http://www.aspt.org/WebNewstext.htm. Accessed November 29, 2003.

20. Bachman A. HIPAA and the POL. *Adv Adm Lab.* 2003;12(6):19.

21. American Hospital Association: Patient's Bill of Rights. Chicago, AHA, adopted 1973, approved 1992. See http://www.patienttalk.info/AHA-Patient_Bill_of_Rights.htm. Accessed February 28, 2011. A 2008 update of this document is available at http://www.aha.org/aha/issues/Communicating-With-Patients/pt-care-partnership.html.

22. Hall MA, Bobinski MA, Orentlicher D. *Health Care Law and Ethics.* 7th ed. New York: Wolters-Kluwer; 2007.

23. Smith V McClung, 161 SE 91 (S. Ct. NC 1931).

24. Chamberlain RT. Chain of custody: its importance and requirements for clinical laboratory specimens. *Lab Med.* 1989;20:477—480.

25. Wilcox KR, Baynes TE, Crable JV, et al. Laboratory management. In: Inhorn SL, ed. *Quality Assurance Practices for Health Laboratories.* Boston: American Public Health Association; 1978.

26. Rose SL. *Clinical Laboratory Safety.* Philadelphia: JB Lippincott; 1984.

Answers to Chapter Review Questions

CHAPTER 1

Review Questions

1. Diagnosis; treatment
2. On the job
3. Physician office laboratories, blood collection centers, research institutes, and veterinary offices
4. To assure employers that the phlebotomists they hire meet a minimally acceptable standard of practice
5. American Society for Clinical Laboratory Science
6. Increased; Although there is no guarantee, it is likely there will be increased work for phlebotomists, especially considering the overall aging of the population.
7. Acting in an ethical manner means to always act professionally and honestly. Always conduct yourself with the patient's care in mind.

CHAPTER 2

Critical Thinking Case Studies

1. Sally, the morning phlebotomist, was paged "stat" to the intensive care unit to collect blood from Mrs. Smith. Among the tests requested are a complete blood count, blood urea nitrogen and creatinine, amylase, and troponin. The respiratory therapist also asks Sally to transport an arterial blood gas sample he has just collected to the laboratory. What organ systems are being evaluated by these tests?
   Answer: The complete blood count and troponin evaluate the cardiovascular system. The urinary system is evaluated by the blood urea nitrogen and creatinine tests. Amylase is used to evaluate the digestive system, particularly the pancreas. The arterial blood gas will evaluate Mrs. Smith's respiratory function.

2. Mr. Black is receiving a unit of blood for a low hemoglobin level when Jim, the phlebotomist, is called "stat" to the floor to collect samples. Mr. Black is partially unresponsive when Jim arrives at his room. Mr. Black has also spiked a temperature and appears to have labored breathing.
   1. What could be causing Mr. Black's rise in temperature and unresponsiveness?
   2. Why might this type of reaction occur?
   3. Why was Jim called "stat" to the floor to collect blood?
   1. Mr. Black could be having a transfusion reaction to the unit of blood he is receiving.
   2. The blood may not be compatible for Mr. Black and may possess a foreign antigen to which he makes an antibody.
   3. Hemolytic transfusion reactions, although uncommon, may be life threatening. It is very important to collect blood samples quickly so the laboratory can determine what type of reaction Mr. Black is experiencing, and treatment can begin.

Review Questions

1. Cell
2. System
3. Cardiac
4. Gonads
5. Platelets
6. Small intestine
7. Oxygen; carbon dioxide
8. Lymphatic
9. Kidneys
10. Arteries, veins, capillaries
11. Transverse/horizontal, frontal/coronal
12. Integumentary
13. Neurotransmitters

14. Neutrophils, eosinophils, basophils, lymphocytes, and monocytes
15. Energy
16. Muscular
17. Cardiovascular
18. A
19. C
20. D
21. B
22. D

CHAPTER 3

Critical Thinking Case Studies

1. A phlebotomist goes to the emergency room to draw a patient. She finds out the patient is a child who has a widely spread skin rash. The emergency room clerk said the doctor mentioned that the child may have meningococcemia. What type of personal protective equipment should the phlebotomist wear and why?

    Answer: Meningococcemia is a severe, systemic infection with *Neisseria meningitidis*. This organism is transmitted by respiratory droplets, so the proper personal protective equipment includes a mask or face shield. Gloves would also be appropriate if the health care worker was drawing a blood specimen.

2. A fellow phlebotomist confides in a colleague that they were stuck with a dirty needle about a month ago. The phlebotomist tells you that they are feeling really tired lately and their urine looks like tea. The individual didn't bother to go to the Employee Health Department when it happened because they were embarrassed. What advice would you give to the phlebotomist? What disease does the phlebotomist appear to have contracted? What treatment is available for the disease?

    Answer: I would be very mad at my fellow phlebotomist for not reporting this to employee health. I would urge them to go to the Employee Health Department immediately to report this occurrence and receive medical care for the symptoms. The symptoms are consistent with hepatitis B. There is only supportive treatment for hepatitis B.

Review Questions

1. A blood-borne pathogen is a pathogen that is acquired from blood and body fluids. It is important for phlebotomists to learn about these organisms so that precautions can be taken to prevent the phlebotomist from becoming infected.

2. Exposure to infectious diseases is an occupational hazard for a phlebotomist. During the course of their duties, phlebotomists will come in contact with sick people. Phlebotomists can help prevent themselves from becoming infected if they know how the diseases are spread and techniques used to break the chain of infection.

3. Direct contact transmission, indirect contact transmission, droplet transmission, and airborne transmission.

4. Malaria is a mosquito-borne illness that is caused by the *Plasmodium* parasite.

5. Human immunodeficiency virus, the primary virus that causes AIDS.

6. Acquired immune deficiency syndrome.

7. If the person having their blood collected had tuberculosis, the most noticeable symptom would be a cough. However, a phlebotomist would not be able to tell if the person had the flu or if they had tuberculosis.

8. The symptoms for meningitis include fever, headache, and stiff neck. If a person had a very severe case of this disease, they would also have sepsis and a characteristic rash. The severe form of the disease has a high fatality rate as well as deafness, mental retardation, and loss of limbs.

9. MRSA and VRE can cause severe infections in people. They are hard to treat because they are resistant to many common antibiotics. Most of the time, physicians will use several powerful antibiotics to kill these organisms.

10. Standard precautions are a strategy or a culture for preventing the health care–associated transmission of infectious agents to anyone, regardless of the infectious agent and its route of transmission.

11. Transmission-based precautions are used in addition to standard precautions for diseases that have multiple routes of infection. The three types of transmission-based precautions include contact, droplet, and airborne. Contact precautions help prevent the spread of pathogens by cutting off

direct and indirect contact with the pathogen. This includes wearing gowns and gloves. Droplet precautions prevent the spread of pathogens that are spread through respiratory secretions. This includes wearing a mask when coming into contact with these patients. Airborne precautions involve preventing the spread of pathogens through the air for long distances. This includes placing patients in a room equipped with special air handling systems to cleanse the air from the patient's room before it enters the atmosphere.

12. It is important to disinfect the patient's environment to minimize the number of pathogens that can infect a person in that environment. It is important to disinfect patient care equipment to prevent patient-to-patient transmission of diseases.
13. Phlebotomists should wear gloves whenever they are drawing blood or handling blood or body fluids. They should also wear gloves when patients are on specific transmission-based precautions. If in doubt, put on a pair of gloves.
14. Gowns should be worn when directed by a nurse or if a patient is on contact precautions.
15. Masks should be worn when directed by a nurse or whenever a patient is on droplet precautions. More recently with the advent of COVID-19, masks are nearly always worn for all patients.
16. This regulation required employers to provide certain safeguards to help their health care workers prevent occupational exposure to hepatitis B, HIV, and other blood-borne pathogens.
17. The Needlestick Safety and Prevention Act updated the definition of engineering controls, exposure control plans, input from front-line workers for identification, evaluation, and selection, and a sharps injury log.
18. Hepatitis C causes a mild inflammation of the liver and people infected with the virus usually find out they are infected after repeated liver function tests come back abnormal.
19. Patients in the ICU are severely ill, and their bodies are trying to heal and fight off infections. Their body is trying hard to overcome the current situation and cannot handle another pathogen causing more disease in the body.
20. Handwashing is the single most important factor in reducing the transmission of infectious agents in a health care setting.

CHAPTER 4

Review Questions

1. A combining vowel
2. A prefix
3. Latin and Greek
4. a. cyt-o-penia: decreased cells
   b. oste-o-pathy: disease of the bones
   c. lip-ase: Fat enzyme
   d. intra-renal: within the renal (kidney) gland
   e. phleb-itis: inflammation of veins
5. a. Fever of unknown origin
   b. Electrolytes
   c. Quantity not sufficient
   d. Partial thromboplastin time
   e. Postprandial
   f. Fasting blood sugar

CHAPTER 5

Critical Thinking Case Study

1. During a routine venipuncture phlebotomists must remember many things about performing a proper procedure. They should not need to worry about the equipment. However, occasionally a phlebotomist is not successful when attempting a venipuncture. Discuss the possible ways that equipment may lead to an unsuccessful venipuncture.
   Answer: It is possible that the evacuated tubes are expired and have lost vacuum. It is also possible that they are in date but may have been previously used and were not properly disposed of.

Review Questions

1. The anticoagulant is EDTA, and it binds or chelates calcium and prevents clotting.
2. Lancet or semiautomated microcapillary puncture device
3. The entire needle and holder are disposed into a puncture-resistant container.
4. The tourniquet is used to assist in locating the vein.
5. Splashguard
6. Density
7. Goggles
8. Alcohol and iodine, povidone-iodine, and chlorohexide gluconate

CHAPTER 6

Critical Thinking Case Study

1. You are just starting your phlebotomy collection rounds at 7 AM. You have been assigned the maternity ward, and you have a total of 22 patients from whom to collect. When you enter Room 345, you greet your patient properly and explain why you are there. She is your sixth patient. While you are putting on your gloves, you ask the patient to state her name. The patient replies, "I am Mary Jones." You look at your requisition slip and notice that the name the patient just gave you does not match your requisition. What should you do?

   Answer: This should immediately send up a red flag, and you should not proceed until this discrepancy is clarified. You should ask her to repeat her name; perhaps you did not hear it correctly, then check her wristband. Assuming she is correct in identifying herself and you have no requisitions for a Mary Jones, you need to inform the nurse in charge. Perhaps your patient has been relocated or discharged.

Review Questions

1. Patient identification
2. 70% isopropyl alcohol
3. Tourniquet
4. Wash your hands and change your gloves
5. Strenuous exercise
6. 15
7. Butterfly
8. Empty or dummy (to be discarded)

CHAPTER 7

Critical Thinking Case Studies

1. You are collecting blood from a patient undergoing a glucose tolerance test (GTT). After the 2-hour collection, you notice that the container with the glucose solution is in the trash can and is still about half full. There have been no other GTTs performed on this day. What should you do if anything?

   Answer: It is suggested that you ask the patient if they, in fact, did drink the entire amount of glucose solution. Accurate results depend on this. If they admit to not drinking all of it, inform the doctor. The test should probably be discontinued because the results will not be valid.

2. The supervisor of the phlebotomy unit has received a call from the microbiology laboratory. They are reporting that a recent specimen is demonstrating the presence of a very common skin bacteria. How could this happen, and what should be done in the future?

   Answer: Most likely, the microbiology laboratory suspects that the specimen is contaminated with normal flora (bacteria that is commonly present on the skin). Proper venipuncture site preparation should be reviewed with the phlebotomist.

Review Questions

1. Blood gases
2. 450 mL
3. Septicemia
4. Glucose tolerance test
5. Increased levels of FDPs are generally associated with such conditions as myocardial infarctions, pulmonary emboli, certain complications of pregnancy, and disseminated intravascular coagulation.
6. Yellow
7. To eliminate the chance of skin normal flora from contaminating the culture tubes.
8. There are several types of venous catheters:
   - *Central venous catheters* are threaded into the right atrium or the superior vena cava.
   - A *percutaneously placed catheter* is inserted directly through the skin and in a large vein of the neck, usually the internal or external jugular or subclavian.
   - *Peripherally inserted central catheters* (PICC lines) are inserted through large veins of the antecubital fossa and threaded into the tip of the right atrium.
   - A *midline catheter* (MLC) may be placed between the antecubital fossa and the head of the clavicle
9. Intravenously
10. Face masks

CHAPTER 8

Critical Thinking Case Studies

1. It is the first time you are asked to go to the neonatal unit to collect blood on a premature infant. Your orders say to collect blood for a hemoglobin and hematocrit assay and a bilirubin assay. When you are done, you notice a notebook labeled "log of blood collected" where the amount of blood you just collected is recorded. What purpose does this log serve?

   Answer: One cause of anemia in newborns is because of repeated blood collections (iatrogenic anemia); therefore it is important to document the amount of blood collected during each draw.

2. While preparing to collect blood from a 78-year-old man, you gather your tubes, needle, and other equipment while you are asking him his name and requesting that he roll up his sleeve. When you have collected your equipment, you realize that he did not state his name and did not begin to roll up his sleeve. What should you do now?

   Answer: It is easy to forget that you may be working with a patient that is hard of hearing. When you realize that he did not respond to your question or directive, repeat the question by facing the patient and speaking clearly (but not overly loud). This will probably resolve the situation and you can proceed with the venipuncture.

Review Questions

1. Phenylketonuria (PKU), galactosemia, and hypothyroidism
2. Osteomyelitis
3. Gown
4. It may be diluted with tissue fluid.
5. Because there are repeated blood draws, a bandage may do more harm than good to the infant.
6. 25%
7. Vision, hearing, and skin changes, as well as mental and emotional changes
8. The loss of elasticity in the skin (and veins) makes it more susceptible to "rolling" and excessive bleeding after the venipuncture is complete.
9. Winged infusion sets or pediatric size Vacutainer tubes are appropriate. Both of these are less traumatic on veins.
10. Infant's body weight

CHAPTER 9

Critical Thinking Case Study

1. Joseph was preparing to collect a fasting specimen on Albert. Just before Joseph was going to perform the venipuncture, Albert said he was feeling lightheaded. Joseph did not continue with the phlebotomy but asked for a nearby technician, Jane, to get a cold compress. Joseph had Jane hold the compress on the back of Albert's neck. When he was feeling a little better, Joseph helped Albert to a nearby bed, gave him some apple juice, and continued with a successful phlebotomy. Please discuss Joseph's handling of this situation.

   Answer: Joseph did a good job in dealing with a lightheaded patient whom he suspected might faint. He did not try to complete the phlebotomy, nor did he leave the patient unattended and eventually got the patient to a bed. However, he did give the patient apple juice, which means that the specimen he was to collect could no longer be considered a fasting specimen. Joseph should inquire whether he should continue with the phlebotomy.

Review Questions

1. Petechiae
2. Hypovolemia
3. Edema
4. Hemolysis
5. Hematoma
6. Syncope
7. Mastectomy
8. Platelet function

CHAPTER 10

Critical Thinking Case Study

1. You are required to obtain glucose readings on five patients before 8 AM. Before testing your patients, you test the quality-control samples, and the results are outside the acceptable range. Should you proceed with patient testing? Why or why not?

   Answer: Patient testing should not be done until the out-of-range quality control results are resolved. Quality control specimens are run to ensure the testing system is working properly. If you proceed with testing patients before resolving the issue, you will not be able to determine if your results are accurate.

Review Questions

1. Oral, rectal, axillary, aural, and temporal
2. Medulla oblongata
3. To decrease turnaround time
4. Electrocardiography
5. Decreases
6. CPR
7. Stethoscope
8. True
9. Waived
10. Any two of the following are acceptable: convenient for the patient, having a quick turnaround, and/or using a smaller volume of sample.
11. Any of the following are acceptable: blood gases and electrolytes, cholesterol, coagulation tests, drugs of abuse, Group A strep, glucose, respiratory viruses, hemoglobin and hematocrit, occult blood, urinalysis, and urine pregnancy testing.
12. With regard to POCT, to ensure that the testing device is working properly
13. Cardiopulmonary resuscitation (CPR), assessing vital signs, electrocardiograms (ECG), direct patient care, donor center/clerical duties, CLIA '88, and waived point-of-care testing

CHAPTER 11

Critical Thinking Case Studies

1. You are returning to work after a day off. While you were off, a colleague, who usually collects blood only from outpatients, used your phlebotomy tray and left it in disarray. Luckily you came in a few minutes earlier than normal so you could restock and straighten out your tray before starting morning collections. When you get back to the laboratory, the colleague that used your tray the day before is collecting blood from an outpatient. You want to address the issue of using your tray. How should you approach the subject with your colleague?
   Answer: You should wait until your colleague is finished with the patient. Then, if both of you have time, you should politely and professionally tell your colleague what your expectations are when someone else uses your tray and that when it is left

unstocked or cluttered, that may delay you getting started on your rounds or you may find that you are missing something once you are up on the floors. Your colleague should be understanding if you deliver your message appropriately.

2. When you are returning from afternoon rounds on the fourth floor, you overhear a doctor and nurse discussing a patient while you and some visitors are with them in the elevator. One statement you overhear is, "I can't wait until Mr. Jones gets discharged; he is such a needy patient!" What is wrong with this exchange and what should you do about it?
   Answer: This exchange is a HIPAA violation in that it breaks the patient's right to privacy. It may be awkward for you to say something to the individuals (please do so if you are comfortable). You should report the incident to your supervisor; presumably the hospital or clinic you work for will have a protocol in place to deal with this situation, which is a violation of the Patient Care Partnership.

Review Questions

1. Life skills
2. Empathy
3. Reference gap
4. Profession
5. Continuing education
6. These are the rights and responsibilities shared between the patient and the health care provider.
7. Continuing education is important for phlebotomists to remain current with changes in the field and profession of phlebotomy.
8. It is important to always conduct yourself professionally.

CHAPTER 12

Critical Thinking Case Studies

1. You have been instructed to create a Quality Improvement Program for your department. What steps should be taken to develop the program? List three indicators that can be used.
   Steps: Ask staff for input, explain why the indicators are being monitored, and give feedback. **Indicators:** Specimen rejection rate, STAT response time, patient satisfaction, patient identification

2. You are planning an outpatient collection station in your facility. Where should this be located and how would you design the area?

Answer: The area should be easily accessible to the registration area and exit. There should be a centralized area to greet patients and process the request. The blood-drawing stations should be private.

Review Questions

1. True
2. To receive orders, obtain patient information, and print laboratory orders
3. Children, mentally handicapped patients
4. Wages and benefits, materials, and equipment

CHAPTER 13

Critical Thinking Case Study

1. You have been asked to review your laboratory's procedure manual. Under the section for specimen rejection, it states only, "Specimens may be rejected if they are not labeled properly." What feedback are you going to give to the supervisors?

Answer: Specimens may be rejected for improper labeling, but they may also be rejected if collection is not timely (such as within a certain number of hours after treatment); if the sample volume is insufficient for the test being ordered, especially when the specimen container includes an additive; if the wrong collection tube or container is used; if a collection tube is used after its expiration date; if the sample is transported incorrectly (for example, not sent on ice); and if the specimen is found to be hemolyzed.

Review Questions

1. Facts
2. Errors
3. Specimen collection manual
4. Assurance
5. Satisfaction
6. Attempts
7. Often, the phlebotomist is the only contact between patients and the laboratory.
8. It is everyone's responsibility to ensure the quality of the phlebotomy service.

CHAPTER 14

Critical Thinking Case Studies

1. Susan Jones, a phlebotomist, was assigned to draw blood from a 46-year-old man. All appropriate patient identification and consent procedures were followed. But during multiple venipuncture attempts, the patient complained of pain. The draw was finally completed on the fourth attempt. Three months later, the man was diagnosed with a median nerve injury that caused partial paralysis. He believed that his injury was related to the multiple, painful venipunctures. He filed a lawsuit against the phlebotomist and her hospital. On what basis do you think the lawsuit was filed against the phlebotomist and why?
   A. Administrative (regulatory) law
   B. Negligence
   C. Assault and battery
   D. Product liability
   Correct Answer: B

Explanation of Incorrect Answers

A. Administrative/regulatory law encompasses federal, state, and local statutes, as well as regulations implementing such laws. Of importance here is that regulations such as the Clinical Laboratory Improvement Amendments of 1988 (CLIA '88) establish *minimum* standards to which laboratories and laboratorians must comply.
C. *Assault* is any active, willful attempt or threat to inflict injury on another person. *Battery* can be viewed as an active intent to cause harm or injury to a person without that person's consent that actually does harm the person. *Technical battery* is sometimes used to describe those situations in which a physician or other health care worker, in the course of treatment, exceeds the consent given by the patient, although no harmful purpose was intended.
D. Products liability focuses on the liability of manufacturers or suppliers for defective products that cause physical harm, in this case the needle. In this case, there is no evidence that the needle itself was defective.

2. During a busy morning of blood draws, Brian, a phlebotomist, collected blood from three patients, left the collection station for another call, and

then returned to the station to apply the patient identification labels to the tubes. Because of the distraction, he misidentified the specimens, which were sent to the laboratory where they were typed and crossmatched according to the incorrect patient information on the tubes. As a result of the incorrect identifications, one of the three patients received incompatible blood and subsequently died. The patient's family filed a negligence lawsuit when they found out about the incorrect identification. Can Brian successfully defend his actions in misidentifying the patient samples?

A. *Yes* because he didn't intentionally mislabel the specimens.
B. *Yes* because there is no standard of practice for phlebotomists that states that all specimens must be properly identified and labeled. If there is no standard, there is no legal basis for negligence.
C. *No* because he did not meet the phlebotomy standard of practice for ensuring that specimen labeling, patient identification, and matching patient to specimen occur at the point of care.
D. *Yes* because it is only the phlebotomist's supervisor who is responsible for a phlebotomist's mistakes.

Correct Answer: C

Explanation of Incorrect Answers

A. Negligence actions do not require that an individual intend to act (or not act) in a careless manner. Legally negligent actions are almost always a result of carelessness, inattention, or otherwise acting unreasonably in a given set of circumstances.
B. Phlebotomy Standards of Practice, as well as CLIA '88 laboratory regulations, require that all patients and patient specimens be completely and accurately identified.
D. The phlebotomist's supervisor as well as the health care facility may indeed be included as defendants in this lawsuit. However, it was the phlebotomist's actions that were the proximate cause of the misidentification leading to the patient death. Thus the phlebotomist must shoulder some responsibility for the outcome of this testing situation.

Review Questions

1. Food and Drug Administration (FDA)
2. Vicarious liability
3. Informed consent
4. Products liability
5. Contributory negligence
6. Health Insurance Portability and Accountability Act of 1996 (HIPAA)

Practice Examination for Certification

1. Blue-stoppered tubes are used primarily for the following assay:
   a. Complete blood count (CBC)
   b. Glucose
   c. Prothrombin time (PT)
   d. Rapid plasma reagin (RPR)
2. Sodium heparin is the anticoagulant most commonly found in which of the following tubes?
   a. Blue
   b. Green
   c. Lavender
   d. Red
3. Yellow-stoppered tubes are generally used for:
   a. Blood cultures
   b. Compatibility testing
   c. Cholesterol assays
   d. White blood cell differential
4. The liquid portion of the blood collected from a red-stoppered tube after centrifugation is:
   a. Anticoagulant
   b. Plasma
   c. Serum
   d. Sodium citrate
5. A phlebotomy quality assurance program may include each of the following EXCEPT:
   a. Abnormal glucose quality-control results
   b. Customer satisfaction surveys
   c. Number of hemolyzed specimens
   d. Number of mislabeled specimens
6. Which of the following defines quality control?
   a. Delivering the right product or service
   b. Doing it right the first time
   c. A process that validates final results and quantifies variations
   d. Treating every customer properly
7. Hemolysis is a reason for specimen rejection. It may be caused by all of the following EXCEPT:

   a. Clotting, because of insufficient mixing with the anticoagulant
   b. Transfusion reactions
   c. Shaking the vacuum tube too vigorously when mixing
   d. Using a small-gauge needle and a large vacuum tube
8. The following procedures should be performed in the nursery when a phlebotomist collects a capillary specimen from an infant EXCEPT:
   a. Applying a bandage when bleeding has stopped to prevent infection
   b. Keeping a log of how much blood has been collected
   c. Wearing a gown and gloves
   d. Wiping away the first drop of blood
9. The order of filling tubes once blood has been collected in a syringe is:
   a. Blue, red, green, yellow
   b. Red, light blue, yellow, green
   c. Yellow, dark blue, green, red
   d. Yellow, light blue, red, purple
10. The term that describes the interrelationship of the law and medicine is:
    a. Forensic science
    b. Litigation
    c. Medical-legal
    d. Standard of care
11. What is not a benefit to multiskilling?
    a. Job security
    b. Marketability
    c. Increased pay
    d. Specialization
12. Which of the following pertains to the absence of oxygen?
    a. Aerobic
    b. Anaerobic
    c. Arrhythmic

d. Tachycardic

13. Medical malpractice lawsuits are most often brought under the legal theory of:
    a. Contacts
    b. Criminal law
    c. Equity
    d. Negligence

14. Laws passed by the US Congress are called:
    a. Cases
    b. Ordinances
    c. Regulations
    d. Statutes

15. *Standard Precautions* is the practice of treating _____ as if they are known to be infectious for hepatitis B virus (HBV), human immunodeficiency virus (HIV), and other blood-borne pathogens.
    a. All people
    b. All body fluids
    c. All body substances
    d. All human blood and other potential infectious material (OPIM)

16. The legal term for the intent to cause harm or injury to a person without the person's consent, and which actually harms that person, is:
    a. Battery
    b. Breach of contract
    c. Negligence
    d. Product liability

17. When a patient refuses to have their blood drawn, the phlebotomist should do the following EXCEPT:
    a. Contact the patient's nurse.
    b. Force the patient to have their blood drawn.
    c. Return the requisition to the laboratory.
    d. Try to convince the patient to have their blood drawn.

18. Equipment error(s) causing no blood to be collected include:
    a. Missing the vein
    b. Needle goes through the vein
    c. No vacuum in the tube
    d. All of the above

19. Which of the following is NOT a reason to avoid an area of the arm to perform venipuncture?
    a. Edema
    b. Obesity
    c. Petechiae

d. Scarred veins

20. What is the first course of action if a patient has convulsions?
    a. Call for help.
    b. Notify a physician.
    c. Offer juice to help revive the patient.
    d. Remove the tourniquet and needle.

21. All of the following statements are true EXCEPT:
    a. Gray-stoppered tubes are used for blood glucose tests.
    b. Gray-stoppered tubes are used for complete blood cell (CBC) and white blood cell (WBC) tests.
    c. Lavender-stoppered tubes are used for CBC, WBC, and platelet testing.
    d. Red-stoppered tubes are used for many tests including serum enzymes.

22. Spurious laboratory results can be caused by:
    a. Hemolysis and lipemia
    b. Improper blood-to-anticoagulant ratio
    c. Improper handling of sample during or after blood collection
    d. All of the above

23. Normally the serum produced after spinning blood in a red-stoppered tube is:
    a. Anticoagulated
    b. Clear or straw colored
    c. Milky white
    d. Pink

24. What gland regulates the pituitary gland?
    a. Hypothalamus
    b. Medulla
    c. Renal
    d. Cerebellum

25. This structure houses the vocal cords:
    a. Adrenals
    b. Hypothalamus
    c. Larynx
    d. Thyroid

26. Which of the following is considered to be a noninfectious bodily substance according to the Centers for Disease Control and Prevention (CDC) guidelines known as the Standard Precautions?
    a. Amniotic fluid
    b. Blood
    c. Semen
    d. Tears

27. Which of the following diseases requires the use of Respiratory Precautions?
    a. Hepatitis B
    b. Salmonella
    c. Staphylococcal skin abscesses
    d. Tuberculosis
28. All of the following are vaccine-preventable diseases EXCEPT:
    a. Acquired immunodeficiency syndrome (AIDS)
    b. Hepatitis B
    c. Polio
    d. Mumps
29. These blood vessels generally carry blood that is high in oxygen:
    a. Arteries
    b. Veins
    c. Venules
    d. All are equally oxygenated.
30. This system gives the body structure and protects vital organs:
    a. Integumentary system
    b. Muscular system
    c. Skeletal system
    d. Vascular system
31. The sebaceous glands are associated with the:
    a. Endocrine system
    b. Integumentary system
    c. Skeletal system
    d. Vascular system
32. All of the following may be required of a phlebotomist EXCEPT:
    a. Donor blood collections
    b. Injections
    c. Specimen preparation
    d. Therapeutic phlebotomies
33. Which of the following is NOT a professional attribute?
    a. Professional appearance
    b. Flexibility
    c. Usually on time
    d. Effective communicator
34. This collection round is routine in all hospitals:
    a. Early morning
    b. Late afternoon
    c. Midmorning
    d. Noon

35. Which of the following is NOT an example of expendable equipment?
    a. Alcohol swabs
    b. Blood pressure cuffs
    c. Gloves
    d. Tubes
36. Which of the following represents normal body temperature?
    a. 37°F
    b. 37°C
    c. 42°C
    d. 99°C
37. Venipuncture should be avoided in the arm on the same side on which a mastectomy was performed, because:
    a. Patients may be embarrassed.
    b. Patients are more susceptible to infection.
    c. Venipuncture is more painful.
    d. It is acceptable to collect blood from either arm.
38. The standard operating procedure manual for specimen collection contains each of the following EXCEPT:
    a. Information about how to prepare the patient for the test
    b. Notes on timing requirements
    c. Specimen labeling requirements
    d. The laboratory supervisor's name and home phone number
39. The quality of blood specimens is best summarized by which of the following statements?
    a. Phlebotomy technique is not critical to test results.
    b. Specimen handling has no effect on the laboratory results.
    c. Specimens of low quality can produce inaccurate and potentially dangerous results.
    d. The laboratory will detect any problem with the specimens.
40. The primary measure for prevention of hepatitis B in the occupational setting is:
    a. Infection control
    b. Jaundice
    c. Avoidance of the occupational setting
    d. Immunization
41. The glucose tolerance test:
    a. Is a monitor of blood glucose after ingestion of 300 g of glucose

b. Is performed to aid in the diagnosis of diabetes mellitus
c. Lasts 1 hour
d. May be collected in a blue-stoppered tube

42. The specimen for fibrin degradation products is collected in a:
    a. Lavender-stoppered tube containing sodium citrate
    b. Syringe containing heparin
    c. Tube containing an enzyme inhibitor and thrombin
    d. Red-stoppered tube

43. The rule of legal evidence that requires documentation of the location and integrity of any laboratory specimens used as evidence in a trial is called:
    a. Accreditation
    b. Chain of custody
    c. Learned treatise
    d. Professional liability insurance

44. Policies that some hospitals have adopted that incorporate the patient's constitutional rights to privacy, confidentiality, and informed consent in medical treatment are referred to as:
    a. Patient Care Partnership
    b. Protest of assignment forms
    c. Statutes of limitation
    d. Technical guidelines

45. When a hematoma is forming, all of the following are acceptable EXCEPT:
    a. Adjust the depth of the needle.
    b. Ignore it and collect the specimen.
    c. Remove the needle and apply pressure to the site.
    d. Try another site.

46. Technical errors causing a short draw include:
    a. A collapsed vein because of too much vacuum in the tube
    b. No vacuum in the tube
    c. The needle bevel against the vessel wall
    d. The syringe plunger withdrawn too quickly

47. Hemoguard is a type of:
    a. Anticoagulant
    b. Lancet
    c. Needle
    d. Splashguard

48. A full sharps container should be:
    a. Emptied into a biohazard bag
    b. Reported to the supervisor

c. Disposed of into a properly lined, leak-proof, puncture-proof container
d. Emptied by recapping the needles and then flushing them down the toilet

49. A retractable sheath is part of a:
    a. Disposal container
    b. Lancet
    c. Multiple-draw needle
    d. Single-draw needle

50. A common site for arterial punctures is the:
    a. Femoral artery in the upper thigh
    b. Radial artery in the wrist
    c. Jugular vein in the neck
    d. None of the above

51. Which of the following neonatal tests is required by law?
    a. Bilirubin
    b. Creutzfeldt-Jacob
    c. Hemoglobin
    d. Phenylketonuria

52. Green-stoppered tubes may be used for the following laboratory tests EXCEPT:
    a. Ammonia
    b. Complete blood count (CBC)
    c. Chromosome analysis
    d. Human leukocyte antigen (HLA) typing

53. Which of the following is NOT classified as a barrier precaution?
    a. Hepatitis B virus (HBV) vaccine
    b. Gloves
    c. Goggles
    d. Gown

54. The most common cause of blood culture contamination is:
    a. Collection of too much blood
    b. Collection of the sample from below the intravenous (IV) line
    c. Improper skin preparation
    d. The use of a needle and syringe for collection

55. Nosocomial infections are those that are:
    a. Acquired during a period of hospitalization
    b. Acquired in the womb before birth
    c. Symptomatic at the time of admission
    d. Transmitted by pets in the home

56. Which of the following viruses are transmitted primarily through contact with infected blood?
    a. Hepatitis A virus and *Rubella* virus

b. Hepatitis B virus (HBV) and human immuno-deficiency virus (HIV)

c. Influenza virus and HIV

d. Polio virus and hepatitis C virus

57. The most effective preventive measure to elimi-nate the transmission of disease in health care in-stitutions is:

a. Use of masks

b. Surveillance

c. Hand washing

d. Use of gowns

58. Which of the following are characteristic of a profession?

a. Distinct field of knowledge

b. Full-time occupation

c. High degree of autonomy

d. All of the above

59. Continuing education in the laboratory profes-sion is generally characterized by:

a. Formalized classroom study after high school that will result in an academic degree

b. Education acquired from workshops and sem-inars attended after formal education has ended

c. Formal education resulting in a post baccalau-reate degree

d. None of the above

60. Which of the following cells contribute most to blood clotting?

a. Lymphocytes

b. Platelets

c. Red blood cells

d. White blood cells

61. Another name for erythrocytes is:

a. Lymphocytes

b. Platelets

c. Red blood cells

d. White blood cells

62. The tricuspid and bicuspid valves are associated with the:

a. Heart

b. Liver

c. Spleen

d. Stomach

63. During exhalation:

a. Oxygen is taken into the lungs.

b. The diaphragm descends.

c. The lungs expand.

d. Carbon dioxide is removed from the lungs.

64. Which of the following is the acceptable order of draw for evacuated tube collection?

a. Gray, yellow, red

b. Yellow, light blue, green

c. Red, light blue, yellow

d. Green, yellow, gray

65. Perhaps the single most important step in phle-botomy is:

a. Cleansing the site

b. Patient identification

c. Using a clean needle

d. Using the proper evacuated tube

66. Which of the following is the vein of choice for venipuncture?

a. Basilic

b. Cephalic

c. Median cubital

d. Pulmonary

67. The bevel of the needle should be in which posi-tion before entering a vein?

a. Facing down

b. Facing toward the side

c. Facing upward

d. It really does not matter as long as the veni-puncture is performed quickly.

68. Which of the following steps are in the proper order?

a. Remove the needle, release the tourniquet, apply pressure

b. Apply pressure, release the tourniquet, remove the needle

c. Remove the needle, apply pressure, release the tourniquet

d. Release the tourniquet, remove the needle, apply pressure

69. Which of the following is NOT a physiological condition that may cause variation in the basal state?

a. Diet

b. Exercise

c. Gender

d. Trauma

70. Striving for quality requires:

a. Commitment

b. Enthusiasm

c. Time

d. All of the above

71. Being a quality-oriented phlebotomist, what would you do when encountering a combative patient?
    a. Attempt the venipuncture anyway; after all, you have a job to do.
    b. Be empathetic.
    c. Immediately tie the patient to the bed rails or chair.
    d. Play psychological games with the patient.

72. When performing an arterial puncture, the phlebotomist should:
    a. Apply pressure on the site for 15 minutes after the collection.
    b. Collect only from patients who have fasted for 12 hours.
    c. Tie the tourniquet tight to obtain good blood flow.
    d. Use the thumb to palpate.

73. Medical screening for blood donors includes all of the following EXCEPT:
    a. Blood pressure
    b. Cholesterol
    c. Hemoglobin
    d. Weight

74. Therapeutic phlebotomy is performed as a treatment for patients with:
    a. Diabetes mellitus
    b. Hepatitis
    c. Lymphocytic leukemia
    d. Polycythemia vera

75. This is a four-chambered organ:
    a. Liver
    b. Stomach
    c. Kidney
    d. Heart

76. Blood pressure measures:
    a. The contraction and relaxation of the heart
    b. The number of heart beats per minute
    c. The force exerted on the walls of the arteries by the blood
    d. Pressure in the arteries when the heart relaxes

77. These prevent aerosol from contaminating phlebotomists' eyes:
    a. Gloves
    b. Goggles
    c. Needle caps
    d. Sharps containers

78. Blood smears:
    a. Are used to count red blood cells
    b. Are used to differentiate white blood cells
    c. Must be made from a drop of blood from a fingerstick
    d. Should be made very slowly and carefully

79. Blood cultures may NOT be collected:
    a. Directly into aerobic and anaerobic culture bottles
    b. In a red-stoppered tube
    c. In a syringe
    d. In a yellow-stoppered tube

80. Which term is NOT one of the four elements that must be proved in a legal action for negligence?
    a. Analyte
    b. Breach of duty
    c. Causation
    d. Duty

81. A patient sitting in a chair has fainted. Possible acceptable actions by the phlebotomist include the following EXCEPT:
    a. Going quickly for help
    b. Placing a cold compress on the back of the patient's neck
    c. Putting the patient's head between his knees
    d. Calling for help

82. All of the following will cause clotting in an anticoagulated tube EXCEPT:
    a. Blood collected in a syringe that is not added quickly to tubes with anticoagulant
    b. Hemolysis of red blood cells
    c. Improper blood-to-anticoagulant ratio
    d. Insufficient mixing of blood and anticoagulant

83. "The degree of skill, proficiency, knowledge, and care ordinarily possessed and employed by members in good standing in the profession" is the legal definition for:
    a. Certification
    b. Damages
    c. Standard of care
    d. Testimony

84. The sagittal plane divides the body into

    _____.
    a. Right and left sides
    b. Anterior (Front) and posterior (back) portions
    c. Superior and inferior portions
    d. Two parts: the head and the rest of the body

85. When a patient is absent from their room, the phlebotomist should do all of the following EXCEPT:
    a. Check with the nurse to locate the patient.
    b. Draw blood from the patient in a new location if possible.
    c. Make a note on the requisition if unable to collect the specimen.
    d. Try to find the patient after lunch.

86. Gloves should be worn:
    a. During all venipunctures and capillary punctures
    b. For human immunodeficiency virus (HIV)–positive patients only
    c. Only in cases of isolation
    d. Only when in the laboratory

87. The type of isolation or precaution category that would be the most important for phlebotomists is:
    a. Blood and body fluid precautions
    b. Enteric precautions
    c. Respiratory precautions
    d. Strict isolation

88. Where does the electrical impulse start in the heart?
    a. Sinoatrial node
    b. Atrioventricular node
    c. Bundle of His
    d. Purkinje fibers

89. Key(s) to providing quality phlebotomy is (are):
    a. Professional behavior
    b. Use of the specimen collection manual
    c. Reporting problems to the supervisor
    d. All of the above

90. This is where patients with the most severe conditions are located:
    a. Maternity ward
    b. Surgical ward
    c. Psych ward
    d. Intensive care unit (ICU)

91. All of the following anticoagulants inhibit the clotting process by binding calcium EXCEPT:
    a. EDTA
    b. Potassium oxalate
    c. Sodium citrate
    d. Sodium heparin

92. Cytology is the study of:
    a. Cells

    b. Muscles
    c. Organ systems
    d. Tissues

93. The epidermis is a very important part of the:
    a. Cardiac system
    b. Integumentary system
    c. Nervous system
    d. Skeletal system

94. The substance in erythrocytes that carries oxygen is:
    a. Albumin
    b. Glucose
    c. Hemoglobin
    d. Sodium chloride

95. The procedure manual for specimen collection should include:
    a. Dress code policies
    b. Details about how to stock the phlebotomy tray
    c. The type of tube or container for each laboratory test
    d. Tips on how to cope with the stress of a difficult patient

96. An individual is considered Rh positive or negative depending on the presence or absence of:
    a. A antigen on their red cells
    b. B antigen on their white cells
    c. D antigen on their red cells
    d. D antigen on their white cells

97. Which of the following is the primary source of information for labeling a specimen?
    a. Nurse
    b. Patient's family
    c. What the patient tells the phlebotomist
    d. Wristband

98. Which of the following is true about microcapillary collection?
    a. It is not necessary to wear gloves.
    b. One can usually collect as much blood as in venipuncture.
    c. The first drop of blood should be wiped away.
    d. The tourniquet needs to be tighter than in venipuncture.

99. Which of the following can lead to an increase in the level of enzymes present in the circulation?
    a. Heart damage
    b. Mild exercise
    c. Normal diet

d. Rapid change in posture

100. Which of the following is a biological condition that may affect the results of blood testing?
    a. Diet
    b. Posture
    c. Pregnancy
    d. Trauma

101. Which of the following is part of being a professional?
    a. Dressing appropriately
    b. Having patience
    c. Being well groomed
    d. All of the above

102. Which of the following is released from the pancreas and has a major effect on blood glucose levels?
    a. Adrenocorticotropic hormone (ACTH)
    b. Insulin
    c. Thyroxine
    d. Renin

103. Which of the following is NOT true:
    a. Needles may be covered with a safety device that is part of the needle holder.
    b. It is acceptable to recap used needles after a routine venipuncture.
    c. The tube holder and needle are discarded.
    d. Disposable needles can never be reused.

104. When performing a venipuncture, the tourniquet should never be on for more than:
    a. 15 seconds
    b. 30 seconds
    c. 1 minute
    d. 4 minutes

105. The ability to understand someone else's perspective is known as:
    a. Intrapersonal communication
    b. One-way communication
    c. Interpersonal communication
    d. Empathy

106. Which of the following is a barrier to effective communication?
    a. Being a good listener
    b. Both parties paying attention
    c. Mutual understanding
    d. Reference gap

107. Which of the following is true?
    a. A phlebotomist must use both verbal and nonverbal communication.

b. It is acceptable to show displeasure with a patient when their family is present.
    c. Looking at your watch is an acceptable way to communicate to a patient that you have more work to do.
    d. It is acceptable to tell a patient that you are a student and just learning.

108. Nutrients are absorbed into the bloodstream to:
    a. Keep blood from clotting
    b. Be excreted in the urine
    c. Be used for the body's chemical reactions
    d. None of the above

109. Which of the following is NOT capital equipment?
    a. Blood pressure cuffs
    b. Centrifuges
    c. Syringes
    d. Timers

110. Which of the following is an example of consumable equipment?
    a. Tourniquet
    b. Printer
    c. Computer
    d. Phlebotomy chair

111. The study of tissues is known as _____.
    a. Anatomy
    b. Physiology
    c. Cytology
    d. Histology

112. Osteomyelitis occurs when:
    a. An infant's heel bone is damaged with a lancet
    b. A patient passes out
    c. A vein collapses
    d. Swelling occurs from blood leakage around venipuncture site

113. When collecting blood with a syringe, it is best to add the blood to:
    a. The EDTA tube first
    b. The plain red (no anticoagulant) tube first
    c. The sodium citrate tube first
    d. Whichever tube you happen to pick up first

114. Hypoglycemia is a condition of:
    a. High blood sugar
    b. High cholesterol
    c. Low blood sugar
    d. Low cholesterol

115. Which procedure is generally done by a nurse or respiratory therapist?

a. Arterial puncture
b. Glucose tolerance test
c. Heel stick on an infant
d. Ivy bleeding time

116. Blood gas analysis measures:
a. Na^+ and K^+
b. CO_2, Na^+, and $Cl-$
c. CO_2, O_2, and pH
d. $Cl-$ and HCO_3

117. HIPAA is:
a. A new health insurance organization
b. Designed to keep personal health information private
c. Designed to allow public access to a person's health information
d. Only applicable to doctors

118. Which of the following needles has the largest bore opening?
a. 14 gauge
b. 20 gauge
c. 21 gauge
d. 22 gauge

119. The procedure for prepping the puncture site for this procedure is similar to that for blood donor collection.
a. Blood culture collections
b. Duke bleeding time
c. Earlobe microcapillary puncture
d. Routine phlebotomy

120. Which test will require the phlebotomist to perform routine venipuncture but use a special collection tube provided by the manufacturer?
a. Blood donor phlebotomy
b. Clotting time
c. Fibrin degradation products
d. Therapeutic phlebotomy

121. Which of the following factors generally does NOT contribute to syncope?
a. Cardiac arrhythmia
b. Fatigue
c. Hyperglycemia
d. Sudden decrease in blood volume

122. Which of the following is generally the most common complication from phlebotomy?
a. Convulsions
b. Fainting
c. Hematoma
d. Hyperventilation

123. A collapsed vein may result in:
a. Convulsions
b. Hematoma
c. Hypovolemia
d. Short draw

124. Which of the following is a technical error in phlebotomy?
Convulsions
Fainting
Hematoma
Missing a vein

125. Which of the following occurrences is NOT a cause for specimen rejection?
a. Clot in a "tiger-top" tube
b. Clot in an EDTA tube
c. Hemolysis in a blood bank specimen
d. Short draw in sodium citrate tube

126. This area of the laboratory often has the strictest specimen collection requirements.
a. Bacteriology
b. Blood bank
c. Chemistry
d. Hematology

127. Which virus accounts for the majority of post-transfusion cases of hepatitis in the United States?
a. Hepatitis A virus
b. Hepatitis B virus
c. Hepatitis C virus
d. Hepatitis D virus

128. OSHA regulations require all health care service providers to provide:
a. Safety and engineered sharp devices
b. Optional Hepatitis B virus immunization
c. Required Hepatitis E virus immunization
d. None of the above

129. Which of the following is NOT measured or recorded for routine blood donation?
a. Weight
b. Temperature
c. Age
d. Eye color

130. Phlebotomists often have many duties and tasks. Which of the following is the primary duty?
a. Specimen processing
b. Specimen accession
c. Collecting venous blood specimens
d. Collecting arterial blood specimens

131. In the word *phlebotomy*, the letter *o* after the *b* is a:
    a. Prefix
    b. Suffix
    c. Combining vowel
    d. None of the above
132. What does the common suffix *itis* mean?
    a. Enlarged
    b. Inflammation
    c. Pain
    d. Reduced
133. What does the word root *ven* mean?
    a. Artery
    b. Bronchi
    c. Capillary
    d. Vein
134. Most medical terms can trace their roots to these two languages.
    a. English and Latin
    b. Greek and English
    c. Greek and Latin
    d. Latin and German
135. This is a sugar deficiency that is included in newborn screening tests.
    a. Fructosemia
    b. Galactosemia
    c. Glucosemia
    d. Lactosemia
136. Screening tests for hemolytic disease of the newborn include testing for this compound.
    a. Bilirubin
    b. Blood urea nitrogen
    c. Galactose
    d. Phenylalanine
137. Iatrogenic anemia is caused by which of the following?
    a. Blood loss for laboratory testing
    b. Hemolytic disease of the newborn
    c. Incompatible transfusion
    d. Internal bleeding
138. This is the fastest-growing age group in the United States.
    a. 18–24 years of age
    b. 85 years and older
    c. Baby boomers
    d. 5 years and younger
139. This condition is often observed in older adults and results in stiff and painful joints.
    a. Arthritis
    b. Dementia
    c. Osteoporosis
    d. Phlebitis
140. Initially, the best way to overcome a patient with difficulty hearing is to:
    a. Be sure the phlebotomy collection area is well lit
    b. Shout
    c. Speak directly to the patient
    d. Write everything down
141. A body system consists of _____.
    a. all of the organs of the body together that perform the function of life
    b. several related tissues that together perform a common function
    c. several related organs that together perform a common function
    d. the process of making larger molecules from smaller ones.
142. Which of the following is not a peripheral venous device?
    a. Central venous catheter
    b. Midline catheter
    c. Peripherally inserted central catheter
    d. Brachial arterial catheter
143. This is a procedure used to revive patients found unconscious and without a heartbeat.
    a. CPR
    b. Heimlich maneuver
    c. Cold compress placed on the back of the neck
    d. Phlebotomy
144. The loss of this in the skin of older adults may make phlebotomy more challenging.
    a. Fat
    b. Epidermal cells
    c. Elasticity
    d. Sebaceous glands
145. Dementia is the loss of:
    a. Vision
    b. Mental capacity
    c. Hearing
    d. Bone density
146. This is the recommended depth of a heel puncture on an infant.
    a. 1 mm
    b. 2 mm
    c. 3 mm

d. 4 mm

147. This test on infants involves blotting blood on specially prepared paper:
    a. Glucose
    b. Hypothyroidism
    c. Complete blood count
    d. None of the above

148. A blood transfer device is used to:
    a. Transfer blood between a syringe and another container
    b. Transfer blood from one patient to another patient
    c. Transfer blood from an evacuated tube to a syringe
    d. Transfer blood from blood culture bottle to an evacuated tube

149. Which of the following generates revenue?
    a. Wages
    b. Equipment
    c. Volume of work
    d. Benefits

150. In the human body, organs combine together to make:
    a. Cells
    b. Beautiful music
    c. Systems
    d. Tissues

ANSWER KEY

1. C
2. B
3. A
4. C
5. A
6. C
7. A
8. A
9. D
10. C
11. D
12. B
13. D
14. D
15. B
16. A
17. B
18. C
19. B
20. D
21. B
22. D
23. B
24. A
25. C
26. D
27. D
28. A
29. A
30. C
31. B
32. B
33. C
34. A
35. B
36. B
37. B
38. D
39. C
40. D
41. B
42. C
43. B
44. A
45. B
46. B
47. D
48. C
49. C
50. B
51. D
52. B
53. A
54. C
55. A
56. B
57. C
58. D
59. B
60. B
61. C
62. A
63. D
64. B
65. B

66. C	109. C
67. C	110. A
68. D	111. D
69. C	112. A
70. D	113. C
71. B	114. C
72. A	115. A
73. B	116. C
74. D	117. B
75. D	118. A
76. C	119. A
77. B	120. C
78. B	121. C
79. B	122. C
80. A	123. D
81. A	124. D
82. B	125. A
83. C	126. B
84. A	127. C
85. D	128. A
86. A	129. D
87. A	130. C
88. A	131. C
89. D	132. B
90. D	133. D
91. D	134. C
92. A	135. B
93. B	136. A
94. C	137. A
95. C	138. B
96. C	139. A
97. D	140. C
98. C	141. C
99. A	142. D
100. C	143. A
101. D	144. C
102. B	145. B
103. B	146. B
104. D	147. B
105. D	148. A
106. D	149. C
107. A	150. C
108. C	

Helpful Spanish Terms and Phrases

Effectively communicating with a non–English-speaking person is critical to successfully collecting a blood specimen. Spanish is the most prevalent language spoken in the United States after English. Although it is preferable to have someone who can translate for you, there may be times when you need to communicate directly with your patient. The following is a list of phrases that should assist a phlebotomist with Spanish-speaking patients. The website Google Translate, http://translate.google.com/translate, is free and allows you to listen how to pronounce the phrases. It is recommended that you use the pronunciation guide and the website and practice the phrases several times before trying to communicate with them.

English	Spanish	Pronunciation
Hello	Hola.	O-la
Do you speak English?	¿Hablas inglés?	A blas een-gles
I only speak a little Spanish.	Sólo hablo un poco de español.	So-lo a-blo oon po-coo day es-pa-nyol
Please	Por favor.	Por-fa-bor
Thank you.	Gracias.	Gra-syas
You are welcome.	De nada.	Day-na-da
Good morning.	Buenos dias.	BWE-nohs DEE-ahs
Good afternoon.	Buenos tardes.	BWE-nos tar-des
Good evening.	Buenos noches.	BWE-nos no-ches
Sir, Mr.	Señor	Se-nyor
Madame, Mrs.	Señora	Se-nyo-ra
Miss, Ms.	Señorita	Se-nyo-ree-ta
My name is . . .	Me llamo . . .	Me ya-mo
I am from the laboratory.	Soy del laboratorio.	Soy DEL la-bo-ra-to-ryo
What is your name?	¿Cuál es su nombre?	Cwal es su nom-bre
Mother, father	Madre, padre	Ma-dre pa-dre
Child	Niño	Nee-nyo
Baby	Bebé	be-Be
May I see your identification bracelet?	¿Puedo ver su pulsera de identificación?	Pwe-do ber su pul-ser-a day ee-den-tee-fee-ca-syon
Your doctor has ordered some laboratory tests.	Su doctor le ha prescrito algunas pruebas de laboratorio.	Su doc-tor le ah pre-scree-to al-goo-nahs pru-e-bas dayla-bo-ra-to-ryo
Are you fasting?	¿Si es usted el ayuno?	See es oos-ted EL ah-yoo-no
When time did you last eat?	¿A qué hora la última vez que comer?	A ke ora la ul-tee-ma bes ke co-mer

Continued

English	Spanish	Pronunciation
Have you had anything to eat or drink in the last 12 hours?	¿Ha tenido algo de comer o beber en las últimas 12 horas?	Ah tay-nee-do all-go day co-mer oo be-berr n lahsul-tee-mas do-say o-rah-s
I need to take some blood for testing.	Tengo que tomar un poco de san-gre para la prueba.	Tay-ngo ke to-mas oonPo-coo day san-gre par-ahLa pru-e-bah
Please make a fist.	Por favor, haga un puño.	Por-fa-bor a-gah oonpooh'-nyo
Please roll up your sleeve.	Por favor, levantará la manga.	Por-fa-bor le-ban-tar-ahLa man-ga
Is the tourniquet too tight?	¿Es el torniquete demasiado apretado?	Es el tor-no-kay-tayDay-mah-seah'-do ah-pray-tah-do
You are going to feel a small prick.	Usted va a sentir un pequeño pinchazo.	Oos-ted ba a sen-teer oon pay-kay-nyo pin-chah-so
Please keep your arm straight.	Por favor, mantenga el brazo estirado.	Por-fa-bor man-tay-gah el bra-so es-te-rah'-do
You can now relax your arm and fist.	Ahora puede descansar su brazo y el puño.	Ah-o'-rah pwe-deh des-can-sar' soo bra-so ee elpooh'-nyo
You need to give us a urine sample for testing.	Es necesario que nos dan una muestra de orina para su análisis.	Es nay-say-sah'-re-o ke no-s dan oo'-nah mod-ays'-trah day o-ree'nah pah'-rah soo ah-nah'-le-sis
Do you feel okay?	¿Te sientes bien?	Te syen-tes byen
Tourniquet	Torniquete	Tor-ne-kay-tay
Blood	Sangre	San-gre
Arm	El brazo	El bra-so
Right arm	Brazo derecho	Bra-so de-re-cho
Left arm	El brazo izquierda	El bra-so ees-kee-er-da
Needle	Aguja	A-gu-ha
Test, analysis	Prueba, análisis	Pru-e-ba ah-nah'-le-sis
Urine	Orina	o-ree'-nah
Urinalysis	Análisis de orina	Ah-nah'-le-sis dayo-ree'-nah
Sample	Muestra	Moo-ays'-trah
Finger stick	Dedo palo	Day'-do pah'-lo
Prick, stick	Pinchazo, palo	Pin-chah-so, pah'-lo
Finger	Dedo	Day'-do
Blood test	Análisis de sangre	Ah-nah-le-sis day san-gre
Glucose level	Nivel de glucosa	Ne-vel' day gloo-co'-sah
Blood count	Sangre cuenta	San-gre cuen-ta
Electrolytes	Electrolitos	Ay-lec-tro'-le-tos
Cholesterol	Colesterol	Co-les-tay-role'
Pregnancy test	Prueba del embarazo	Pru-e-ba del em-barr-a-so
Liver enzymes	Las enzimas hepaticas	Las en-thee'-mahs je-pa-ti-ka
Relax	Relajese	Ray-lah-hay-she
Do you understand?	¿Entiende usted	En-tyen de oos-ted
Have you been exposed to anyone with COVID in the last 14 days?	¿Ha estado expuesto a alguien con COVID en los últimos 14 días?	Ha es-ta-doe pwesto al-gu-en con COVID en los ul-ti-mos dias

INDEX

Page numbers followed by *f* indicate figures; *t*, tables; *b*, boxes.